Evidence-based Research

Evidence-based Research

DILEMMAS AND DEBATES IN HEALTH CARE

Brian Brown, Paul Crawford and Carolyn Hicks

Open University Press

Open University Press
McGraw-Hill Education
McGraw-Hill House
Shoppenhangers Road
Maidenhead
Berkshire
England
SL6 2QL

email: enquiries@openup.co.uk
world wide web:www.openup.co.uk

First published 2003

A catalogue record of this book is available from the British Library

ISBN 0 335 21164 X (pb) 0 335 21165 8 (hb)

Library of Congress Cataloging-in-Publication Data
CIP data applied for

Typeset by RefineCatch Limited, Bungay, Suffolk
Printed in the UK by Bell & Bain Ltd, Glasgow

Contents

1 Introduction: theories of science and theories of society   1

2 Epistemology I: positivism – 'they don't build epistemologies like that any more'   19

3 Concepts and theories I: what is a concept in the health sciences?   46

4 Concepts and theories II: operationalism and its legacy   78

5 The philosophy of experimentation   109

6 Experiments in medicine and the health sciences   141

7 Epistemology II: interpretation and hermeneutics   174

8 Philosophies of description   199

9 The post-modernist challenge   234

10 Philosophy and research design in practice   260

Index   285

For Pat

Acknowledgements

Some of the arguments concerning postmodernism in Chapters 7 and 9 draw upon our earlier publications, namely Crawford et al (1998) Communicating care, Cheltenham, Stanley Thornes, and the discussion of autobiography and self follows the argument presented in Crawford et al (1995) Linguistic entrapment, Journal of Advanced Nursing 22, 1141–1148.

In addition, there are many others we would like to thank. The impetus for this volume came from the students on the MSc. in Health Sciences at Birmingham University who took part in the 'Philosophy of Research' course. Without their enthusiastic response this volume would not have appeared in the first place. You know who you are. Finally thanks are due to Babe, Luci, Jo, Nikki, Amanda, Julie and Chloe. Once again, you know who you are and you know what you've done.

1

Introduction: theories of science and theories of society

At the start of the new millennium, health care is in a state of transition. In the English-speaking world, there are a number of strong political and scientific currents pulling practitioners and clients into new and unfamiliar territories where their skills, practices and even their identities will be challenged. Health care organizations, policies and funding arrangements are rapidly being restructured. New challenges are emerging from new health problems. HIV, Gulf War Syndrome, the proliferation of severe and life-threatening allergies, the resurgence of diseases such as leprosy in nations from which it was previously believed to have been eliminated, the problems presented by warfare, global migration, hunger and even iatrogenic problems originating in health care itself, all are being increasingly brought into focus for health professionals.

At the same time – and this is where we come in – in Europe and America there is an increasing emphasis on research in health care. There has been a massive shift in the policy arena towards evidence-based practice. Everyone in health care, from the consultant surgeon to the volunteer care assistant, is being urged to become research literate, to read research and apply it to their practice, and even to do research themselves.

A further development – and another on which we can help – is the change in focus in health care provision. More and more policy is emphasizing the needs of the patient. Indeed, they are increasingly seen not as patients but as 'clients', 'users', 'consumers' or even 'customers'. They are consulted, surveyed and assessed, via health needs surveys, user involvement in service planning and devolution of decision making to local level. This process of inclusion and consultation, in the UK at least, is built into the statutory framework for health care providers such as the newly formed 'trusts' which administer an increasingly large part of the UK's health care. This policy context has already been written about extensively. What interests us is the conceptual shifts that many of us will have to make to keep abreast of these changes. The shift from 'patient' to 'consumer' is, in some ways, just as profound as the change in thinking from 'demonic possession' to 'illness', or from an 'imbalance of the humours' to 'bacterial infection'. Thus, we would argue that there are lessons to be learned from previous revolutions in the way we think about health and illness. Like these earlier conceptual, theological and political shifts, the new climate in health care changes the way practitioners practise, how they are trained, how they do research and, just as importantly, what it means to be a patient.

Philosophy can also help us make sense of what we are trying to do whatever role we take, perhaps as health care researchers, health care providers, or even as concerned relatives or patients ourselves. A philosophical orientation might make us reflect on some questions that we often leave unasked. What do health and disease mean and how might we best conceptualize them? How do we tell whether someone has anything 'wrong' with them? The classic 'What seems to be the trouble?' is far from simple. Once we try to do research on the issues it gets more complex still. What balance should we give to the biological, social or spiritual aspects of health care practice? How can we tell if the patients got 'better'? Do we take their word for it? This list is not exhaustive. Even worse, philosophy can't answer these questions anyway. However, we can begin to sketch in some of the things that might help us think about them more effectively.

The first question to answer is why do research at all? Many of the world's major civilizations have risen and fallen without doing much organized science. The present-day species of scientists doing research that assists health care is a relatively new breed in historical terms. The natural philosophers of the Euro-American enlightenment were in most cases not concerned with health care issues in their scholarly work. The scientific work of medicine got most fully under way in the mid-nineteenth century in Europe's great laboratories, pioneered by the likes of Robert Koch (1843–1910), who discovered the bacteria responsible for cholera and tuberculosis, or Claude Bernard (1813–1878), whose pioneering work on many of the organ systems of the body was accompanied by his maxim 'why think when you can experiment?'.

Bernard's influence on health care was profound. Ironically, this is precisely because he thought so little of it. His contempt for clinical medicine – which he felt was little better than alchemy – was manifested many times during his career. His desire was to develop a laboratory discipline of physiology and medicine that looked like physics and chemistry. Thus, the real action of medicine was progressively re-engineered so as to make it seem like it took place in the laboratory rather than in the ward or the consulting room. The image of the pre-nineteenth-century surgeon as a primitive 'sawbones' and the midwife as the drunken 'Mrs Gamp' was built at this time. As we shall see later, judging from the seventeenth-century works of Jane Sharp, midwives had access to a sophisticated genitourinary medicine some 200 years before this. From the Greeks onwards, surgeons practised a careful and nuanced regime of battlefield wound care. These earlier healing practices were systematically downgraded by a number of intellectuals as medicine was respecified as a scientific enterprise. Again, perhaps this was a revolution in ideas. From our point of view, it was an especially important one because it put science into medicine, and dragged medicine into science. Indeed, so solid was Bernard's commitment to laboratory work that he was even hostile to Darwinian notions, when he became aware of them, because they were not founded on experimental or histological evidence.

What we are suggesting, then, is that health care looks the way it does because of a particular set of historical events and processes. The apparently natural seamless relationship between published research, the clinic and the laboratory that has characterized late twentieth-century health care has not come about purely by accident or because of some underlying unity in nature. Recently, scholars of science and society have considered the role of assumptions, values, world-views and paradigms in knowledge and how these contribute to the structure of scientific revolutions.

We shall deal with some of the major trends in thinking about science and research in the later chapters. Our intention here is to 'set out our stall', so to speak. The history of human enquiry, we believe, is full of shifts, changes, accidents and dead ends. Nature itself is sufficiently untidy for it to be difficult to grasp. If, indeed, we believe in an underlying reality at all. The problem, then, as far as we are concerned is to make sense of the business of research and health care science as a human activity. It is a little difficult to say that late twentieth-century Euro-American knowledge is unproblematically better than anybody else's. The fact that so many people in our contemporary evidence-based technological civilization are rediscovering and exploring spiritualities, alternative health care and ancient healing practices suggests that it would be difficult to find any consensus about what the best kind of health care knowledge is.

As a way of beginning to make sense of these variations and shifts, let us spend a few moments thinking about how we might conceptualize the process of scientific revolution. One of the key texts here is Thomas Kuhn's famous *The Structure of Scientific Revolutions*, originally published in 1962. Kuhn argued that scientific research and thought are defined by 'paradigms', or conceptual world-views, that consist of formal theories, classic experiments, trusted methods and a variety of tacit theories about what's important, what happens and what matters. Scientists typically work within a prevailing tacitly accepted paradigm and try to extend the scope of knowledge by refining theories, explaining puzzling data and establishing more precise measures of variables, standards and phenomena. Eventually, however, their efforts may generate insoluble theoretical problems or experimental anomalies that expose a paradigm's limitations or contradict it altogether. At first, scientists may try to explain away the oddities, leave them unresearched or address questions that fit most comfortably into the existing paradigm. One day, however, this accumulation of difficulties may trigger a crisis that can only be resolved by an intellectual revolution that replaces an old paradigm with a new one. The abandonment of Ptolemaic cosmology and its replacement with Copernican heliocentrism, and the displacement of Newtonian mechanics by quantum physics and general relativity, are both examples of major paradigm shifts.

Kuhn's work is important also because he questioned the traditional conception of scientific progress as a gradual, cumulative acquisition of knowledge based on rationally chosen experimental frameworks. Previously, this rather complacent 'up the mountain theory of knowledge' had pervaded most attempts to understand scientific enquiry. Instead, he argued that it is the paradigm that determines the kinds of experiments scientists perform, the types of questions they ask and the problems they consider important. A shift in the paradigm alters the fundamental concepts underlying research and inspires new kinds of research questions, new standards of evidence, new research techniques, and new pathways of theory and experiment that are radically at odds with the old ones.

In the 40 years since the publication of Kuhn's book, his concept of paradigm shifts has been something of a cliché. It has been extended to disciplines such as sociology, political science, economics and, importantly, health care. It is common for people to talk about a dominant paradigm in research, but very often nobody really knows what it is. Is it biomedical reductionism? Possibly, but usually this is mentioned only to criticize it and present alternative psycho-social models of health care. Is it empiricism or positivism? Again, possibly, but very few people would admit to being positivists these days, even though it flourished in the nineteenth and early twentieth centuries. We shall see more of what positivism involves later on, but for the moment let us note that it usually appears as a kind of straw figure to be ridiculed. Is the dominant paradigm individualism? Certainly, a good many assumptions are made about the site of problems and interventions being the individual client. On the other hand, some of the debates about methodology in the caring disciplines have challenged this focus on individuals and many authors have tried to encourage thinking about how individual physical and mental distress is linked to broader social structures, processes and inequalities (e.g. Smail 1997). Thus, at the specific level of actual research and writing, it is often difficult to detect a dominant paradigm in any simple sense.

A further reason why we would want to encourage scepticism of an overly simple model of health care research and experience is because of the variety of world-views and belief systems that can be detected in contemporary health care. For example, a good many authors emphasize spirituality in health care (e.g. Brencick and Webster 2000). This, it is argued, involves interacting with people on a plane of reality that is distinct from the reality that is scrutinized by scientific enquiry. This kind of issue is not simply ghettoized into the territory of the hospital chaplain, but is blossoming on the pages of scientific journals devoted to health care.

Given this diversity, it is difficult to take the idea of a dominant paradigm too literally. Often, in explaining ideas to the reader we will have to make use of meta-phorical devices. The idea of a 'dominant paradigm' is one of these. It evokes the idea of a kind of scientific researcher or clinician who probably has never really existed. One who, perhaps, is overly concerned with biomedical models, reductionist reasoning and quantifiable experimental evidence at the expense of psychological, social or spiritual perspectives. This is a stereotype, a cartoon if you will. However, it is a useful one in making sense of the different trends in science and thinking about health care.

Let us try to characterize some of the tendencies in the so-called dominant paradigm more fully. One of the major ways of making sense of traditional scientific enquiry is to see it as manifesting an orientation that has been called 'positivism'. Positivism has involved a belief that there is a real universe out there, which is revealed to us through our senses and which we can come to know more precisely through scientific enquiry, the techniques of which are broadly similar in both the social and natural sciences. The universe is seen as being a lawful place where relations of cause and effect determine the organization of events. Whereas the universe is very real to the positivist, he or she would be willing to accept that scientific ideas are somewhat tentative and need not always literally reflect the reality they seek to describe. They are always open to challenge by new data, which may result in their rejection or revision.

The mid-nineteenth-century variety of positivism envisioned by Auguste Comte also firmly rejected metaphysics and speculation. Moreover, to the positivist the idea that there is a grand design to the universe – that it has first causes and ultimate ends – is not acceptable either because these ideas are not verifiable via the scientific method.

This vision of positivism has more recently been supplanted by realist theories of science. These tend to accept the idea that there is a reality 'out there' and we can achieve successively better approximations to it through scientific endeavour. Modern realism, especially that which is influenced by Roy Bhaskar (1998), pitches itself as an alternative to traditional positivism and the newer constructivist approaches to the philosophy of science. As well as an external reality, contemporary realisms assert that there is a kind of deep generative structure to the world. Rather than the superficiality of facts and their accumulation, these realisms seek to discover a 'deep' or 'generative structure' to events. This, then, is one of the purposes of science. As one of the anti-positivist realists of the nineteenth century Karl Marx put it, 'all science would be superfluous if the outward appearances and essences of things directly coincided' (Marx, 1933, p. 817). In modern, so-called 'critical' realism, the natural and social sciences are related though not identical. There are, in this view, discoverable generative structures governing the world. The natural sciences enable us to discover a world that has a relatively independent existence, whereas human social phenomena – within which a good deal of health care research is conducted – are more complex. Social structures are themselves the result of human interaction, but they, in turn, influence the kinds of actions that take place. They enable human action but also might constrain it. The famous sociologist Anthony Giddens calls this the 'duality of structure'.

Our discussion of realism and positivism as if they were related would probably horrify some people. Especially those who see 'critical realism' as a kind of radical alternative to positivism. However, we have put them together to highlight the differences between these notions that emphasize scientific realism and some of the perspectives that challenge it.

There are a number of challenges to the notions of science embedded in realist approaches. Some of these challenge mainstream science on political grounds – in terms of the interests it promotes and whether the sectional interest groups who perform science, or pay for it, are constructing knowledge. This kind of thinking is perhaps exemplified by some strands in Marxism, where it could be argued that science and culture turn out in ways that are broadly congenial to the economic interests of a society. These approaches tend to assume, however, that there is a real world that we can think about and know. Marxists are usually happy to talk about 'false consciousness' and 'false needs', as if it were possible to know what the real ones were. Maybe they're right. Let's take the argument a little further and shift a bit more deeply into the kind of intellectual territory that is sceptical of scientific realism and positivism. Where, in other words, the challenge to positivism and realism is at its most acute. Some of these challenges question the foundations of human knowledge itself. In the 1980s and 1990s, some social scientists, scholars of health care and the humanities turned to an even more radical interpretive perspective on social phenomena, culture and health care, namely postmodernism. This perspective questions whether an objective understanding of other people and their role in health and illness is at all possible. It has been termed postmodernism because it represented a reaction to modernism, at least as this took the form of a scientific, rational approach to understanding the world found in most branches of European and North American scholarship from the eighteenth to the late twentieth centuries. Allied to this is the approach to philosophical thinking known as 'deconstruction', which derives from the work of Jacques Derrida. This work focuses on language, and originates with the idea that the traditional way of seeing the language in which scientific or academic ideas are expressed is mistaken. Positivistic and realist models have to assume that it is possible to talk and write about the world as if it existed independently of language. Put crudely, to make realism viable you've got to believe that language is able to express ideas about the world without changing them too much. In the traditional model of language, writing describes speech and speech describes the world, as if it were possible for language to clearly describe a reality which was external to language. Moreover, the author of a text is the source of its meaning. Derrida's work, on the other hand, tried to mount a challenge to these assumptions. He promoted a deconstructive style of reading that attempted to subvert these assumptions and undermine the idea that a text has an unchanging, unified meaning which the reader can discover. Reality is not something that texts can easily describe. They do not allow us to discern the writer's intentions or the reality which the writer could see. There are many legitimate readings of a text. The interesting question, then, is not whether the text – a scientific paper or report perhaps – corresponds to reality, but how it constructs truth *in situ* within its pages. To many of us in health care and in the education system, this might be an appealing position. One of us (B.B.) has tried for a number of years to get his host institution to buy him an MRI scanner or a particle accelerator, but sadly these devices are well beyond the budget of most universities. It is therefore very difficult to see what nature is made of in any fundamentalist or foundationalist sense. It is not possible for most of us to see inside the body or inside the molecule. Derrida's maxim is often taken to be 'there is nothing beyond the text'. Some scholars of nursing have found the idea that health care itself is a 'textually mediated reality' to be very attractive (Cheek and Rudge 1994). If we take the message of Derrida, and other deconstructive and postmodernist writers in a strong form, it means that it would be very difficult to make decisive claims about nature – the atoms, the cells, the structures and processes – because most of us only encounter them through language. This tendency to accord language a central place is often found in studies of health care that are intended to be critical, transformative or revolutionary. This encourages us to be sceptical of any text that makes claims about truth, reality or nature. From the deconstructionist position, a reader might be most interested in the rhetorical devices that make a piece appear true, and be less concerned with whether it literally is, because, in this perspective, there is 'nothing outside the text'. Within postmodernism and a postmodern view of the world the progress of science, health care and human welfare is acknowledged to be a process that is not necessarily straightforward. A pharmaceutical firm may add to the infant mortality rate in Central America by causing pollution, yet may dramatically lower the mortality rate for cancer patients in Oklahoma by importing drugs at a cost low enough to satisfy the company's shareholders. The geometry of good and evil is not simple in the postmodern paradigm.

Returning to our earlier point about what kind of paradigm might be found dominating health care research, our brief tour has illustrated some of the differing perspectives on the philosophy of science that we might find and some of the viewpoints that might also be found when researchers in health care turn their attention to conceptual matters. This list is not exhaustive and, as the book unfolds, we will see more of these perspectives. The point is that it is difficult to see a single paradigm that is dominant in conceptual terms, as all of these points of view happily – if somewhat argumentatively – exist in contemporary academic life. Thus, we would argue that a universal paradigm for health care enquiry that is one day going to shift, is probably an oversimplification. It is certainly possible to see vast sums of money and highly prestigious researchers doing experimental work in the laboratory and in the form of clinical trials. Much of this would be eminently familiar to the likes of Comte, Bernard and their ilk from over a hundred years ago. But we can see also a variety of other techniques and conceptual orientations flourishing, even if they are not usually so well funded.

Nature's untidiness and its tendencies to resist easy classification do not necessarily lead to regular paradigm shifts. Novel phenomena are often readily reinterpreted in line with the prevailing scientific world-view at the time. Accounts of alien abductions are seen as examples of delusion, hallucination or the 'fantasy prone personality', creatures such as the giant panda were supposed to be quaint mythical folktales until they were captured by Western naturalists in China in the 1930s, the sense of moving towards a light which people report in near death experiences is seen to be, say, the result of anoxia, and so on. Most good 'paradigms' give us the tools to deal with anomalies.

Let us explore the kinds of difficulties we might face in making sense of 'strange' things by means of a few examples. In the first of these, concerned with cutting holes in the skull, we hope to illustrate the way that science and scholarship might grapple with novelties and how they might try to reformulate phenomena so as to bring them into line with what is known at the time.

'Like you need a hole in the head': trepanning and the reconstruction of health care histories

Why would people believe it was a good idea to cut holes in their heads? Let us spend a moment or two examining medical and theological explanations and their philosophical assumptions. How can we as researchers interpret the past and learn from it? This will illuminate the issues of how researchers, historians and archaeologists interpret the way that other cultures make sense of their own bodies. It will enable us to introduce the idea of Euro-American, secular, late-modern conceptual frameworks and how they influence our understanding of other peoples and cultural milieus.

In the nineteenth century, archaeologists were puzzled by the discovery of skulls with holes that appeared to have been bored or scraped into them. The first examples seem to have been presented in the work of the fanatical American skull collector Samuel Morton in his Crania Americana (1849). As more specimens of these so-called 'trepanned' skulls came to light (around a thousand have been discovered from Bolivia and Peru alone (Verano and Ubelaker 1992)), it became apparent that this practice must have occurred commonly in the area over a period of 2000 years, from around 500 B.C. to A.D. 1500. In Europe, too, the intellectuals of the day with an interest in medicine and anthropology were puzzled by archaeological finds involving skulls with holes in them. Gradually over the late nineteenth and twentieth centuries the history of trepanation has come to light and the discovery of these skulls prompted scholars to re-read the history of medicine and examine the classic texts from Greece and China to see what the authorities of the ancient world had to say about the procedure. The European variants of trepanning are estimated to have originated 10,000 years ago. The practice seems to have reached a peak among the Neolithic 'battleaxe people', who constructed a series of chambered tombs in France about 4000 years ago, enormous numbers of whose skulls are perforated in this way.

The concept of trepanning is interesting because it highlights how we go about making sense of issues in the past through our own frameworks of experience. We've chosen to include it because the sight of a skull with a hole in it and the knowledge that people were doing this successfully in the pre-modern era has often fascinated and revolted our students. The whole issue of how we make sense of what might have been a health care practice illustrates some important themes in how we make sense of the body and what people do with it.

Let us look at the history of the practice in a little more detail. This is a history which is difficult to find in mainstream textbooks and from our early twenty-first-century vantage point it is difficult to appreciate just how much these skulls with holes in mesmerized our intellectual forebears in the nineteenth century. Lipowski (1967) reminds us that at first it was believed that these skulls had received the holes either after the skull's owner had died or that the patient would have died very shortly after the operation. Eighteenth- and nineteenth-century surgeons had abandoned pro-cedures that involved breaching the skull entirely because of the 100 per cent mortal-ity rate. So it was inconceivable to these early scholars that these apparently primitive people could have fared any better. More recently, it became apparent that this initial pessimism was misconceived. Not only had this hazardous procedure been widely performed but the 'patients' had survived. The nineteenth-century scientific and medical belief in their own proficiency was severely dented by the fact that they had been outperformed by so-called 'primitive tribesmen', 'savages' and 'heathens' working without instruments, antiseptics or operating theatres.

The South American skulls suggest that the survival rates from these operations were relatively good, and exceeded the survival rate achieved by European doctors until much later. If the patient survives, the edges of the bone around the hole lose their sharp, recently cut appearance and begin to round over, rather like a tree grow-ing over the stump where a branch has been cut off. Judging by the presence of these signs of long-term healing, Verano and Ubelaker (1992) estimate that as many as 70 per cent of the people trepanned during the Inca period survived the operation, and even the earliest skulls from the coast of Peru show a 40 per cent survival rate. By contrast, neurosurgery patients in the nineteenth and early twentieth centuries, even after the development of antiseptic procedures and anaesthesia, rarely even achieved survival rates of 25 per cent.

The interest in trepanation generated over the past 150 years is instructive because it mirrors a good many of our modern concerns. The aim of our discussion, then, is to show how the lenses of our present scientific framework enable us to make sense not only of present-day phenomena, but to make sense of the past as well.

Even though medicine had been revolutionized by the turn to dissection in the Renaissance, people were still (as they are now) interested in the medical texts of early Greek authors. Just count how many references there are to the ancient Greeks in any contemporary textbook. On studying the original works of Greek scholars in the classical period, it became apparent that trepanning was known to the Greeks. Hippocrates (c. 460–355 B.C.) advised trepanation as a treatment for head wounds for example. More recently, medieval authorities such as Roger of Salerno (1170–1200) in his treatises on head injuries makes reference to the use of trepanation as a treatment and the conditions for which it might be indicated. In China there are accounts that Thai Tshang Kung (205–150 B.C.) used to 'cut open skulls of patients and arrange their brains in order' (Lipowski 1967).

Making sense of trepanation has exercised the minds of many prominent nineteenth-century scholars. Why on earth would people embark on such a procedure? Paul Broca (1876), one of the leading authorities on the brain and skull in the mid-nineteenth century, and the originator of the classic study of brain damage in a patient who had lost his powers of speech, which led to the identification of Broca's area in the brain, maintained that trepanation represented an early attempt to deal with diseases of the skull and brain. The early peoples of Europe and South America were thus, in this view, 'inept technologists'. This view was supported by the accounts from Greek and medieval doctors of the use of trepanation to deal with head injuries. Moreover, trepanation, according to Lipowski, has been performed in many parts of the world for headaches, epilepsy and insanity. This process of reasoning by means of what he called ethnographic parallels still exists in anthropology and archaeology. One finds a group of people who one knows about and uses them to interpret the traces left by lesser known cultures.

The surgical theory, however, runs into difficulties with the observation that most trepanned skulls do not show other evidence of fracture or trauma – bad news for those who believe that it was an operation done to relieve the effects of battleaxe and slingshot wounds. Thus perhaps the operations were performed to relieve a non-traumatic condition or maybe to deal with something else, for example spiritual malaise. The fact that many of the French finds of perforated skulls were recovered from near elaborate burial sites with a presumably ritualistic function led to some speculation that this might apply to the cutting of holes in the skull. This is a much more difficult issue to clarify. We do not, of course, know what the people in question might have thought they were doing. The use of the cut-out fragments or 'roundels' of bone as decoration, charms or amulets in South America supports this possible interpretation. Some believe that cutting holes in the skull might be done to release evil spirits. This kind of speculation tells us as much about present-day ideas of spirituality as it does about pre-historic ones. Notions of a separate and largely ethereal spirit realm of autonomous beings who might wish to interfere with us are a relatively recent idea, possibly originating with the Greeks and reaching a peak in medieval Europe. We don't know whether Neolithic people had these beliefs, and if so, whether they were related to trepanation. Even though ethnographers and anthropologists have discovered beliefs in evil spirits in many developing nations, this still doesn't literally tell us what ancient peoples might have believed. Indeed, the idea that ancient Europeans might resemble contemporary Africans or South Americans has recently been treated with suspicion. It is part of a post-Enlightenment intellectual strategy that puts the Europeans and North Americans at the top of a pyramid of development and places people from less developed nations at the bottom. As if they were a kind of unevolved living fossil.

Thus, to make sense of this piece of history, we need to understand not only the artifacts that remain – whether they look as though healing had occurred or not, for example – but also how the intellectual communities who have striven to understand them made sense of the phenomena too, and what their cultural and historical reference points were.

The day the earth moved: Renaissance anatomies

The European Renaissance revolution in the arts and sciences, including the invention of gross anatomy and the re-invention of medicine, is usually taken to represent a change in perspective and world-view. Why did so many intellectuals suddenly turn to dissections as a way of understanding the body and to astronomy as a way of understanding the celestial sphere? This also invites the question of how revolutions can happen in knowledge. Do these events help explain changes in research orientations in the present? This illustrates the importance of history when studying knowledge systems and in tracing the historical links between different formats of knowledge and how revolutions sometimes enable things to stay the same. Here, one of us (BB) takes up his personal story.

When I was at school, we were taught a kind of 'received view' of the Renaissance in Europe. It went along the lines that Galileo had challenged the orthodoxy of the Catholic Church, was censured and subject to threats and a period of house arrest. Some of the more lurid (but less historically verifiable) accounts described him as being tortured as well. Despite the vagueness that sometimes accompanied these accounts, the impression was given that some part of this challenge involved seeing satellites orbiting Jupiter.

This is sometimes depicted to children as a kind of morality play of scientific triumph. Observation triumphs over prejudice, empirical evidence triumphs over dogma and the stage is set for the flowering of late Renaissance science in its full glory, with the likes of Newton, Leibniz, Gauss and their imitators just around the corner. Moreover, it is almost as if the founders of the Renaissance scientific revolution received their credentials by the sufferings they underwent. As if science, too, could have its martyrs. Science then, was a heroic, challenging, iconoclastic and ultimately liberating enterprise.

As I grew up, I found out more about the ideas and conflicts in Medieval and Renaissance theology and philosophy and saw far more of the diversity of views which it encompassed. The sense of perfection of the heavenly bodies apparently so dear to Catholic theologians derived from much earlier thinkers such as Aristotle. The idea of a stationary, central earth with the wandering heavenly bodies – the planets – orbiting around it, which was supported by the Church, derived from Claudius Ptolmaeus-Ptolmey (A.D. 90–168), a Greek astronomer working in Alexandria. The planets moved in small 'epicycles' as they orbited, such that they then would follow a path rather like a long coil spring stretched out into an arc. He believed, like Aristotle, that these orbits of the heavenly bodies were defined by crystal spheres.

Even in the modern era of physics, the relationship between science and religion is by no means clear-cut. The foundations of contemporary 'big bang' theories of the universe were laid by a Belgian Catholic priest, Georges Lemaitre.

Even to astronomical observers at the time, it was clear that the models proposed by Copernicus and defended by Galileo were difficult to square with the observations. Their insistence on circular orbits for the planets made it difficult for such a model to make accurate predictions, and it was only once the idea of elliptical orbits, introduced by Kepler, that theory fell more closely into line with observations. Many members of the Catholic Church were themselves enthusiastic astronomers. Copernicus was a Catholic priest and it was the Jesuits who, in Galileo's lifetime, were credited with discovering sunspots.

Roger Bacon – 'Doctor Mirabilis' himself – was reported to be using glasses at Oxford in the 1200s and some of his writings suggest that he had grasped the use of multiple lenses for projecting images of the heavens. It is not known whether he actually made such an instrument successfully. Some of the earliest instruments for which there is better evidence come from a Dutch inventor called Lipperhay in 1608, whose devices were soon improved upon by Galileo in 1609.

Flat earth astronomies are certainly not always intellectually inferior. The Greek astronomer Thales believed in such a system and yet was able to predict a solar eclipse in the sixth century B.C.

The theologies of the Middle Ages, Renaissance and Enlightenment are often thought of as somehow backward looking, hidebound, locked into outmoded and primitive ways of thinking. Yet there are a number of features of theological and scholastic thought in the Middle Ages that were very like the sciences developed by later generations of intellectuals. The philosopher Alfred North Whitehead (1861–1947) suggested that the Middle Ages 'trained' the intellect in a 'sense of order' and created the 'faith in the possibility of science'.

One of the puzzling things is why Galileo's views should have attracted such hostile attention from church officials. The idea of a moving earth had been previously – and uncontroversially – proposed by Nicholas Orseme (*c.* 1325–1382) and Nicholas of Cusa (1401–1464). Copernicus (1473–1543), the Catholic priest whose heliocentric theory was expounded in his book *On the Revolutions of the Celestial Spheres*, published in the year of his death, was not censured by the church, as far as we know. Indeed, it was at the urging of Pope Clement VII in 1536 that Copernicus's book was eventually published, and it contained a dedication to Clement's successor, Pope Paul III. The Catholic Church was much more friendly to heliocentric theories than the newly active Protestants. Copernican cosmology was most strongly opposed by Martin Luther and Protestant scepticism of heliocentric astronomy extended to the English Puritan reformer Dr John Owen (1616–1683), who declared that the Copernican system was 'a delusive and arbitrary hypothesis, contrary to scripture', and even the British founder of Methodism, John Wesley (1703–1791), argued that these ideas 'tend towards infidelity'.

The very fact that the deceptively simple story of Galileo versus the Church is told at all gives us a few clues about the nature of scientific storytelling, which we must be mindful of. First, look at what it's about: astronomy, mathematics and physics. It helps to establish them at the head of the scientific table. And, at least until the closing decades of the twentieth century, they have continued to enjoy that kind of prestige. Moreover, there's a notion embedded here that sciences such as physics are somehow more basic and fundamental to nature, that atoms, say, are the precursors of the more complex systems studied by other disciplines like medicine. Yet to understand this, we need to go back to a pre-Enlightenment idea, a Medieval notion that microcosm – our insides – reflected the macrocosm. The secrets inside us, so to speak, were mapped out in the heavens. Hence, the study of physics, astronomy and mathematics can tell us about apparently unrelated matters such as the palpitations of the heart, the motions of the blood and the balance of the humours. This idea has been good for physics. Overwhelmingly, philosophers and historians of science, ourselves included, have been mesmerized by the ways in which scholars have grappled with physical phenomena. Conflicts between science and religion, paradigm shifts, hypothesis testing – many of the standard features of the philosophy of science canon – take the physical sciences as their model.

In this book, we intend to get away from this physicalist model. As we shall argue, health care disciplines present a particularly interesting case for the philosophy of science as they are based in a more immediately practical set of concerns – life, death, suffering, curing – and their nostrums are often verified not through precise observation and geometrical plotting, but through a subjective sense that something has improved.

Gross anatomy: the discovery of the human body

The famous artist and inventor Leonardo da Vinci (1452–1519) provides some interesting illustrations of how the body was reconceptualized in the Renaissance. In earlier art, the body was often depicted as a relatively smooth, undifferentiated mass. The musculature and anatomical detail of classical statues seemed to have been forgotten. Bodies were either nondescript or, in the case of mythical or horrific creatures, they were monstrous and grotesque. In Leonardo's work, however, we can see a new vision of the body emerging. Now, most interestingly, this emerged first of all not from his famous dissections but from his attempts to paint saints. Saints, moreover, whose bodies were so often distressed, torn apart, pierced and wounded. It is with Leonardo's work that what we now call the 'striped muscles' were first drawn with stripes. His early painting of Saint Jerome, for example, suggests some close observation of the head and neck muscles.

Leonardo da Vinci was interested in applying natural analogies to the study of the human body, drawing on his wide-ranging interests in hydraulics, mechanics and painting to make sense of the body. At the time, the representation of the body was coming on by leaps and bounds. Leonardo's contemporary and rival Michaelangelo was revolutionizing the external perceptions of musculature. Leonardo himself, in his later studies, was examining the deep structure of the human body. To record this for himself and for posterity, he developed a whole new visual notation to convey a sense of what he was looking at. Whereas representations of skeletons had been common, at least since Roman times, it was Leonardo who originated cross-sections, cutaways and see-through diagrams to represent what he thought he had seen. It was he who originated exploded diagrams and who represented muscles as if they contained lines of force. All of a sudden the body was something that could be represented graphically and pictorially. It was mappable.

One of his famous illustrations of the human body was familiar to a generation of TV viewers in the UK as part of the title sequence of the documentary series 'World In Action'. This picture, the so-called 'Vitruvian Man', shows how the human body fits neatly into both a square and a circle. The human body was thus a geometrical entity rather than simply a fleshy one. Like the ancients, Leonardo used animal models to make sense of human functions. He provided detailed accounts of horses' entrails and frogs' spinal cords.

Leonardo was responsible for mapping the contents of the human torso and changing the way that they were seen. His principal studies of anatomy seem to have been done in the early 1500s and, in addition to dissection, he was successful in making wax models and plaster casts of the chambers of the heart and the ventricles of the brain. To give some examples of how he re-interpreted the body, previously the womb had been thought of and drawn as an organ with several chambers, and multiple pregnancies were believed to occur with each foetus in a different compartment. Leonardo 'invented' the single chambered womb which we see today. His drawing of a foetus in a single chambered uterus marked a fundamental shift in the way the reproductive apparatus was seen. Likewise, his discovery of the uterine artery and the vascular system of the cervix shifted the way we see these organs.

At the same time, Leonardo's vision of human anatomy differed from the kind that we might see today in, for example, classic textbooks like *Gray's Anatomy*. His wombs do not have fallopian tubes. These had to wait for Gabriele Fallopius (1523–1562) to map them some 50 years later. The placenta in his drawing of the foetus looks more like that of a cow than a human being. The spleen and liver are drawn as being roughly of equal size – nowadays the spleen is represented as being much smaller. Perhaps this relates to how the spleen was seen to be connected with the emotions during the Renaissance. In women's anatomy, a tube links the uterus and the breasts, while the penis is depicted as having two tubes running down its length – presumably one for urine and the other for semen – rather than the single urethra we see today.

Perhaps, as well as his classic illustrations of the body, the most important legacy of Leonardo is to do with the way we think about the body. For him, although the body was created by a 'supreme master', it was possible to understand it as if it were a machine. The heart had, from the ancient Greeks onwards, been seen as a source of the vital spirit and as the organ that heated the blood. To Leonardo, however, the heart was a mechanical, muscular device and the movement of the blood through it exhibited the same sorts of qualities as any other fluid flowing through tubes, with vortices and turbulence being created as it passed through the valves. Indeed, he lent his weight to an intellectual movement that sought to argue that the seat of our consciousness was not in the heart itself, but in the brain. This was consolidated by later scholars such as Descartes, who located a structure in the brain which they saw to be the actual seat of the soul. Throughout the body, Leonardo believed, the muscles expanded and contracted as a result of air being passed through the nerves. Causal chains were thus elaborated in his work, which, while not quite the same as those we believe in today (for example, we now believe nerves to convey electrical impulses rather than 'air' or 'spirit'), helped to set the stage for contemporary medical knowledge.

At the time Leonardo was working on his anatomy, a man was being born who would shift the paradigm of how we understand the body even further. The impact of Andreas Vesalius (1514–1564) on modern medicine and health care is perhaps equally as revolutionary as Leonardo's. It is not just that he was another pioneer of dissection, but he introduced the artistic and literary motifs of medicine which have stayed with us right through to the present day.

For example, rather than the vernacularized Latin that other scholars were using at the time, he modelled his text on the artistic prose of Cicero. This would be difficult to understand, even for the classically literate intellectuals of his day. However, it was believed that this kind of presentation was important. Vesalius himself believed that it was important to recollect and restore not only the knowledge which he felt had been lost since classical times, but that it was also important to recollect the language. Thus, in 1543 (the year of Copernicus's death) he published the first edition of his magnum opus *De Humanis Corporis Fabrica*, in seven volumes. Lavishly illustrated, possibly by students of the famous artist Titian, Vesalius hoped that these volumes, and their associated textbook for students – a kind of Renaissance study guide – would guide physicians away from rote memorization of the Greek texts of Galen and Hippocrates towards active dissection and observation of the human structure. Trainee physicians, he believed, would benefit from this practice. Rather than leaving the dissection to their servants, as had been the practice in the past, Vesalius believed in the importance of physicians and surgeons doing the dissections themselves.

This kind of anatomical investigation was regarded with suspicion. Anatomists were often distrusted because of their suspicious alliance with hangmen and executioners, whom they bribed so as to secure their supply of corpses. The classic depiction of the human head, which shows the neck twisted and the head tilted back, originated with Vesalius. The head is in this position because he would be dealing with people who had been hanged. The judicial technologies of the time influenced how we still see the body – this illustration has been stylized and reproduced as the cover art for twentieth-century editions of Gray's anatomy.

Moreover, the anatomy in Vesalius's work looks a lot more familiar than Leonardo's. His illustrations do not contain the peculiar arrangements of tubes and connections that Leonardo's did. His is an anatomy that looks reassuringly modern.

Despite his revolutionary status in the history of anatomy as it is conceptualized and taught nowadays, Vesalius's own notion was that he was going back to the ancients and he saw himself in a long historical line that went back to the Greeks. Anatomy, he said, 'should be recalled from the dead, or that if it did not achieve with us a greater perfection than at any other place or time among the old teachers of anatomy, it might at least reach such a point that one could with confidence assert that our modern science of anatomy was equal to that of the old, and that in this age anatomy was unique both in the level to which it had sunk and the completeness of its subsequent restoration' (*De Fabrica*, praefatio, 3r, 11.22ff). Thus he thought he was going back to restore or offer a rebirth to the spirit of enquiry which he felt had been lost since the ancient Greeks. So what does all this mean? Is it a paradigm shift? Or a reconstruction of history to make novelty look more respectable and appease the powerful religious interests that prevailed at the time? Of course, it is difficult to tell at this distance. However, what we are keen to point out is that even revolutionary movements are sometimes remarkable for leaving a good deal of the history intact. Revolutions, paradigm shifts and so on may be remarkably conservative.

Returning to Vesalius for a moment, just as interesting as the scientific content, perhaps, is the way that the pictures were presented. For example, the first picture we see in his books is of a theatre of dissection, where the anatomist – possibly Vesalius himself – performs an autopsy on a female corpse in front of a crowd of spectators, students and others, about 70 strong. A figure of a skeleton is also prominent, possibly because Vesalius used one in his teaching, but there are allusions to the figure of the Grim Reaper that would be familiar to audiences at the time. Dissection, then, was not just a furtive candlelit activity as it had been for Leonardo da Vinci, but a public spectacle – a surgical 'theatre'. This performative aspect of medical illustration and explanation can be seen in other ways too – the flowery classical Latin, for example. His famous series of 'musclemen' – depicting the arrangement of a person's muscles – are drawn walking around in rural landscapes or resting on ruined bits of classical architecture. Another feature of Renaissance anatomical drawings is that they often represent a 'self-disclosing' figure. That is, the corpse in the picture is putting its hands into its abdomen to open it up for the viewer. As well as being an artistic flourish, this was also important because of the way that many people, including some senior church figures, were suspicious of the new science. The 'self-disclosing' corpses, on the other hand, were showing how natural it all was.

The 1500s, then, were an important period in refashioning what was believed about the body. In the space of less than 100 years, the discipline of medicine changed from being one that was largely based on texts to one that was based on observation. From being a divine and spiritual creation, the body was turned into something that was made of frameworks, levers and tubes. In this respect, it anticipated the slightly later vogue for mechanical models, systems of fountains and mechanized statues that entertained the wealthier classes in Europe and inspired the youthful René Descartes (1596–1650) to speculate about how reflexes were achieved by the body. This dream – that mechanical models can tell us how human beings function – is prevalent in studies of cognitive science and artificial intelligence today. The idea is that if we can convincingly model a process on a machine, then maybe this tells us about how it works in 'real life'.

There are some interesting points to make about this whole period in the history of anatomy. On the face of it, it looks like a paradigm shift. Ideas, concepts, images and practices changed rapidly. On closer inspection, however, this picture is complicated by several issues. First, it is clear that Vesalius didn't necessarily want to be a revolutionary. He described what he was doing – the anatomy, the language and the pictures – as a kind of return to classical times. Retrospectively, he might have looked like a paradigm shift, but he doesn't necessarily look that way from his own perspective. Whose vision of scientific change, then, do we believe? Secondly, we might well ask what impact all this had on health care for ordinary people in Europe and elsewhere. It is difficult to detect a similar revolution in the regime of bleeding, purging or vomiting that persisted in Europe through all this rapid change among Europe's intellectuals. These treatments were based on Galenic and Hippocratic theories of the humours, which had a lasting influence on health care until much more recent times, arguably into the twentieth century.

Following the expansion of knowledge and human enquiry in the Renaissance, this set the stage for late Renaissance and early Enlightenment philosophers to try to characterize and develop a rationale for the new natural philosophies which were rapidly developing in Europe. A common theme which unites the work of Descartes, Locke and Hume is the primacy they attached to perception, observation and experience as the foundations of knowledge. Rationalist notions that we could understand the physical and spiritual worlds through contemplation and prayer were explicitly rejected, even though the Medieval concern with thinking, introspection and reason remained intact. European intellectual life was thus newly shot through with empiricism and became progressively secularized. These developments went hand in hand with changes in politics, economics and society as English political life underwent a major phase of secularization in the Civil War and the foundations of the Industrial Revolution were laid.

The virtues of history

In this volume we will be using history a great deal. In a sense, it is easier to understand the construction of human knowledge if you know how people built it, what problems it was designed to solve and why people thought they were interesting at the time. History is also useful because it teaches us about how people's ideas about nature and what it means to be human often emerge through struggle and conflict. Sometimes this conflict is of a largely scholastic or academic nature, as with the question of how many angels can dance on the head of a pin, whereas at other times contested ideas are intimately bound up with warfare, revolution or other large-scale conflict. History, then, can sometimes give us a sense of the building blocks of knowledge, or what some contemporary students of the stream of scientific consciousness call 'the genealogy of ideas', a phrase which borrows from Michel Foucault's teaching.

There are, however, some dangers in taking this flirtation with history too seriously. First, it tends to give us the sense that we somehow know more than people did in the past. This is sometimes called the 'up the mountain' story of knowledge. Now, our contemporary technologies certainly allow us to tackle issues which our ancestors would be powerless to master, but this does not necessarily mean that they somehow knew less than we do. Nor does our present-day science lead to solutions that everyone would agree are beneficial.

Second, another trap for our thinking into which we may fall with our penchant for history is to see ideas as if they were entirely the product of the economic, social or theological crises of the time. For example, think of the Greek notion that the human condition is related to the balance of the four humours – blood, phlegm, yellow bile and black bile. This derived from the work of Galen and Hippocrates and it is perfectly possible to argue convincingly that it suited the political and theological spirit of the times in ancient Greece. Yet in making sense of this idea we need to understand how it persisted through a further 1500 years of political and spiritual revolution, crossed geographical, cultural and climatic boundaries and was probably one of the most persuasive, long-lived and successful notions in medicine. Indeed, treatments based on it, such as bleeding, purging and vomiting, fell into disuse only relatively recently. Bleeding fell into disrepute in the early nineteenth century and purging, in the form of laxatives, remained popular in the UK until well into the twentieth century. This occurred despite medicine having undergone a number of major intellectual paradigm shifts through the previous 600 years or so. Thus, ideas are sometimes considerably more than byproducts of the cultural periods that produced them.

To span the period in history from the Norman Conquest of Britain to the present day would require only 13 70-year-olds' lifetimes. Yet as we shall see, during these 13 lifetimes, the picture of the world, the place of humanity within it, notions of morality and consciousness itself have undergone some dramatic shifts.

To give a fairly well-known example of this process, let us consider the history of opiate use. Throughout much of the nineteenth century, opiate drugs were freely available in Britain – they were cheap and, by all accounts, very widely used. Yet more recently, these have been redefined as exotic 'Class A' substances, the pleasures and pains of which are now known only to a small minority. Without wishing to lapse into a crude pharmacological determinism, it is possible to argue that the consciousness of our nineteenth-century forebears would differ in important respects from our own. Moreover, most of us whose families have lived in the UK for several generations are descended from people who would nowadays be called 'smackheads', complete with its connotations of criminality, fecklessness and poor parenting skills. Likewise, contemporary readers of Arthur Conan Doyle's famous 'Sherlock Holmes' stories are sometimes puzzled at the blatant and sometimes prodigious cocaine use of the hero. Nowadays, of course, in our modern narratives of crime and punishment, the miscreants rather than the detectives are depicted as the drug users.

The point to note is the dramatic shift not only in social practice but also in the legal and moral connotations of self-administered drug use. Any understanding of what it means to consider human beings and their fleshy embodiment needs to take account of such shifts. The apparent indifference of some nineteenth-century surgeons to the pain and suffering of their patients during childbirth or amputations was not necessarily because they were brutal or insensitive as we would nowadays understand it. It simply wasn't their job to worry about this, as it was assumed that the patient could take care of their own anaesthetic needs via a few pennyworth of laudanum.

Thus, history, even when it is the stuff with which we are familiar, is often worth a second, more critical look. The alleged revolution of the Renaissance and the alleged brutality of nineteenth-century medicine are cases in point. We need to understand what was going on at that time to make sense of the impact on knowledge, moreover, we need to understand the process of creating histories in the present day to make sense of what our vision of the past means. The past is important to contemporary scholars. In the host discipline of two of us (B.B. and C.H.) it is customary to intro-duce pieces of academic writing with some allusion to what the ancient Greeks (or perhaps a more recent originator) thought about the issue. History is itself part of the process of constructing a regime of truth. It has played a part in the construction of theories of knowledge from positivism to postmodernism, so it will come as no surprise to the reader to see history in the present volume.

However, we are not plundering history to support a particular world-view. Rather, it is to show the peculiar changes and constancies in the business of ideas and to examine how ways of knowing have come about. Ideas, concepts and research strategies that appear commonsensical and part of the bedrock of science often have quite specific genealogies and their invention and adoption was shot through with controversy. The present contours of scientific knowledge, with the mines of informa-tion, factories of facts, frameworks of clinical governance, and border guards in the form of grant-awarding panels and referees of publications, were, like the political and economic map of the world, often formulated through struggle and warfare. It is to these struggles, then, that we shall turn in the forthcoming chapters.

References

Bhaskar, R. (1998) *The Possibility of Naturalism*. London: Routledge.

Brencick, J.M. and Webster, G.A. (2000) *Philosophy and Nursing: A New Vision for Health Care*. New York: State University of New York Press.

Cheek, J. and Rudge, T. (1994) Nursing as textually mediated reality, *Nursing Inquiry*, 1(1): 15–22.

Lipowski, F.P. (1967) Prehistoric and early historic trepanation, in D. Brothwell and A.T. Sandison (eds) *Diseases in Antiquity*. New York: C.C. Thomas.

Kuhn, T.S. (1962) *The Structure of Scientific Revolutions*. Chicago, IL: University of Chicago Press.

Marx, K. (1933) *Capital* (with an introduction by G.D.H. Cole). London: Dent.

Smail, D.J. (1997) *Illusion and Reality: The Meaning of Anxiety*. London: Constable.

Verano, J.W. and Ubelaker, D.H. (1992) *Disease and Demography in the Americas*. New York: Smithsonian Institution Press.

2

Epistemology I: positivism – 'they don't build epistemologies like that any more'

The facts that began to speak for themselves.

(Quetelet 1840)

Introduction

This chapter will get us started in the philosophy of science proper. That is, we will deal with one of the standard set pieces of the philosophy of science, namely positivism. The persistence of positivism in books about the philosophy of science is peculiar, in that it flourished relatively briefly in the nineteenth century and again in the early twentieth century, and hardly anyone would now admit to being a positivist. Indeed, it is a kind of insult in the present day, being used largely to describe work one does not like, especially if it is considered to be particularly mindless and inhumane. Indeed, positivism is increasingly excluded from attempts to philosophize about health care (Polifroni and Welch 1999; Hussey 2001). However, the impact of positivism on the shaping of modern scientific enquiry and scientific attitudes has been profound. Most alternative philosophies of science have originated as a kind of dialogue with what their makers thought of as positivism, or as an attempt to clarify, extend or transcend positivism.

This chapter will consider some of the important aspects of the intellectual and social context in which positivism emerged and try to show how it made sense relative to the sciences and scholarly currents at the time. Positivism gained in stature because it enabled its adherents to speak very flatteringly of the sciences of the day. It has been suggested that the positivists were 'science intoxicated'. It also provided a rationale for the obsessive accumulation of facts, especially from the unsavoury crevices of nineteenth-century civilization. Positivism provided a rationale for the shifts in patterns of knowing, types of knowledge and the development of knowledge in the nineteenth and early twentieth centuries and provided a protocol for the way in which this new-found knowledge should impact on practice, policy and education. Its founder, Auguste Comte's vision of sociologists as a new priestly caste may seem amusing, but it reflects a much more durable idea that social problems could be addressed via research, which has left its imprint on present-day approaches to human welfare, such as the vogue at the time of writing for so-called 'evidence-based practice'.

Epistemology – towards a definition

The term 'epistemology' is made up of the Greek-derived terms *episteme*, 'knowledge' or 'science', and *logos*, 'knowledge', 'information', 'theory' or 'account'. It is the theory of knowledge, or as it is sometimes taken to mean, an analysis of the conditions, possibilities and limits of our knowledge-gaining processes (Johnson and Cassell 2001). A good deal of contemporary epistemology is concerned with the analysis of propositional knowledge ('knowing that') and has not, by and large, focused on pro-cedural knowledge ('knowing how') and acquaintance knowledge ('knowing who'). Epistemology is often concerned with the nature, sources and justification of the major kinds of knowledge, for example how we may come to know things through the senses in the form of empirical knowledge, or *a priori* knowledge that we may have from other sources or via logic. The philosopher Richard Rorty (1979) notes that epistemology is appealing because it appears to offer a vantage point from which we can evaluate other claims to knowledge. A kind of Archimedean point from which we can ask 'how do you know that?'. Epistemology, in this view, is pivotal to science.

However, it does have some difficulties. As Otto Neurath (1944) pointed out, any theory of knowledge has to presuppose knowledge of the conditions under which knowledge takes place. It has a self-defeating circular quality. You have to use some sort of knowledge to evaluate other claims to knowledge, even if it is merely know-ledge about research methods. Epistemology in science often involves using science to evaluate scientific claims. For Neurath, it is not possible to avoid philosophy and detach ourselves from our epistemological commitments to evaluate epistemological rules, because we would need to depend on them to perform this reflexive task. Thus, there are no secure foundations from which we can begin our evaluation of know-ledge. This is not a very unusual philosophical claim. Many philosophers have been concerned with how we can know things or how we can be persuaded that anything in the so-called real world is indeed real. However, what is extraordinary about this claim from Otto Neurath is that he was a core member – a striker, if you will – of what has been called the Manchester United of positivism: the Vienna Circle. This group is usually famous for its rabid empiricism, its fanatical devotion to the hard sciences as a model for human enquiry, and a strongly foundationalist approach, involving a belief in an external reality which science can help us to discover. However, as we shall see, there are a number of surprises in store when we explore positivism and empiricism a little more deeply.

To begin with, let us consider for a few moments what was special about positiv-ism and why it was different from a good many other philosophical perspectives. In addition, we shall show how many of the apparently dispassionate empirical enquiries into the human condition of the nineteenth and early twentieth centuries were not strictly empirical at all, but were lurid with moral, sentimental and political values. The positivists' repertoire of scientific rhetoric allows these values to be smuggled into a research programme, yet gives us very few tools to analyse them or dig them out once they have been embedded.

Histories of reason: the precursors of positivism

Let us begin our quest with a little history of ideas. Whereas the story of positivism in this chapter begins in the nineteenth century, the previous 300 years had seen intellectuals struggling to accommodate the shifts in world-view and strategies of enquiry prompted by the Galilean and Newtonian revolutions. Despite these profound changes, the implications of radical empiricism had yet to be worked through fully within philosophy. The piecemeal attempts to make sense of nature and human enquiry within it are cumbersome to catalogue in detail, but a brief tour of its edited highlights might include the legacy of Plato (429–347 B.C.) in the form of rationalism, consisting of a belief that it is possible to obtain knowledge of what exists by reason alone. Plato highlighted the importance of ideas and concepts, in the form of ideal forms or archetypes. The permanent, disembodied forms or ideas were perfect spiritual entities and the physical world was a poor and imperfect copy.

Plato, then, thought that we were all born pre-programmed with certain kinds of knowledge, an idea that has variously been described as innatism, idealism or rationalism. He viewed ordinary people as like prisoners trapped in a dark cave, forced to watch a shadow puppet show which they think is 'real' and only those trained to a high level of logic will see the more real world of ideal forms – a kind of permanent and disembodied view of knowledge. Aristotle's (384–322 B.C.) understanding of knowledge was more down to earth. He saw the scientist's job as observing particular phenomena and generalizing from that – called induction – for example, by looking at swimming frogs, concluding that all frogs can swim.

These thinkers, then, asserted the primacy of thought and ideal forms – hence the terms idealism and rationalism. One way of thinking of this is to see it as a kind of 'top-down', theory-driven variety of processing, where the ideas strongly determine the outcome.

This insistence on the primacy of thought is also to be found in René Descartes's (1596–1650) work where his systematic doubt produced his famous axiom *cogito ergo sum* – 'I think therefore I am' – from which he satisfied himself that God existed, and hence everything else. His philosophy asserted that true knowledge can only be derived from reason and that empirical knowledge – based on observation – was flawed.

The concept of a realm of ideas or reason that was relatively independent of reality found its way into a good deal of pre-nineteenth-century thought. Kant (1724–1804), for example, concluded that although we acquire knowledge of the world from our experiences (*a posteriori*), unless we as sentient beings had some kind of pre-existing or *a priori* conceptual apparatus to begin with, no experiences would ever be possible. He thus blended the rationalist or idealist tradition with the empirical one. Although his epistemology is anti-empiricist in denying that all knowledge is derived from experience, he joined with the empiricists that knowledge is limited to the world of experience.

The perceiving mind and its role in supporting sensations and perceptions was also central to Berkeley's (1685–1753) theories of perception. Bishop Berkeley insisted that our experiences are mental – that there is no 'out there' and everyday experience is just an illusion. In this sense, his philosophy was a variant of idealism in that only ideas exist. Thus when things are not perceived they do not exist, so that when the proverbial tree falls in the forest when no-one is around, it does indeed make no 'sound', for sound is a human sensation. For Berkeley, it was possible to take this even further – in such a situation, the tree may not exist either.

The social impact of ideas was appreciated by Francis Bacon (1561–1626) when he declared that 'knowledge is power', giving idealism an altogether more political flavour, a point appreciated by Machiavelli (1469–1527) too. Bacon, like many of those who asserted the primacy of ideas and rationality, believed in induction – that is, generalizing from specific examples or phenomena to form a universal conclusion or truth and predicting what would happen in the future. Previous experience is thus a useful guide to future experience. These two thinkers, in their way, proposed that knowledge is a way of solving social or diplomatic problems and thus began the idea that philosophy could be used to understand and manipulate the 'body politic' – the social body or the state.

In contrast to this trend in European thought, which asserted the primacy of ideas and human or divine organization of experience, there was a countervailing trend that emphasized the sensory impressions or experiences themselves. This is known as empiricism and more formally stated it asserts that all knowledge of matters of fact is based on experience. The name of John Locke (1632–1704) is associated with this trend, though ironically he probably wasn't an empiricist himself, strictly speaking. His enquiries were directed at 'what God has fitted us to know' – again emphasizing the pre-formulated and pre-figured nature of human understanding. However, he is well known for his insistence that the content of human knowledge is not innate and that the infant at birth is like 'white paper' – the famous *tabula rasa* or blank slate – on which experience 'writes'. This assertion of the importance of sensory impressions and experiences was at the time a minority point of view in European intellectual life and it is doubtful if even Locke believed in empiricism fully. However, this is taken as one of the key starting points of the line of thinking which led to the development of positivism in the nineteenth century. Although Locke insisted that fundamental knowledge must come from the senses, he was complicit with rationalism in that he agreed with Descartes that our minds only achieve representations of the 'world' – we cannot have direct knowledge of the external world that we know to be 'out there'. Empiricism was pushed further away from rationalism by David Hume (1711–1776), who disagreed with Francis Bacon that induction was a reliable foundation for science. He argued that all scientific findings based on observation and induction must remain temporary. It does not offer the certainty of deductive logic. He gives the example of the induction that all swans are white until you find out that there is a black one in Australia. He was also sceptical about causation – and saw causes as merely metaphysical human beliefs based on past experiences. However, like Locke and Bacon before him, Hume considered that the search for knowledge started with 'direct sensory experience, and it was this latter branch of the epistemological divide that was carried forward by positivist philosophy'. There are seven species of swans, all white except for the Australian Black Swan and the South American Black-necked Swan. The first European to see a Black Swan is believed to be the Dutch sailor Antonie Caen, who described the species during his visit to the Shark Bay area in 1636. Later, the Dutch explorer Willem de Vlamingh captured two birds on the Swan

River, Western Australia in 1697, but many people in Europe did not believe him. An example of induction leading them astray, perhaps.

The point of this short history lesson is to show that there was a great deal of emphasis – even among those who are usually thought of as empiricists – on notions of divine influence, the primacy of ideas, and reason. Even though Locke and Hume had laid the foundations, there was a strong desire for an epistemology equal to the Enlightenment developments in 'natural philosophy', as science was then known. The 'age of reason' was not about reason alone, it was about experiments. Electricity coursed through the body, crackled through Benjamin Franklin's kite string and Luigi Galvani's frogs' legs. Changes in pressure and temperature caused rain to fall, dew to form and pistons to pump the mineshafts dry and turn the wheels of Samuel Crompton's spinning mules in the textile mills. Moreover, the political revolutions reconstructing Europe and the new world fed the hunger for a new secular philosophy uncontaminated by the religious sentiments of the old order.

This begins our story of positivism itself. The basic idea – that it was possible to develop knowledge systems that avoided theology, speculation and metaphysics and that rely exclusively on what can be observed – was most thoroughly developed in the mid-nineteenth-century work of Auguste Comte (1798–1857). Even so, Comte's dream of a positive philosophy based on observation that would liberate humanity from the failures of tradition was only one of a number of important but lesser known strands in nineteenth-century thinking.

What was happening in connection with the industrial and political revolutions taking place in the Western hemisphere at that time is that scholars and policy makers were seeking new ways of making sense of the new civil and economic body politic. For example, to raise money by selling annuities (a kind of early form of pension scheme), entrepreneurs and governments would need to know how long their clients were likely to live, and the widely used Northampton mortality tables overestimated the morality rate to such an extent that this money-raising venture instead cost the British Government as much as £8000 per annum. In this context, the measurement of the 'social body' became particularly urgent, and it was Comte's near contemporary Lambert Adolphe Quetelet (1796–1874) who first propelled statistical methods into the human sciences. Originally working as a statistician and meteorologist for the Belgian Government, Quetelet became fascinated by tables of mortality rates, crime rates and illnesses, such as were newly available from the governments of Europe. Rates of crime, illness and death obeyed a curious stability from one year to the next, which puzzled intellectuals of the day – surely the decision to commit murder, perpetrate a robbery, or whether one succumbed to illness was a profoundly individual matter? The discovery of these regularities was a source of great excitement to Quetelet, who believed they revealed information of great interest to governments and business people (Murphy and Cooper 2000). In addition, Quetelet pioneered the measurement of human beings themselves as well as the body politic. One of his techniques, the calculation of a body mass index (weight in kilogrammes divided by height in metres squared), is still widely used today. He was fascinated by such data as the chest circumferences of Scottish army recruits and the heights of French ones and dedicated himself to mapping human physical and moral characteristics. He called this new science social mechanics. He was also one of the first to borrow probabilistic notions and import them into this science of social mechanics. In particular, the idea of a normal distribution, first invented in 1733 by DeMoivre and popularized by Gauss in 1809 to describe the pattern of error in astronomical measurement, could, Quetelet discovered, describe the pattern of variability in measurements of human characteristics and human activity. All of a sudden, the human sciences had become statistical disciplines (Hankins [1908] 1968). This tradition was, of course, carried forward with the attempts by Emile Durkheim to use suicide rates to tell one something about the kind of society where the suicides take place. The measurement and systematic comparison of people and their characteristics led, through the work of Francis Galton, to the development of twentieth-century psychology. One of the important features of Quetelet's thinking was that facts could 'speak for themselves' or rather 'speak loudly of their own accord'. As well as pushing statistical techniques into the human and moral disciplines, Quetelet made the fact–value distinction a central feature of his new social mechanics – the idea that is was possible to have knowledge, especially of a quantitative kind, from which morality and values had been excluded.

These technical developments were accompanied by a philosophical reconfiguration of knowledge. Auguste Comte was developing his theory of the history of science and was proposing the new discipline of sociology, which had a lot in common with Quetelet's social mechanics. Comte is credited with coining the term 'positivism' and he influenced figures as diverse as Karl Marx, Charles Darwin, John Stuart Mill and even the novelist George Eliot, who believed herself to be a positivist.

Comte believed, optimistically, that human knowledge, indeed the human mind itself, evolves through three stages as it moves from superstition to empirical science:

1. First, the theological stage where people view nature as having a mind or will of its own. This may take the form of: (i) animism, where objects themselves are viewed as having their own will; (ii) polytheism, where a variety of divine wills are seen as imposing themselves on objects and on people; and (iii) monotheism, where the will of a single god imposes itself on objects and humanity.

2. Second, human knowledge passes through a stage of metaphysics, where instead of wills, desires and minds, people see nature as full of forces and causes.

3. Finally, a third positive phase is entered where (according to Giddens 1995; Porter 2001) scientific enquiry has a number of important characteristics: (i) The adherence to scientism – that is, scientific knowledge is the only true and reliable knowledge, gathered through careful and systematic observation, which will enable the observer to generate theories about the causal relationships between them. (ii) The belief in phenomenalism – that reality is made known to us through sensory impressions. (iii) The rejection of speculative philosophy, such that the pursuit of knowledge should be, in this view, anchored to the pursuit of reality and utility. A positive philosophy should not attempt to see behind appearances and should restrict itself to being the handmaid of science by helping to set out the principles of scientific knowing. (iv) The rejection of metaphysics. Comte's philosophy was an avowedly secular one – he did not believe that knowledge could be arrived at by means of divine revelation or speculation, and we could not know about the origins or ultimate ends

and purposes of the universe or human life in it. (v) The rejection of epistemological absolutism, in that knowledge is always seen as provisional and does not emerge from any grasp of absolute essences. However, as time goes by, our knowledge will get closer and closer to the truth, but probably never get there – that is, it approaches truth 'asymptotically'. (vi) Determinism. Unlike Quetelet, Comte did not place very much importance on chance. The relationships between events are determined and invariable. (vii) The separation of facts and values. This involves the contention that empirical knowledge of the world is separable – and, moreover, should be kept separate – from morality. This is where the ideas of 'value neutral' knowledge, 'neutral facts' and 'objectivity' come from, as well as the idea that facts can speak for themselves. (viii) The belief in naturalism – that is, the idea that there is an essential unity between the natural and social sciences, and that the social world is governed by empirically discoverable causal relationships in the same way that the natural and social sciences share a common logical foundation. This last point should not be taken to suggest that Comte thought that the natural and social sciences should be identical – indeed, he believed that each science should develop a unique and appropriate methodology.

Today, Comte is best remembered for his invention of sociology, the new science *par excellence*, which would encompass and surpass the sciences that had gone before, outstripping the mere 'social physics' of his contemporaries. On the one hand, sociology would study social statics; that is, it would measure the current state of socio-political systems. On the other hand, there was social dynamics, which would examine how far humanity had come through the three stages of theology, meta-physics and positivism. Moreover, once a science of society had been achieved, order and progress could be achieved in a rational and humane manner. Influenced by the revolutionary and socialist sentiments of the new Republican France and his mentor and friend Saint-Simon, his aim was for a society in which human beings would 'live for others', aided by the knowledge that would emerge from the new positivistic sciences. Under such conditions people would not be willing to fight over political or religious ideas as they had in the past and conflict would be replaced by a new spirit of cooperation for the common good.

In practical terms, these philosophical movements undergird the conviction that 'The truth is out there' as they say on the popular science fiction series the 'X Files'. Positivism has informed science, but most importantly it has informed popular culture. Positivism thus has a legacy in everyday and scientific thinking. Arguably, positivism has been implicated in the rise of reductionism, the ascendancy of the medical model and the late twentieth-century resurgence of genetic and evolutionary paradigms for explaining health and social behaviour, of a kind that some have argued is overly reductive and politically reactionary. At the time of writing, many would see positivism as a socially conservative trend in science. This is particularly ironic as Comte himself saw positivism as a kind of liberation from the political and religious dogmas that stunted humanity in the past. Comte saw positivism as being a suitable replacement for religion, He had visions of new, secular saints replacing the old sacred ones – Adam Smith, Frederick the Great, Dante and Shakespeare, for example, would have their holy days. There was a positive Catechism, and he even got as far as designing the costumes for the positivistic sociologist-priests of the new religion.

The story of positivism does not stop there, however, because the ideas within this influential way of looking at the relationship between science, society and the natural world were very attractive to several other European thinkers. In particular, a group of intellectuals from the University of Vienna began to meet to discuss ideas about science, from about 1907. They included Otto Neurath, a sociologist, Hans Hahn, a mathematician, and Philipp Frank, a physicist. Later, in the 1920s, Moritz Schlick became the leader and arranged for Rudolf Carnap to join them in 1926. The so-called Vienna Circle ceased to function as a coherent group in the 1930s with the rise of Nazism, especially as many of its members were Jewish, or had Marxist sympathies, or both. Their leader, Moritz Schlick, was shot and killed on the steps of the main university building by one of his students in 1936 (Sarkar 1996).

Although they are thought of mainly for their contributions to the philosophy of science, in the form of 'logical positivism', the members of the Vienna Circle were especially interested in language, and were concerned with how we could know the truth about statements which were made about the world. Their overarching concern was with verification. A statement was meaningful in so far as it could be challenged against facts that might verify or refute it. Probably most Vienna Circle members would have concurred with Carnap's idea that the essential problem faced by the scientist was to do with verifying statements about the world using immediately given sense data. In his 1928 magnum opus, 'The logical structure of the world', Carnap argued that all terms suited to describe empirical facts are definable in terms referring exclusively to elements of immediate experience (Sarkar 1996).

Subsequently, this approach to making sense of statements about the world has run into difficulties. For example, there has been increasing concern with the way that human beings make sense of the world in an active, constructive fashion, and the way we assign these experiences to human-constructed categories. This means that it is very difficult to imagine what a description of experience purely in terms of sense data would look like. However, this insistence on empirical verification led the philosophy of science towards Karl Popper's later development of falsificationism, which we shall deal with later. There were other statements that the Vienna Circle believed were meaningful but did not have to do with empirical verification, namely statements that were *a priori* true on logical or mathematical grounds. Of particular interest to the Vienna Circle were so-called protocol statements. These were statements about basic empirical sense data or records of scientific observation. Carnap insisted that they should record experience directly and contain nothing which resulted from induction. This idea of verifying our knowledge by comparing it to a set of basic statements about the world can be found also in Wittgenstein's idea of elementary propositions, Russell's atomic propositions and Ayer's basic statements, and has been a very influential idea in empiricist theorizing.

Interestingly, the Vienna Circle, while it included sociologists, mathematicians and physicists, as far as we are aware did not include anyone with a background in medicine or any other health care discipline. This may explain why health care has not figured very prominently in the twentieth-century philosophy of science, which has focused on either physics (famously undergoing revolutions and transitions), or sociology (one of the more philosophy-friendly social science disciplines). Medicine might occasionally climb into bed with moral philosophy, especially where ethics are concerned, but it is not typically a site where epistemological battles are fought out. However, the relationship between the health care disciplines and the kinds of issues tackled by investigators of a positivistic bent is more complex. The social body was emblazoned and made visible in a similar way to the physical body in the Middle Ages. Moreover, the qualities of the social body came to be understood in much the same way as those of the physical body. Durkheim is credited with the phrase 'crime is a disease', yet he was merely repeating a commonplace phrase from the intellectual life of his day (Durkheim 1973). The ills of the physical body became the model for the social body or body politic. Nowadays, it is common to contrast the 'medical model' with psycho-social approaches, yet both of these apparently contrasting perspectives have a common heritage.

At the same time as the members of the Vienna Circle were advancing philosophy deeper and deeper into a deliberately mindless empiricism, this suspicion of mentalist and metaphysical concepts was driving much American and British psychology towards behaviourism, following Watson's (1914) statement, and was flourishing with the kind of analysis that sought to establish logical and mathematical laws of behaviour. In the meantime also in England, a kind of analytical language philosophy was being practised in the early twentieth century by Russell and Wittgenstein (e.g. Russell 1914, Wittgenstein 1922). Here, in Russell's formulation all our statements can be analysed into elementary propositions that directly picture states of affairs. Thus not only was scientific enquiry dominated by this spirit of challenge against reality, but any kind of language, scientific or otherwise was meaningful and truthful in so far as it pictured states of affairs.

The association between positivism, mathematics and the human sciences itself was not inevitable but was carefully cultivated in the human disciplines. We have already mentioned Quetelet's efforts early in the nineteenth century, but this tendency was at work in psychology too. In 1891, Joseph Jastrow commented:

> To anyone impressed with the importance of objective results it is always gratifying to throw into numerical form the result of subjective or partially unconscious operations. The difficulties of introspective observations are many and obvious; such observations are warped, not only by the thought-habits of the individual observer, but they labour more particularly with the difficulty that if we allow our mental processes to go on in their natural trend, our memory of them soon fades away and becomes distorted, while in so far as we turn about to stare at them as they pass through the mind their original purity passes from them and leaves them artificial; they are like children romping about unconcernedly and expressing themselves freely in the privacy of the family circle, but bashful, silent, and conventional before strangers.
>
> (Jastrow 1891, p. 559)

This kind of concern, common among intellectuals in the late nineteenth and early twentieth centuries, may seem quaint by contemporary standards. In our present age of palmtop personal computing, voice recognition and live streaming web-cam feeds, when everything is so compellingly and immediately visible, the concern with the possibility that thoughts might be distorted if not expressed in an immediately mathematical form might seem obtuse. However, in an age that relied much more heavily on face-to-face communication, when papers and books had to be written out laboriously in longhand, checked through and sent to the typesetter to be meticulously set, cast or etched before printing, when the development even of viable tape recorders was 50 years away, the attraction of a relatively permanent mathematical summary of one's intellectual endeavours grasped the thinking classes with ferocity that is now difficult to imagine. In the 1880s, Alphonse Bertillion was measuring criminals in the hope of devising a unique set of measurements that would enable individual offenders to be recognized. This was especially apposite at the time because the numbers obtained could readily be transmitted by telegraph, whereas expensive photographs could only be sent through the slow and unreliable postal systems between the police forces of Europe (Bertillion 1941).

'Spectacular impoverishment' – making the body politic visible in the nineteenth century

This idea of exploring, recording, quantifying and reporting the state of humanity and the state of society itself was a common theme in nineteenth-century intellectual and public life. Societies were not obvious, even to their own members. It took pioneering investigators and collectors of statistics to demonstrate the level of poverty and the conditions affecting the 'labouring classes' whose filth, criminality, profanity and disorderliness preoccupied Victorian policy makers and intellectuals. Edwin Chadwick, in his report 'The Sanitary Conditions of the Labouring Population' in 1842, disclosed that the labouring classes lived in rubbish, excrement and offal, and was able to demonstrate that in 1839 less than two out of three infants born in England would reach their fifth birthdays.

Researchers were struggling to make visible the fleshy mysteries of the body, and this spirit of exploration also inspired the investigations of the social fabric in which these bodies were embedded. Why, for example, were these bodies so often undersized, malnourished and suffering from rickets? In the mid-nineteenth century, the work of Henry Mayhew (1851) became famous as he published his four-volume work on the condition of the poor, *London Labour and the London Poor*. This ethnographic excursion into the *terra incognita* – the unknown world of poverty in London, based on his journalism for the *Morning Chronicle* – disclosed to the literate classes a world of whose existence they had little comprehension, where, for example, people foraged in the sewage for objects that could be re-used, including the occasional set of false teeth that could be washed off and sold; where people subsisted on a diet of street refuse; or followed occupations such as that of the 'pure finder', who collected dog dirt and sold it to tanneries. Here it was used for preparing the leathers for bookbinding and making kid gloves. Even Mayhew, with his emphasis on lived experience, was fascinated by the numbers who followed these occupations and the incomes they made. One of his contemporaries, Thackeray, described this work in the following terms:

A picture of human life so wonderful, so awful, so piteous and pathetic, so exciting and terrible, that readers of romances own they never read anything like to it;
and that the griefs, struggles, strange adventures here depicted exceed anything
that any of us could imagine. Yes; and these wonders and terrors have been lying
by your door and mine ever since we had a door of our own. We had but to go a
hundred yards off and see for ourselves, but we never did . . . We are of the upper
classes; we have had hitherto no community with the poor. We never speak a
word to the servant who waits on us for twenty years.

(From *Punch*, 9 March 1850, p. 93; quoted in Himmelfarb 1984,
p. 350)

The imagery of exploring and heroic adventure is rife in these pages. At the same
time, the sensibilities of Victorian middle-class propriety are left curiously intact.
They might be troubled by the wretchedness and abject poverty, but they are not
transformed. The spectrum of suffering, from the microbes to the abject poverty, is
laid out before us, yet the moralities are not subject to the same rigorous scrutiny as
the stigmata of disease.

In similar vein, the late nineteenth-century businessman Charles Booth and his
wife Mary undertook a prolonged investigation into the condition of the labouring
classes. They and their collaborators succeeded in surveying approximately 100,000
families and provided information on around 18,000 streets, represented on their
famous poverty map of 1891, where houses and streets were coloured to represent the
different classes of people living there, from black for the vicious semi-criminal to
yellow for the relatively wealthy streets and dwellings (O'Day and Englander 1993;
Bradshaw and Sainsbury 1999). Not only were large-scale maps showing individual
dwelling plots relatively unfamiliar at that time, but Booth and his team were innov-
ators in that they originated the practice of using themed maps to show the topography of various aspects of city life. This 'spectacular' poverty, from being invisible,
was made graphically apparent to the middle and upper classes, to specialists in
public health and policy makers. Positivism then flourished at a time of great efforts to
make things visible, both in the social body and in the mind. At the same time, as we
have seen earlier, there were revolutions taking place in physiology and microbiology
and pioneers such as Claude Bernard found in positivism the ideal philosophical
laboratory assistant. Moreover, the possibility was emerging that disease in cities
spread not from the 'miasma' of stagnant water (as Chadwick had originally
believed), but from specific, individuated microbes, visible in the best laboratories of
Europe.

Thus, with these examples, we have hoped to demonstrate how the frenetic
accumulation of facts – Charles Booth's work alone is estimated to have cost him the
equivalent of £1.3 million at current prices – formed part of a new way of compre-
hending the condition of humanity. This, in spirit, was very much consonant with
Quetelet's social physics, Comte's sociology and Durkheim's social facts. Aligned
with the spirit of accumulating facts, explorations and verification in the sciences, the
full horrors of urban life were beginning to disclose themselves. This voyeurism and
thrill of terror at the condition of the labouring classes found its voice in a number of
popular outlets, including Charles Dickens's 'Household Words'. Despite the vigour

with which reform was attempted, a sense of hopelessness sometimes supervened. For example, trying to teach the families of the East End domestic skills was hampered by the fact that they had no cooking facilities and no utensils, apart perhaps from a single pot that was used for boiling crusts on the open fire, bathing the babies and overnight sanitation.

The depths of depravity: mapping the interior landscape

Even in the twentieth century the horror of feeble-mindedness gripped the early researchers who sought to measure the intelligence of the lower orders. The drive to obtain the facts of the human condition was not a task for the meek or the faint-hearted. The early pioneer of intelligence testing in the United States, Lewis Terman (1916), catalogued in his book *The Measurement of Intelligence* the high levels of what he called 'feeble-mindedness' in delinquents, children in reformatory homes, those from slum areas and immigrants from Europe, and concluded that this lack of intelligence, originating largely in hereditary factors, was a major cause of America's social ills.

> But why do the feeble-minded tend so strongly to become delinquent? The answer may be stated in simple terms. Morality depends upon two things: (a) the ability to foresee and to weigh the possible consequences for self and others of different kinds of behavior; and (b) upon the willingness and capacity to exercise self-restraint. That there are many intelligent criminals is due to the fact that (a) may exist without (b). On the other hand, (b) presupposes (a). In other words, not all criminals are feeble-minded, but all feeble-minded are at least potential criminals. That every feeble-minded woman is a potential prostitute would hardly be disputed by any one. Moral judgment, like business judgment, social judgment, or any other kind of higher thought process, is a function of intelligence. Morality cannot flower and fruit if intelligence remains infantile.
>
> (Terman 1916, p. 11)

Human welfare, then, depended on our relentless investigation and measurement of the factors which might threaten social order. The sentimental Victorian notion of the moral failings of the lower orders and labouring classes was, in the early twentieth century, replaced with the idea that one could examine and measure their inner workings to ascertain the cause of their failings and to make sense of why they had not flourished in the land of opportunity and instead continued to commit crime and spread syphilis.

No matter how horrific the social conditions, the poverty and the moral depravity were, these facts had to be brought to the surface. We can see here the fact–value distinction so beloved of positivism in action. Using and developing methods of studying and transforming the human condition required that one's personal values be put on one side, no matter how sordid and wretched you found the conditions. The researcher, then, was like an explorer and there are parallels to be drawn between the imperial adventures of the European powers abroad and the rapacious spirit of these societies to know themselves inside and out. Although difficult matters were brought up by these investigations, the optimistic spirit of positivism suggested that once we know the conditions, rational scientific management of them will yield the solution.

So far we have been speaking of scientific activities that sought to describe the world using methods which, while innovative, left intact the conceptual terrain that they were studying. Certainly, reform might be overdue, but this was conceived of as something that would come later once the facts had been laid on the table.

Let us now turn to another aspect of nineteenth-century science and medicine, the study of sexuality. Here the fearless spirit of enquiry was doing something a little different. With both physiology and sociology the desire for knowledge and the terrain over which the investigators gazed was self-evident. In sexology, however, something different was happening. First, science – particularly medicine – was reconfiguring the private, moral conduct of individuals along medical lines. Second, in tandem with this, scholars were actively reaching out to plant their flags on this new territory. Poverty, mortality or physical illness were, to most liberal thinking people, 'bad things'. Sex, on the other hand, required a certain amount of work to be done to bring it under the rubric of illness.

The medical discovery of sex is the story of how concepts and activities were colonized by scientists and physicians and matters such as masturbation, female sexuality, and the forms of sexual activity that were possible and desirable were all brought under scientific and moral scrutiny. The nineteenth-century medicalization and regulation of a number of aspects of human sexuality has been documented by several authors (Weeks 1985; Laqueur 1990; Porter and Hall 1995). The 'making of the modern homosexual' has been extensively catalogued (Plummer 1981; Weeks 1985), as has the discovery and treatment of the infamous masturbatory insanity (Hare 1962). Our illustration here will deal with nymphomania, to illustrate how sciences branch out, spread over new surfaces and bring fresh scrutiny to bear on aspects of the human condition. Now, we do not wish to assert that all those who studied sexuality were self-confessed positivists. Neither do the deductions made by doctors at the time adhere to the strict criteria of positivism. However, the discovery of sex yields a number of important images and motifs for the student of late nineteenth-century science. The importance of penetrating the *terra incognita*, and the dispassionate collection of facts no matter how morally or aesthetically repugnant, outweighed fears for one's own moral safety. The legacy of this aspect of how women were formulated as a problem in nineteenth-century medical discourse has stayed with us and translated itself into late twentieth-century accounts of relationship problems. To make sense of many professional and lay accounts of the human condition, and in particular sexuality and its difficulties in the present, we need to see how the problems were formulated in the intense nineteenth-century scrutiny of sexuality.

Carole Groneman (1994) takes up the story of this fearless seeking out of nymphomania:

> the mother of a seventeen-year-old girl contacted Dr. John Tompkins Walton in 1856 because the girl, Catherine, was having 'a fit.' 'This paroxysm,' according to Walton, 'was peculiar and specific . . . in the lascivious leer of her eye and lips, the

contortions of her mouth and tongue, the insanity of lust which disfigured [her], . . . as well as in the positions she assumed and the movements which could not be restrained' (Walton 1857, p. 47). He judged her to be 'in a condition of ungovernable sexual excitement' and was convinced that the primary cause of the disease was seated in her 'animal organization,' which he deduced from her small eyes, large, broad nose and chin, thick lips, and the disproportionate size of the posterior portion of her head (Walton 1857, p. 47).

An enlarged cerebellum was believed by some doctors to indicate increased 'amativeness' or sexual desire. Moralism and science – and class bias – combined in Walton's belief that Catherine was infected by 'the exposure and contagion incident to several families living in one house, with a hydrant and water closet shared by all the court, and [by] the immorality of the youths who lounged about the place' (Walton 1857, p. 48). Ultimately, the girl admitted that she was a 'wanton' and that her sexual appetite was insatiable. Walton rendered her 'emasculate for a time' (although he does not describe his method), prescribed a 'vegetable diet, various drugs, cold hip baths, and leeches to the perineum' (Groneman 1994, p. 338).

By means of this and other examples, Groneman documents how nineteenth-century scientists and doctors addressed the issue of women's sexuality. In this case, note how the good doctor Walton is proceeding. Like any good scientist he carefully notes the significant features of the case, the postures undertaken by the girl, the shape of her face and head – for phrenology and physiognomy were very important intellectual disciplines of the day – and deduces that the underlying cause is sexual excitement, which is suitably treated by means of diet, baths and leeches. Note also the notions of contagion – translated from the latest theories of disease and lurid with the memories of major outbreaks of cholera in the West through the nineteenth century. As well as providing the conceptual apparatus, medical science and positivistic philosophy also provide the guise of dispassionate neutrality. Positivism thus provides the stalking horse behind which the parlour moralities of the Victorian age can be smuggled into play.

The debate around the newly identified organic disease of nymphomania was characterized by a good deal of diversity. It was variously associated with too much desire, too much coitus (either wanting it or having it) and too much masturbation. It was variously theorized as a symptom, a cause and a disease in its own right. In addition, the term, once it had been invented, was broadened to include a variety of other behaviours which parents and the male medical establishment found unpalatable. In the late nineteenth century, European and American doctors were hard at work identifying symptoms of nymphomania, which included committing adultery, flirting, being divorced, or women feeling more passionate than their husbands (Groneman 1994, p. 341). Indeed, in material aimed at a popular audience, some writers identified nymphomania in women who sought to attract men by wearing perfume, adorning themselves and talking of marriage (Talmey [1904] 1912, p. 112).

This discovery of a veritable epidemic of nymphomania went hand in hand with some other significant developments in nineteenth-century health care. Gynaecology became a medical speciality. Prior to this, according to Moscucci (1990), it was

mainly in the hands of midwives. The medicalizing of gynaecology paralleled a growing conviction on the part of most specialists that women's diseases (both of body and
mind) originated with the reproductive organs.

Indeed, to the trained clinical gaze, a good deal could be revealed about women
which they might not themselves be aware of: 'a predominating sexual desire
in women arouses a suspicion of its pathological significance' (Krafft-Ebing [1886]
1965, p. 87). Or, because the causes, signs and symptoms of nymphomania were so
uncertain, physicians were keen to identify physical signs of the disease. Redness,
soreness or itching of the genitalia were identified as signs, and also the size of the
clitoris was assumed to be a major indicator. Hypertrophy of the clitoris or labia was
believed to be the most reliable indicator of the condition, according to theorists like
Churchill (1857).

To many doctors, merely identifying these symptoms was dangerous because
their women patients, they believed, would be sufficiently lust-crazed to attempt to
seduce them. A fear of the insatiable female lurks in other late nineteenth-century
writing about woman and sexuality. As Krafft-Ebing ([1886] 1965) notes, 'Woe unto
the man who falls into the meshes of such an insatiable Messaliona, whose sexual
appetite is never appeased' (p. 403). Indeed, the insatiability of some woman could be
extremely dangerous because 'when they are touched and excited, a time arrives
when, though not intending to sin, they lost all physical control over themselves'
(Heywood Smith, in Routh 1887, p. 505).

The suffering which some women underwent in relation to their assumed nymphomania was extreme. As one case study by Charles Mills (1885) disclosed, the
protagonist, a 29-year-old woman said: 'I inherited from my mother a morbid
disposition' (Mills 1885, p. 535) and 'When I felt tempted, I would kneel and honestly
pray to be kept from doing wrong, and then get up and do it [masturbate] not because
I wanted to but because my life could not go on until the excitement was quieted'
(p. 537). 'At times I felt tempted to seek out the company of men but was too modest'
(p. 535). She was treated by means of clitoridectomy, 'but it grew again ... I
tormented the doctors to operate again' (p. 535). They did, this time removing
the ovaries. 'Since the removal of the ovaries I have been able to control the desire
when awake, but at times in my sleep I can feel something like an orgasm taking place'
(p. 536).

The new spirit of obstetric enquiry was certainly concerned with the gathering of
facts, in best positivistic spirit. But it was not generally accompanied by any reflexive
sensitivity to the moral and political outlook of the scientists and clinicians themselves
or the society within which they were embedded. The separation of facts and values
has yielded a sexual science that is curiously innocent of all the feminist developments
that were going on in the nineteenth century, as the views of Mary Wollstonecraft,
Sojourner Truth, Josephine Butler and even John Stuart Mill became better known.
According to Groneman (1994), making sense of the problems of the women who
found themselves diagnosed with nymphomania involves understanding ideas about
the appropriate forms of sexuality in the nineteenth century. Moreover, this situation
can be understood in relation to the limited opportunities the women had in
nineteenth-century society. When the woman with the re-growing clitoris was
training as a nurse, she 'was not once troubled with nymphomania; but when I had to

give it up and go away, crushed with disappointment, weakness and poverty, . . . when I had to again spend my days in work which held no interest for me, the old morbid depression came back and with it the disease' (Mills 1885, p. 536).

Thus, a territory of female desire is marked out and demarcated also as a problem for those who suffer from it as well as the doctors who treat them. The masterful colonization of this focus of positivistic medicine was deftly accomplished by taking the symptoms, including the subjective reports as well as the physical signs, at face value. Any reflection on the scientists' own inferential process or the cultural context was neatly avoided. The positivist orientation to nature allowed the middle-class front-parlour morality to survive unblemished, and the proponents of these approaches were able to sidestep alternative interpretations of this issue, which seem obvious given the last 150 years of feminism.

There was much more analysis of sexuality in a similar vein as the nineteenth gave way to the twentieth century. Feminist critiques of Freud are well known, but there were a large number of other medical and psychological writers who sought to understand women's sexuality at the turn of the century. Chief among these was the pioneer sexologist Havelock Ellis. According to some recent histories of sex (e.g. Weeks 1985), Ellis's work was progressive in that it admitted that women had sexual desires, but profoundly conservative in other ways in that he subscribed to the view that males are active and predatory and females are passive and wish to be overpowered.

Equally, at the end of the nineteenth and beginning of the twentieth century, as women agitated for the vote, campaigned to be able to study in universities and enter the professions, there was an increasing drift in sexology, biology and medicine to assert the 'naturalness' of female sexual desire. Yet this desire was carefully described by Havelock Ellis and his contemporaries as one which fitted into the 'natural order' of the sexes. Havelock Ellis's work was predicated on the notion that heterosexual sex is based on a power relation that is biologically determined: 'male domination and female submission are therefore not only inevitable but essential to sexual pleasure' (quoted in Jackson 1994, p. 109). If sexual intercourse took place against a women's will, it was usually with the consent of her 'unconscious instinct', which sided with her attacker against her conscious resistance (Ellis 1913, Vol. III, p. 42). As Jackson puts it, in Ellis's scheme of things:

> The male sexual urge was defined as essentially a desire to conquer the female. Female resistance, far from being real, was the manifestation of female sexual desire – the need to be conquered. Conquest and resistance, dominance and submission, were defined as natural. In both sexes, desire manifested itself period- ically and spontaneously; it was thus inappropriate to blame or criticise men for the sexual exploitation of women, or for sexual 'excess'. If the female experienced pain, this too was defined as natural; it was rooted in impulses which were essentially 'innocent', and thus not inherently harmful or problematic.
>
> (Jackson 1994, p. 111)

Ellis's philosophical manoeuvre, then, was made possible by the fact–value distinction so beloved of positivists. He was able to write from a position that appeared to be rooted in the science of sex, embedded within the very best of Darwinian principles, well beyond any superficial contamination from morality. This version of naturalness and the location of the origins of present-day human characteristics in prehistoric utopias is precisely why evolutionary thinking is controversial, then as now. As Donna Haraway (1986, p. 77) famously said, 'primatology is the pursuit of politics by other means'.

One of the important points to appreciate in this historical tale is why the most self-consciously scientific accounts of human nature are so controversial. The discussion of primates, organ systems and social statistics is conducted in scientific terms, yet does not acknowledge alternative perspectives, points of view of other constituencies or interest groups. In so far as the voices of the poor or of patients are heard, they are usually co-opted to the investigators' moral programme. This story of sexuality, then, illustrates why scientific models and methods are often charged with being reactionary. This curious interplay of science with progressive and reactionary ideologies is illustrated in some contemporary therapeutic discourse on relationships and sexuality. The pre-eminently scientific discourse of evolution is deployed to make differences between the sexes appear natural. Whether evolution in the strict Darwinian sense has indeed predisposed us to act as sex-stereotyped men and women is, of course, debatable (e.g. Keller and Longino 1996). However, the interesting feature of these debates is the way they draw not only upon notions of science, but also deploy the fact–value distinction so that the facts are taken to be established and inevitable and the job of the advice seekers is to work around these. A similar process is at work in popular contemporary advice about relationships. Thus, for example, best-selling author John Gray, in his popular *Mars and Venus* books (e.g. Gray 1992, 1995), describes men as Martians and women as Venusians – characters constructed in line with widely held stereotypes that help to naturalize the difference between men and women. The interesting part of this strategy, as Potts (1998) argues, is how it 'surreptitiously encourages the female reader to accept and relax into her position of subordination, to resign herself to the natural/inevitable authority of her man' (p. 171). For example, like her nineteenth-century forebear, the more sexually voracious woman is in need of restriction and control. If women orgasm too frequently or are left hungry for more, Gray suggests, they should limit themselves to only one big one (Gray 1995, p. 143). Thus, female sexuality is legislated into a mould that mimics the male variety as a way of working around what is 'scientifically established' and the male model remains unproblematically setting the agenda. Here again, it does not take a very politically sensitive soul to be drawn to Donna Haraway's assertion that primatology is politics by other means.

Of course, nowhere do popular advice givers identify themselves as positivists, any more than characters in the 'X Files' quote Auguste Comte. What is interesting from our point of view is how the sciences and the accompanying scientific philosophies of the nineteenth century have left their stamp on contemporary culture. The power of positivism is its very invisibility. The positivist can be thought of as doing what Haraway calls the 'God trick', attempting to be invisible and having no influence on the apparently 'objective' facts.

Theorizing visibility: factual anchorage and political slippage

So far we have dealt with empiricism and positivism as if they led inevitably to a certain kind of science – obsessed with facts, reality, truth, quantification, but at the same time somewhat socially conservative. There were a number of ways in which this spirit of enquiry set the stage for the enthusiasm for deductive reasoning strategies in science and medicine. The collection of facts and observations was accompanied by a great deal of classification and category building. The categories of sexual desire, the colour coding of social deprivation, the diagnoses of disease, all facilitated deduction. That is, it allowed those who observed black regions on the map to imagine, with some accuracy, that these would be plagued by social pathology, just like the ones which had been studied intensively. Fresh cases of nymphomania, homosexuality or masturbatory insanity would exhibit the same pathologies as those we already knew. The physician or the social reformer, though he (and it usually was a he) might blench at the horrors involved, knew with a grim scientific certainty that the new cases would exhibit the same tragic degeneracy as the theory predicted.

Deduction, then, goes from the general to the specific and tries to make predictions based on theories. If the theories and the deductive processes are right, the conclusion will always be right. Induction, on the other hand, where we try to build a general model by looking at specific examples, no matter how well it is done, is always suspect and frequently wrong. Deduction, where we use general theories and models to build predictions about specific cases, is a process of logic and is probably not seen very often in its pure form. On the other hand, there are variants of deduction that are more often seen in empirical science. For example, Peirce's notion of abduction (Fann 1990) describes the kind of thinking that scientists may be found performing in their work. This involves a sense of suspicion, a hunch if you will, followed by observations to check whether it is true or not. Peirce's description of this process of suspicion followed by discovery represents an important part of scientific enquiry. When faced with an observation or measurement that is surprising on the basis of previous knowledge, scientists try to find an explanation that makes it less surprising, and then move on to test that explanation as strenuously as they can.

All these scientific developments we have just described set a kind of background for the early twentieth-century development of positivism by the Vienna Circle. The parallels between the social, natural and health sciences had been firmly established by investigations of the kind we have described. This shows that philosophers are not the only ones who contribute to the philosophy of science. It is often the result of curious people trying to solve practical problems and drawing on the cultural, scientific and moral resources of their times.

Following these developments, then, the Vienna Circle tightened the screw of positivism and intensified the respective truthfulness of so-called synthetic, empirical observation by a strong focus on analytic, mathematical and logical propositions that are true by virtue of the rules of the symbolic system they lie within. Religious, moral and aesthetic statements were seen as metaphysical rubbish and discarded. For logical positivists like Schlick and Carnap, truths about the world would be reached by science and not philosophy.

Unfortunately for strong forms of positivism, philosophy (the 'love of wisdom') continues to ask questions that are tricky, such as: What are we? What is reality? What is our relationship to the world? Can we be certain about anything? What is truth? What is meaning? In addressing these questions, many thinkers – including logical positivists – have been forced to conclude that when we research and gather new knowledge, we do so from a particular philosophical viewpoint or basis. In other words, our philosophy shapes or determines how we go about gathering knowledge. The philosophical basis that we come from or adopt will inevitably say something about the trajectory or flight path of our values and beliefs. That is, our research will be informed by such issues as what we hold important in our 'world', what concepts and theories we give weight to, the kind of answers about health care that we are trying to get, how we go about getting those answers, how much control we have over the research process and the politics behind getting answers. Again, some thinkers – including, as we shall see, the occasional positivist – have suggested that our search for answers through philosophy and into research will constitute 'reality', the world, the health care world, in a particular way. It will determine the type of knowledge we build about phenomena. And that knowledge may have very different effects and consequences for people in the 'real' world beyond the academy. In other words, philosophy and the research that philosophy shapes has a bite to it. Of course, as many have argued, the status of the 'real' world, what constitutes it and our ability to derive certainties at one end of the spectrum and interpretations at the other, is by no means clear.

As we have also described above, two key ways in which we construct knowledge are through the process of induction and deduction. To sum these up, induction means that after a large number of observations have been made, it is possible to draw conclusions or theorize about particular phenomena (for example, the oft repeated statement that 'all swans are white'). The inductive method consists of description, classification, correlation, causation and prediction. Or we can formulate a theory or a hypothesis (a mini theory) and then collect data to support or reject it. This second approach to knowledge acquisition is called deduction. In our daily lives, we use both inductive approaches to gather information and draw conclusions and deductive ones – having a 'hunch' about something and then looking for evidence to support our beliefs. Scientific research extends from this general notion of gaining knowledge – it can be defined as the study of phenomena by the rigorous and systematic collection and analysis of data.

All of us will have reason to claim that we know something – through experience or inspiration at one end of the spectrum to experimental methods and analysis at the other. Attempts to secure the best knowledge have been going on for centuries. We seek knowledge to change not only our environment, but also ourselves. Yet it is still far from clear as to which methods and procedures for securing knowledge are the best. This is particularly the case with human sciences, as we shall see. A continuing debate is to be found between the so-called 'real' science, or natural science, and social sciences. Health sciences are caught up in this debate and our own emerging views about this will guide the kind of research we choose to involve ourselves in and, ultimately, the constitution of the care we give to people with health care needs.

Now, there are those who seek a foundational approach to knowledge. Often, though not always, this is associated with a positivist outlook. Just think here of the foundations of a building. Here knowledge is seen to rest

> upon a set of firm, unquestionable . . . indisputable truths from which our beliefs may be logically deduced, so retaining the truth value of the foundational premises from which they follow, and in terms of which our methods of forming further ideas about the world and investigating it can be licensed.
>
> (Hughes and Sharrock 1997, pp. 4–5)

Others, in particular the so-called postmodernists, deny the possibility of foundations to knowledge – such attackers on this notion of firm knowledge and truth are called anti-foundationalists. The scene is set, then, between those such as the 'positivists' who support the notion of accumulated, scientific knowledge, based upon a secure set of truths and those who are sceptical of truth itself, and all that can follow in terms of knowledge.

Foundations for knowledge have been sought in mathematical logic by, for example, Gottlob Frege (1848–1925) and Bertrand Russell (1872–1970) and this emphasis on logical analysis informed the Vienna Circle logical positivists, hence their name. Moritz Schlick (1882–1936), Otto Neurath (1882–1945) and Rudolf Carnap (1891–1970) claimed there was no such thing as 'philosophical knowledge' any more. The road to real knowledge was through science. One important corollary of their 'verification principle' declared that any proposition that cannot be tested empirically is nonsense.

Despite their apparently rabid empiricism, the logical positivists were very interested in Russell and Wittgenstein. Wittgenstein argued that there are limits to the sorts of meaningful thoughts that we can have with language. Meaning, indeed knowledge, is the result of socially agreed conventions produced by 'forms of life' and cannot possibly be established 'outside' of language. This at first might seem to be at odds with the manifest position of the members of the Vienna Circle, who are usually thought of as adhering to a kind of physicalism, where the real world is seen as containing matter and energy and where objects have real physical properties which science can determine. Yet eventually, the Vienna Circle's empiricism drew them closer and closer to Wittgenstein's position.

The knowledge produced by science is very powerful – but why? Philosophers of science have typically concerned themselves with what is so special about this knowledge and how it is different from other forms. Very often, the answer is that science employs some kind of special scientific method that produces a unique kind of knowledge, which is likely to be universal, quantifiable, empirical and to have predictive power. Additionally, many would argue that the key feature of science is not what it keeps but what it throws away. Karl Popper argued that all scientific theories are provisional and the true scientists will always suggest ways in which their theories could be 'falsified' by a new contradictory observation. In this view, the better scientists are not emotionally committed to their theories, but would see scientific 'truth' as provisional and something that can be discarded once data are discovered which do not fit the picture. However, some resist this and stick to their guns that science is more than relativized discourse and is capable of discovering a relatively permanent reality through its focus on rigour, discipline and elaborate precautions against self-deception or prejudice.

What the thumbnail sketch so far in this chapter shows is that the status of knowledge has been contested throughout the centuries and, rather than being a durable thing, knowledge of our world can change with social and historical fashions or outlooks. Certainly, the idea of knowledge evolving towards some ultimate state of truth has been heavily questioned, not least by postmodern thinking. The relativity of knowledge, therefore, in our own time, remains an issue. How far does our knowledge go? When we conduct research we set out to find out something not already known about. But people research from different philosophical bases. For some researchers, research must be carried out in the full spirit of scientific enquiry – with rigour, scrupulousness, and sure method and procedures. The scientific approach to research deploys techniques such as experiments, hypothesis testing, measurement – with results and data placed in the public domain for criticism. This was a model of scientific good practice described and endorsed by Robert Merton in his study of science as a social institution in the 1950s (Merton 1973).

As Hughes and Sharrock (1997, p. 19) write: 'positivism considered science to be very special, to be the embodiment of an authoritative, universal and final understanding of the nature of reality and superior to all other forms of understanding'. As such, positivism is a twin of rationalism – and seeks to provide a universal, definitive, objective account of the nature of reality. In the social sciences, this positivism has sought to promote acquisition of knowledge in a similar way to the natural sciences, such as biology or physics. Thus, it involved the use of the social survey, questionnaires and techniques of statistical analysis with a strong emphasis on quantitative analysis. This positivism has been promoted in trying to make social science a 'hard' or proper science. But since the 1960s there has been increasing criticism of the limitations of 'positivism'. In such attacks, 'science' was seen as but one way of representing reality among many others. The notion of plural versions of reality and not just one has taken a strong grip on contemporary intellectual life. The attack on 'positivism' has often sought to undermine its privileging of scientific, quantitative knowledge and allow for the legitimacy of qualitative or interpretative forms of research work which positivism tends to scorn. This kind of attack attempted to reassert 'understanding' rather than mechanistic 'explanation'.

Despite such attacks, and the widespread scepticism to which it has been subject, the philosophical paradigm of 'positivism' has greatly influenced much research in the health and social sciences. Its great strength in the nineteenth century was its staunch critique of supernatural and metaphysical interpretations of phenomena, grounded in Comte's own atheism. The name itself derives from the emphasis on the positive sciences – that is, on tested and systematized experience rather than an undisciplined speculation.

The key characteristic of 'positivism' is 'empiricism', according to which all knowledge of fact as distinct from that of purely logical relations comes from or derives from 'experience', from what we can observe. Positivists are keen on formal schemes and protocols for research and knowledge acquisition. They do not value diverse, alternative, human-based explanation of such things as 'well-being', 'belonging', 'satisfaction', except inasmuch as these can be measured through ratings scales. Through to the present day a great deal of effort and money has been expended by bodies such as the World Health Organization and the United Nations in trying to develop cross-culturally valid ways of measuring well-being, quality of life and even 'health' itself. These efforts are meaningful precisely because of the legacy of positivism.

Equally, and most importantly for us in health sciences, there is an increasing body of opinion that positivism has failed to appreciate how understanding and knowledge of humans is rarely suited to scientific methods (Polifroni and Welch 1999). Knowledge of the human realm – with its fluid interactions – cannot in this view be attained through the kind of generalizing schemas and explanations of natural sciences. Human activity and communication is of such diversity that only a hermen-eutic or interpretivist stance is acceptable to a growing body of scholars.

Positivism, as we have seen, places great weight on empirical research in the production of knowledge. The view is of accumulated facts, like building blocks, that produce generalizations which we know as scientific laws. As such, data should not come from interpretation but 'brute' facts. Positivists believed that it was possible for there to be a neutral, uncontaminated language of observation, such that what they described had a direct match with observed phenomena. Therefore, the truth of any theoretical statement is to be determined by its correspondence with the observed facts: a so-called 'correspondence theory of truth'. As we shall see later when we look at 'interpretivist' philosophies in more detail, such a neutral, observation language is not attainable in any strict sense. The language of observation is far from being neutral.

There is more to scientific observation than directly observing the world's 'brute' facts. There is a problem in observing humans' mental states because not only are these not directly observable, but also we encounter the problem of how a language of observation can capture the diversity of mind states. Here, positivists generally looked for the outward bodily or physical display of mental states. Bodily, physical behaviours became an index to mental states – this was especially true in psychiatry and criminology. But the question remains, how accurately do physical phenomena or behaviour replicate mental states?

The rhetorical shell of positivism: social issues are physical problems

Perhaps the strongest legacy of positivism is that it has made a certain variety of health care enquiry possible. It has not survived the twentieth century intact, and our ability to apprehend nature in a raw, untheorized form has been severely called into question. However, it has facilitated the very idea that we can measure human experience and has universalized the rhetoric of facts speaking for themselves. What is left of positivism is not its epistemological soft tissues but its rhetorical shell.

A good deal of work in health care and the human sciences proceeds as if positiv-ism was a sufficient and literally true account of knowledge and of the scientific process of knowledge generation. As is clear from any perusal of the more prestigious journals, however, most researchers and authors in the avowedly scientific fields of health care do not reflect on their epistemological presuppositions. While much of this work appears to rely on positivist epistemological commitments, 'a silence reigns around this so that they are forgotten and any reflexivity skilfully avoided (Chia, 1996)' (Johnson and Cassell 2001, p. 127). Perhaps if we were to press them, researchers in these traditions would argue that the assumptions they made were so uncontentious and commonsensical that they were scarcely worth talking about, especially as there were much more important issues – patients' lives, for example – to be concerned with.

One of the major points of departure for the critique of positivistic research in health care is the contention that there are a number of ways of promoting health, feeling healthy or unhealthy, suffering and healing that are not easily included in the range of phenomena that positivism is equipped to study. However, even though they would be hopelessly mentalistic and metaphysical to Comte or Carnap, the literary and rhetorical shell of positivism enables authors in the health sciences to present them as if they were researchable in these terms.

There are some aspects of caring work that do tend to get researched in conventional positivist terms. For example, Weiss (1990) reports a study of the use of touch in the care of patients with heart disease. The study showed that if nurses touched or gently massaged patients, their heart rates were lowered and their blood pressure dropped, more so than simply talking to patients sympathetically. There was also some evidence that by using these touch and massage techniques, nurses could help to adjust patients' irregular heart rhythms. This study used a technique that would look eminently sensible to positivists, randomly assigning the patients to conditions with touching, talking or talking-and-touching and taking quantitative measures of the variables under scrutiny. Thus, it is possible, under some circumstances, to use avowedly scientific – indeed, positivistic – methods to study some aspects of the caring process.

The debate gets more fraught when we examine some of the other claims being made in health. In the view of some recent authors, there are important parts of the health care process which are best understood as reflecting 'constructed reality, mutual process and epistemological notions of description, pattern, interpretation . . . and participation' (Mitchell and Pilkington 1999, pp. 283–4). Moreover, increasing numbers of health care researchers see the kinds of science that comply with positivist thinking as being overly restricted and are instead searching for a new epistemological model which 'reveals the limits of reductionistic cause–effect thinking' and offers the opportunity to 'respect alternative healing modalities and folkways' (Baumann 1998, pp. 89–90). Thus we see a curious case of positivistic methodologies reaching out into the topography of care, while others are frantically defending these enclaves as being beyond the scope of strict scientific enquiry.

As we shall see later in this volume, positivism has been subject to a number of different challenges over the 150 years of its existence. A brief tour of some of the sites of special scientific interest in this landscape of epistemology might include Nietzsche (Nolan *et al.* 1998), who claimed that regimes of truth were enforced rather than allowed to emerge naturally from the facts. Additionally, we should pause over Peirce, who contended that science is a kind of sign interpretation and knowledge as adaptive response to our environment (Brent 1993), an idea which prefigures the models of perception developed later by Gibson (1979). Quine, who was influenced by the

Vienna Circle, argued that it was not possible to challenge individual hypotheses against evidence but that sensory experience challenges the whole body of our beliefs. Any conceivable sentence can be held to be true, in his view, if we make drastic enough adjustments elsewhere in the knowledge system (Quine 1953). Therefore, to understand truth and falsity, we have to examine the whole structure of beliefs, including all the special conditions, modifications, exceptions and qualifications. As Quine (1953, p. 43) argues, 'We can even retain an ordinary belief about our surroundings in the face of contrary experience by pleading hallucination or by amending certain statements of the kind called logical laws.'

The chapter so far should show two things. First, that disagreement about what knowledge amounts to is commonplace. Second, it should give a sense of a movement away from rather optimistic views of capturing knowledge exemplified by positivism, to increasingly sceptical views of the possibility of being certain about our world, and a stronger insistence by many contemporary thinkers that we are instead reliant on 'interpretations' or formulations of the world 'out there'. Indeed, according to some scholars, the 'out there-ness' of factual discourse is itself a socially mediated linguistic accomplishment and tells us next to nothing about whether there might be a world out there at all (Potter 1996).

With respect to the question of the reliability of knowledge, a potent influence in the history of epistemology has been the role of the sceptic in demanding whether any claim to knowledge can be upheld against the possibility of doubt.

Positivism post-modernizes itself

Possibly the most interesting thing about the Vienna Circle's logical positivism is that it led some of its members, and many subsequent thinkers, away from a foundation-alist model of scientific enquiry altogether. Some, especially Otto Neurath, were paralysed by the difficulty of making any statements about the world. He described scientific enquiry in the following terms: 'We are like sailors who have to rebuild their ship on the open sea, without ever being able to dismantle it in dry-dock and reconstruct it from the best components.' This formulation of the task of knowing has been adopted also by Ayer (1959) and Quine (1990). It graphically depicts the anti-foundationalism Neurath ended up with as he followed a strong empirical position doubting everything. This doubt extended beyond epistemology and included the social sciences, society and politics: knowledge and life are built without foundations. In tandem with this, Neurath pushed positivism away from ideas about truth or verification based on sensory experience but on the coherence of our statements. In this way, his work had parallels with Wittgenstein's focus on language. Thus he set the stage for more explicitly anti-foundationalist philosophies, which we shall review in detail later. Following on from the ideas expressed in Neurath's boat analogy, Richard Rorty (1979) expressed profound scepticism that it would ever be possible to judge the truth of our beliefs from an objective or transcendental standpoint.

A final irony of positivism and falsificationism is that they were at their most active after they were obsolete as forms of scientific enquiry. After about 1890, physics – the touchstone science *par excellence* – had taken a turn away from direct observation. It would have been very difficult to identify any direct sensory data that allowed the formation of protocol statements or which could be used to test theories in any simple sense. The science of positivism is the science of the nineteenth century. Once practising physicists abandoned Newtonian mechanics and became interested in relativity and quantum mechanics, the science lost its connection with ordinary sense perceptions. Since the 1890s, physics has been concerned with sub-atomic particles that cannot be seen or with galactic processes that are altogether too distant to be experienced directly. Rather than assuming an 'out there' reality, physicists are just as likely to believe that we cannot observe events without changing them, as the well-known paradoxes of Heisenberg's uncertainty principle and Schrödinger's cat attest (Brown 1979; Zukov 1991). Positivism, then, is about a science of 'medium-sized dry goods', rather than what scientists were actually doing for most of the twentieth century.

At the same time, almost everything we have in our homes and workplaces is based on a kind of science which was at its height in the nineteenth century and which originated theories that attempt to explain the technologies on which our cars, computers and creature comforts depend. Nineteenth-century science was entering our homes and our lives just as the beloved physics was accelerating (at the speed of light) away from positivism and away from intimate engagement with our mundane reality.

References

Ayer, A.J. (1959) *Logical Positivism*. London: Allen & Unwin.

Baumann, S.L. (1998) Nursing: the missing ingredient in nurse practitioner education, *Nursing Science Quarterly*, 11(3): 89–90.

Bertillion, S. (1941) *Vie D'Alphonse Bertillion, Inventeur D'Anthropometrie*. Paris: Gallimard.

Bradshaw, J. and Sainsbury, R. (eds) (1999) *Proceedings of the Conference to Mark the Centenary of Seebohm Rowntree's First Study of Poverty in York*. Cambridge: Polity Press.

Brent, J. (1993) *Charles Sanders Peirce: A Life*. Bloomington, IN: Indiana University Press.

Brown, H.I. (1979) *Perception, Theory and Commitment: The New Philosophy of Science*. Chicago, IL: University of Chicago Press.

Chia, R. (1996) *Organisational Analysis as Deconstructive Practice*. Berlin: De Grutyer.

Churchill, F. (1857) *On the Diseases of Women*. Philadelphia, PA: Blanchard & Lea.

Durkheim, E. (1973) *On Mortality and Society: Selected Writings* (edited by R.N. Bellah). Chicago, IL: University of Chicago Press.

Ellis, H. (1913) *Studies in the Psychology of Sex*, Vols I–VI. Philadelphia, PA: F.A. Davis.

Fann, K.T. (1990) *Peirce's Theory of Abduction*, 2nd edn. The Hague: Martinus Nijhoff.

Gibson, J.J. (1979) *The Ecological Approach to Visual Perception*. Boston, MA: Houghton Mifflin.

Giddens, A. (1995) *Politics, Sociology and Social Theory: Encounters with Classical and Contemporary Social Thought*. Cambridge: Polity Press.

Gray, J. (1992) *Men are from Mars, Women are from Venus*. New York: HarperCollins.

Gray, J. (1995) *Mars and Venus in the Bedroom: A Guide to Lasting Romance and Passion*. New York: HarperCollins.

Groneman, C. (1994) Nymphomania: the historical construction of female sexuality, *Signs: Journal of Women in Culture and Society*, 19(2): 337–67.

Hankins, F.H. ([1908] 1968) *Adolphe Quetelet as a Statistician*. New York: Arne Press.

Haraway, D. (1986) Primatology is politics by other means, in R. Bleier (ed.) *Feminist Approaches to Science*. New York: Pergamon Press.

Hare, E.H. (1962) Masturbational insanity: the history of an idea, *Journal of Mental Science*, 188: 1–25.

Himmelfarb, G. (1984) *The Idea of Poverty*. New York: Knopf.

Hughes, J. and Sharrock, W. (1997) *The Philosophy of Social Research*, 3rd edn. London: Longman.

Hussey, T. (2001) Thinking about change, *Nursing Philosophy*, 3(2): 104–13.

Jackson, M. (1994) *The Real Facts of Life: Feminism and the Politics of Sexuality 1850–1940*. London: Taylor & Francis.

Jastrow, J. (1891) A study of mental statistics, *New Review*, 5: 559–68.

Johnson, P. and Cassell, C. (2001) Epistemology and work psychology: new agendas, *Journal of Occupational and Organisational Psychology*, 74: 125–43.

Keller, E.F. and Longino, H.E. (1996) *Feminism & Science*. Oxford: Oxford University Press.

Krafft-Ebing, R. von ([1886] 1965) *Psychopathia Sexualis*. New York: G.P. Putnam.

Laqueur, T. (1990) *Making Sex: Body and Gender from the Greeks to Freud*. Cambridge, MA: Harvard University Press.

Mayhew, H. (1851) *London Labour and the London Poor*, 3 Vols. London: Author.

Merton, R. (1973) *The Sociology of Science: Theoretical and Empirical Investigations*. Chicago, IL: University of Chicago Press.

Mills, C.K. (1885) A case of nymphomania with hystero-epilepsy and peculiar mental perversions – the results of clitoridectomy and oophrectomy – the patient's story as told by herself, *Philadelphia Medical Times*, 15 April, pp. 534–40.

Mitchell, G.J. and Pilkington, F.B. (1999) A dialogue on the comparability of research paradigms – and other theoretical things, *Nursing Science Quarterly*, 12(4): 283.

Moscucci, O. (1990) *The Science of Woman: Gynaecology and Gender in England, 1800–1929*. Cambridge: Cambridge University Press.

Murphy M.S. and Cooper, B.P. (2000) The death of the author at the birth of social science: the case of Harriet Martineau and Adolphe Quetelet, *Studies in the History and Philosophy of Science*, 31(1): 1–36.

Neurath, O. (1944) *Foundations of the Social Sciences*. Chicago, IL: University of Chicago Press.

Nolan, P., Brown, B. and Crawford, P. (1998) Fruits without labour: the implications of Frederich Nietzsche's ideas for the caring professions, *Journal of Advanced Nursing*, 28(2): 251–9.

O'Day, R. and Englander, D. (eds) (1993) *Mr Charles Booth's Inquiry: Life and Labour of the People in London Reconsidered*. London: The Hambledon Press.

Plummer, K. (1981) *The Making of the Modern Homosexual*. London: Hutchinson.

Polifroni, E.C. and Welch, M.L. (1999) *Perspectives on Philosophy of Science in Nursing: An Historical and Contemporary Anthology*. Philadelphia, PA: Lippincott.

Porter, R. and Hall, L. (1995) *The Facts of Life: The Creation of Sexual Knowledge in Britain 1650–1950*. New Haven, CT: Yale University Press.

Porter, S. (2001) Nightingale's realist philosophy of science, *Nursing Philosophy*, 2: 14–25.

Potter, J. (1996) *Representing Reality*. London: Sage.

Potts, A. (1998) The science/fiction of sex: John Gray's Mars and Venus in the bedroom, *Sexualities*, 1(2): 153–73.

Quine, W.V.O. (1953) *From a Logical Point of View*. Cambridge, MA: Harvard University Press.

Quine, W.V.O. (1990) *The Pursuit of Truth*. Cambridge, MA: Harvard University Press.

Rorty, R. (1979) *Philosophy and the Mirror of Nature*. Oxford: Blackwell.

Routh, C.H.F. (1887) On the aetiology and diagnosis considered specially from a medico-legal point of view for those cases of nymphomania which lead women to make false charges against their medical attendants, *British Gynaecological Journal*, 2(8): 485–511.

Russell, B. (1914) *Our Knowledge of the External World as a Field for Scientific Method in Philosophy*. London: Open Court Publishing.

Sarkar, S. (1996) *Logical Empiricism at its Peak: Schlick, Carnap and Neurath*. New York: Garland.

Talmey, B. ([1904] 1912) *Woman: A Treatise on the Normal and Pathological Emotions of Feminine Love*. New York: Practitioners Press.

Terman, L.M. (1916) *The Measurement of Intelligence*. Boston, MA: Houghton Mifflin.

Walton, J.T. (1857) Case of nymphomania successfully treated, *American Journal of Medical Science*, 33(1): 47–50.

Watson, E. (1914) Reply to a male contributor, 4 July 1912. Watson, J.B. (1913). Psychology as the behaviourist views it, *Psychological Review*, 20: 158–77.

Weeks, J. (1985) *Sexuality and Its Discontents: Meanings, Myths and Modern Sexualities*. London: Routledge.

Weiss, S.J. (1990) Effects of differential touch on nervous system arousal of patients recovering from cardiac disease, *Heart and Lung*, 19(5): 474–80.

Wittgenstein, L. (1922) *Tractatus logico-philosophicus*. International Library of Psychology, Philosophy and Scientific Method. London: K. Paul.

Zukov, G. (1991) *The Dancing Wu Li Masters: An Overview of the New Physics*. New York: Rider.

3

Concepts and theories I: what is a concept in the health sciences?

Introduction: where do concepts come from?

In the first two chapters, we discussed the nature of a number of concepts in health that have waxed and waned over the years. Within the positivistic tradition, concepts are often supposed to be anchored in nature. In this chapter, we will consider some of the concepts that one can encounter in health care in a bit more detail. In particular, we will look at how concepts come to be shared in common by a community of people who are attempting to achieve health, and we will show that a good deal of important social activity goes into making concepts. The concepts we use are intelligible and seem sometimes even to be natural, but we shall show how they depend on a particular sequence of intellectual developments, economic and political circumstances and practical everyday ways of seeing the world.

This can be shown even if we take a very basic concept, that of illness and heath. Our most fundamental ideas about medicine are embedded in culture and language. In the UK in the 1990s, most people would think that they know what a sick person is. However, history suggests that the way illness is defined today depends a great deal on fairly recent changes in patterns of sickness and health:

> The appearance of today's 'sick person' seems predicated on at least three conditions: first, disease must cease to be a mass phenomenon [e.g. plagues and epidemics]; second, illness must not be followed immediately by death; and third, it is probably also necessary that the diversity of suffering be reduced by a unifying general view which is precisely that of clinical medicine.
> (Herzlich and Pierret 1987, p. 23)

In the late twentieth century, everyday complaints like the common cold and gastro-intestinal upsets have a set of symptoms that we expect to co-occur. As sufferers or healers, we tend to look for distinct patterns in illness. For example, in the early twenty-first century, callers to the UK's telephone helpline NHS Direct might well have found themselves being asked a number of questions relating to experience of nausea, headache, aches and pains in the muscles and joints and whether they had a rash which did not fade when pressed. This constellation of features was important at that time as a result of concerns over meningitis and whether such cases would be missed. In this instance, then, the concept, and the fear of what would happen if the illness were undetected, yields a set of screening questions. To take another concept, that of cervical cancer, we can see how the concept, and theories about its aetiology and the development of the disease, have been built into the structure of health care in the UK, such that primary care practices are under financial pressure to screen as many of their female patients as possible. So concepts become embedded in the economic fabric of health care very readily.

Thus, whereas ideas about health and illness might appear to be rooted in biology, they can equally well be argued to be embedded within systems of meaning, social structure and economics. In this chapter, we will attempt to illuminate what concepts are by looking at how some of the concepts in health care emerged and evolved and by examining how we might study them *in situ* as they are used by sufferers and healers. There have been several competing views of the concepts of illness and health and, in describing how these concepts have originated, we will be able to illuminate some of their philosophical implications, their assumptions and the implicit models on which they draw.

In philosophical terms, the sense of the word concept is to do with the product of the faculty of conception, or an idea of a class of objects. The term 'concept' was first formulated in this way in the seventeenth century. In a somewhat less specialized way, the word is used to refer to a general notion or idea. In much intellectual usage, the term 'concept' is used instead of the older term 'idea'. The two differ in that 'ideas' are often more richly adorned with images, yet, confusingly, a concept also might involve images.

A further source of connotations for the term is disclosed when we look at popular language, where a concept is often something that is experimental or novel. A concept car, a concept album or an interior design concept all have connotations of novelty, especially in contexts of marketing and design.

As the *Oxford Companion to Philosophy* reminds us, the notion of a concept is intimately bound up with language. There are many concepts that would lie beyond the grasp of a creature without language. This chapter is being written on a computer, the mastery of which includes the attainment of concepts such as *format*, *debug* and *backup*, most of which are beyond even the most sign-language-fluent chimpanzee.

In terms of the work that concepts do in our thinking, Kitson (1993) attempts to distinguish between facts, values and concepts, looking at issues relating to caring and gender. We might observe a 'fact' that more women are involved in caring for family members than men. This may be tied up with a 'value' such as 'women are more caring than men'. The concept at stake here might be 'caring' itself. Of course, in practice, the facts, values and concepts may not be so easily separated. If we take a phenomenon such as prostate cancer, the concept of 'cancer' is a very loaded one and can lead health care professionals and patients to feel the best course of action is to remove the offending organ, yet these concepts, values, emotions and surgical techniques may also be tied up with research evidence – 'facts', if you like – suggesting that conservative treatment or 'watchful waiting' might yield a better outcome than aggressive surgical intervention. Trying to dissect out the concepts, values and facts into a neat typology would be nightmarishly complex in this situation.

In contemporary health care, the situation is often even more complex as there may be a variety of regimes of truth at work. Health care practitioners and researchers may encounter clients from a variety of cultural and spiritual backgrounds and health care itself may be administered from a number of differing conceptual frameworks as complementary and alternative therapies continue to gain in popularity. In addition, the academic field of research and theory continues to diversify as Marxist, feminist, multicultural, postmodern and user-led perspectives are raised in the discussion of health and illness.

These perspectives will differ in terms of how they construct the truth of illness and disease. Making sense of this diversity might be a little easier if we were able to define what a concept is in health care and examine the role of concepts in framing our perception of the human condition and their use as guides for future action.

The development of concepts in Western heath care has also been affected by the cross-fertilization between medicine and other disciplines. For example, the role of artistic styles in developing concepts of the human body in Renaissance Europe facilitated new ways of thinking about what might go wrong. The role of illustration and photography in nineteenth-century medicine similarly revolutionized the discipline and democratized visions of the human body that had hitherto been available only to an elite audience of health care professionals in training who would be graduating from newly founded universities and teaching hospitals. Knowledge, then, was being democratized and liberated. Much as the development of mass production revolutionized business, the mass production of knowledge, textbooks and health professionals themselves was proceeding apace as the twentieth century began. In this way, we hope to illustrate how technological changes have informed intellectual life and may even have changed the shape of philosophy itself. There is a curious visual similarity between the layout of the machines in the textile mills and the beds in the 'Florence Nightingale' style wards. Each in its own way was a factory for producing something, whether it be wealth or health, and as a result of both of these innovations it is possible to think about human well-being in new ways. The hospital patients were, in a sense, hard at work being cured in what was to become a rationalized, mechanized and technologically infused manufacture of health.

By the end of this chapter, the reader should be able to appreciate the relationship between 'concepts' and 'theories' and the kind of research that is done with them. Furthermore, the reader might be able to identify the epistemological limitations of concepts and theories, and be able to detect the social and historical influence on their formation. This, we hope, will lead the reader towards greater awareness of the role of concepts in theory building and in thus achieving a more sophisticated understanding of the philosophical base of research in health care settings.

We use concepts – or mental images if you like – to inform our everyday understanding and experiences. By this token, almost everything is a concept. Concepts are often demoted by abstract and general words that describe mental images of reality. We might think of concepts such as 'caring' or 'distress' which might have images attached to them but are difficult to pin down to a particular mental image. We have numerous concepts or mental images relating to the world. They help us to keep track of the world of experience and give mental labels to objects, relations and interactions between phenomena.

We share concepts with others. We agree that someone else's concept or mental image that is performed through language is similar to our own or has sufficient similarities for us to ignore the differences. Despite any divergence, there may be sufficient 'family resemblance' between concepts to allow for practical communications and exchange. The divergence will often go unchallenged unless a 'battle for definition' occurs.

Concepts are important to us. We map out our world in concepts. For example, our conceptualizations of fish may differ from our conceptualizations of cats – that one has scales and the other has fur may be just one difference; yet there may also be some blurring or crossover of concepts in terms of, say, both being pets, needing to be fed by us or bearing a physical resemblance as in 'catfish'. Despite occasional blurring, generally concepts help us to put boundaries around words and contain the shared meanings we have of them (Kitson 1993).

When we think of 'concepts', we think about 'words' and their meaning – in a way that we don't perhaps normally do. In this sense, it is easy to become self-conscious about meanings and descriptions, so the process of inspecting our everyday working concepts might change them. There are various ways of conceptualizing concepts themselves. One of the most common and easiest forms of thinking to slip into is to think of concepts as cognitive entities. In this sense, concepts are rather like mental representations: schemas, stereotypes or inferential structures that individuals or groups of individuals can use to interrogate the world. In this sense, it is as if we have our own 'conceptual maps' of the world. For instance, among nurses, there may be a conceptual map about nursing, what it is to be a nurse, what is health, suffering, illness, distress and so on. In the cognitive model we have been outlining, health professionals' concepts affect their practice – in a similar way to our language. The 'conceptual mix' in health care is influenced by other people's mixtures of concepts via personal experience, and may include education, historical, social, political and psychological factors (Kitson 1993).

Concepts can be translated into empirical indicators; for example, the concept of 'ethnic prejudice' as manifest in various indicators of 'prejudice' in the world (Hughes and Sharrock 1997). We look for patterns and interrelationships between indicators of 'concepts' to build up empirical descriptions and to devise theories.

So far we have been talking about concepts as if they were cognitive entities or mental representations. However, it is possible to challenge this notion. First, it is extremely difficult to investigate concepts in this inner mental space. One of the fundamental questions in cognitive science is how we can possibly know that this mental furniture exists, and whether it underlies action. There are alternative positions. A number of scholars, including Jonathan Potter and Derek Edwards, have attempted to reappraise this lexicon of mental concepts so as to emphasize how they are embedded within social action. Edwards (1995, 1997), for example, takes the cognitivist construction of 'scripts' – a sort of memory for orderly, sequenced events such as going to a restaurant. He shows how – analytically and theoretically – we can 'respecify this idea in terms of practical, situated accomplishments in interaction' (Potter 2000, p. 10). Thus, rather than thinking of an entity in memory, we are, in this approach, encouraged to think in terms of a different kind of entity, the *script formulation*, which involves the orderliness or disorderliness of a sequence of events being accomplished by the people doing the interacting, or describing it to others later. The story of events is often done so as to enable the teller to assign responsibility for the events, avoid blame and head off possible negative interpretations of the story. Borrowing from Edwards's and Potter's insights, we should be sensitive to the way that concepts are employed in scientific debate so as to place a favourable gloss on the speaker's position, discredit opponents, secure agreement and marshal evidence. Rather than existing in a cognitive intellectual space to drive scientific action from above, the 'concept formulations' we find in everyday debate among scientists and practitioners are inherently part of the action, involved in the practical and moral work of accountability.

Thus, rather than speaking of concepts, our own preference in this chapter is to discuss 'concept formulations', but we will use the term 'concept' where we are quoting or borrowing from others' use of the term. We have used the term 'concept formulation' also to remind us of how the role of concepts can depend on the kind of scientific work they are being called upon to describe, justify or interpret. To make sense of concepts in science, we need to understand something about the pragmatics of scientific interaction as researchers struggle to make themselves understood by the rest of the scientific community, journal editors and referees and funding bodies. The audience will make a difference to the concept formulation in use at the time.

Concepts: special or just specialized? From gods to vital essences

There are a variety of philosophers, from Paul Feyerabend to Karl Popper himself, who have argued that there is nothing inherently special about scientific concepts and that they are not superior to lay conceptions. To understand why they are special, then, involves our making sense of how and why they are being used. This emphasis on the deployment of concept formulations is tied to our concern with how social reality is harnessed to language, and the concepts and meanings of that language, and how language activity is a kind of performance as individuals act in the world. In this sense, as they collaborate, compete and come into conflict, they create the human 'world'. Scientific concept formulations are bound up with social activity – the activity of language – and are part of the set of conventions, limitations and constraints of that everyday language activity and social construction.

The past 2000–3000 years provide many examples of how there have been a variety of competing conceptions of health and illness and how health may best be enhanced and how illness may best be dealt with. One of the longest struggles is that between natural, physical explanations for health and disease and theological ones. This kind of debate has existed at least since the ancient Greeks. It has been suggested that Hippocrates was one of the first to advance physical explanations and concepts in Western medicine. For example, he believed that epilepsy, rather than resulting from interventions by the gods of the time, was physical in nature. A general manifesto for his position runs something like this:

> Men ought to know that from the brain, and from the brain only, arise our pleasures, joys, laughter and jests, as well as our sorrows, pain, grief and tears . . . It is the brain which makes us mad or delirious, inspires us with dread and fear,

whether by night or by day, brings sleeplessness, mistakes, anxieties, absentmind-edness, acts that are contrary to our normal habits. These things that we suffer all come from the brain, including madness.

(quoted in Howells 1975, p. 15)

At the same time, the Hippocratic version of human well-being contained elements that would appear strange when viewed from the early twenty-first century. For example, he believed that the brain was the primary organ for the production of the nasal secretions.

At the same time in Greece, there were a number of competing accounts, especially of madness. According to Padel (1981), in Greece some thinkers felt that the experience of distress was not a turmoil inside the head but a clash of wills outside. The different deities demanded different courses of action from the unfortunate human subject. Thus, in the fifth century B.C. there are accounts of the mad being isolated from the mainstream of society because they were dangerous. Not necessarily because of what they might do, as is the case nowadays, but because of their proximity to this divine conflict. Madness was the sign of closeness to the gods. The gods ordinarily propel people to act in certain ways. Generally, the gods co-existed peace-fully, but sometimes their interests clashed and this is when problems were believed to occur. Those whom the gods, proverbially, wish to destroy, they can make mad via a process of isolation. This notion of isolation as being a central feature of madness yielded the contemporary word 'idiot' from the Greek *idiotes*, a private person. Greek culture at the time did not generally approve of privacy or solitude and demanded a high level of public, congenial sociability from its members, and the tendency to isolate oneself would appear to be abnormal. On the other hand, notions of seclusion, segregation and retreat have characterized cultural conceptions of madness in the modern period. Tuke's famous 'retreat', for example, or the idea of 'asylum' as a resting place, suggest this kind of treatment process. Thus, when we look at the concept formulations in different regimes of healing, we can see some 'family resem-blances' over the generations, but at the same time we should be sensitive to the fact that these are often accompanied by some diversity once we delve beneath the surface to examine the implicit theories about causation or the theological meaning of the events in question.

The concept formulations of disease in the modern European tradition are difficult to understand without their opposites, health. This linkage between opposites is made especially explicit in the theory of the four humours – blood, phlegm, yellow bile and black bile – which dominated thinking on health and disease in Europe from ancient Greece to the eighteenth century. A balance of the humours was equated with health and an imbalance was implicated in sickness. Consequently, the treatments available – bleeding, purging and vomiting – were devoted to readjusting the humoral balance.

This concept was displaced by a number of developments in the eighteenth century that eclipsed the humoral theory. As these changes in medical thinking took place across a wide canvas of European and American intellectual life, it is difficult to dissect out precise pathways of influence. However, the work of Dr John Brown (1735–1788) revolutionized medicine at that time. His theory of health and disease was based on a relatively simple concept formulation, that of excitability. The body, he reasoned, was continually being excited and stimulated by a variety of agents acting upon it internally and externally. An optimal level of stimulation yielded health, whereas too little or too much would yield debility. For example, poisons and 'typhus contagions' were debilitating because of the smallness of the stimulation they effected on the body. What is important in this concept formulation of health, then, is the idea of a quantifiable, scaleable measure of what is happening to the body.

In Brown's system, this dimensional quality was central to states of illness and disease. This even extended to emotional well-being. Fear and grief are lower degrees of confidence and joy. Of course, this formulation was controversial. There were some, such as his near-contemporary Hufeland, who asserted that there were two scales, one running from indifference to vexation, grief and despair, and the other running from indifference to joy and rapture. However, despite disagreement on the nature of the scales, the crucial feature is that people had started the process of turning the qualities of human existence into dimensions. There is a measurable aspect to all these concept formulations which allows a translation into the quantitative experimental health sciences of the nineteenth century to be accomplished. Although both Brown and Hufeland lived a little earlier than Quetelet, notice how Brown makes this leap. Rather than a typological system, like the humours, Brown's was a measurable system, where optimal levels of stimulation – around 3000–3010 units per day – were believed to be optimal. Thus began the quest for health care information of the kind that can be rated on pain questionnaires, quality of life measures and general health questionnaires. Concept formulations, then, are sometimes crucial in liberating new possibilities for researchers, theorists and practitioners.

This concept formulation also permitted a revolution on treatment. Too little stimulation, in Brown's system, produced direct debility, whereas too much produced indirect debility through exhaustion. A healthy level of excitability was reckoned to be '40 degrees', whereas from 40 to 25 degrees predisposed an individual to direct debility and less than 25 degrees represented 'complete and extreme' direct debility. Likewise, higher levels of excitement, over 40 degrees, increased the risk of indirect debility. What these degrees were and how they were counted are difficult for the present-day reader to determine. However, Dr Brown's regime – the 'Bruonian system' – proved popular, perhaps due to his sovereign remedies, with the power to produce life or excitement. These were opium, 'spirituous liquors' (mainly brandy), Musk and cinchona or 'Peruvian bark' (yielding quinine) for fever. The Bruonian system influenced a great many thinkers, some of whom are better known in the present day, such as the architect of the American medical enlightenment Benjamin Rush, as well as literary men such as Coleridge and Goethe. It gained favour in the New World, as well as in Italy, but was opposed in England. In Scotland, riots took place between supporters and opponents of the system. Moreover, there was a curious timeliness of the relationship between his reassertion of the medicinal properties of opium and the development of the global drug trade at the end of the eighteenth century.

We have mentioned this system because it is important to identify the way that concept formulations from the medical systems of days gone by have left important legacies for latter day conceptions of health and disease. The role of this system is not so much its literal truth, but rather the impetus it had in overthrowing the Hippocratic, 'four humours' medicine, and in replacing it with concept formulations of health that could be quantified and measured.

It was this kind of conceptual work and political controversy in the eighteenth century that enabled nineteenth-century scholars to discourse on health and disease in a way that is familiar to us in the West in the present day. That is, health care providers and scientists in Europe and North America mostly subscribe to a pathogenic concept formulation of disease. Now, this was partly made possible by the debates over Bruonian medicine at the end of the eighteenth century. Once you formulate health and disease in this way, it opens up an 'explanation slot' for some sort of device or entity that is causing the morbidity. According to Lohff (2001), it has developed in tandem with the laboratory sciences through the nineteenth and twentieth centuries. When people speak of the 'medical model' nowadays, it is generally this kind of idea they are alluding to. The pathogenic model, in a sense, contains slots into which the pathogenic agents could be neatly incorporated as they were discovered.

Some of the foundations of our present-day medical model and our understanding of health and disease were laid in the early part of the nineteenth century. For example, Johann Lucas Scholein, Professor of Medicine at the Charite of Berlin, said in 1839: 'Disease as negation of health therefore, is that state of the organism in whom its functions take place in such a way, that there is no accordance with the laws of the species and the individual' (quoted in Lohff 2001, p. 545). That is, disease is somehow a perversion or deflection of nature. In disease, we fail to behave according to the best tendencies of our species. More in the same register flowed from the pen of Rudolf Virchow in 1869, who set out the challenge for medicine and pathology as developing skills in this new technology of health and illness. He expressed his manifesto in the following terms:

> The skilfulness consists therein, that he [the physician] is able to prevent, abolish, remove and neutralise all those unnatural conditions which have developed, the abnormal situations which have arisen, that means the causes of disease and that he because of the knowledge that has been provided by physiology and by the serious study of pathology assures that he by extending this very knowledge himself can intervene and thereby achieve that the organs of the organism can thereby function again regularly.
>
> (quoted in Lohff 2001, p. 545)

Nineteenth-century physicians were thus able to shift the picture of health away from Jacobean notions of the human condition where decay was inevitable, manifested in the works of Webster and Marlowe. This conceptual shift was sudden. The couplet 'Change and decay in all around I see, Oh he who changest not, abide with me' was incorporated into the early nineteenth-century hymn 'Abide with me' by Henry Francis Lyte (1793–1847). Everything decayed except God. However, by the middle years of the nineteenth century nature was looked at a little differently. Disease was the opposite of life and of what was natural. Given the sickliness of Europe's population at the time, with pandemic levels of syphilis and tuberculosis, this was a bold assertion. It has nevertheless been an influential one. Things that are suboptimal according to the standards of the time are readily recast as some sort of pathology, whereas things that are considered desirable are ascribed the status of health. This is something we can see in operation in the present. Tiredness, angst at the human condition, classroom unruliness and adolescent defiance are readily redefined as pathologies and medical interventions are sought. Once again, the concept formulations liberate certain kinds of treatment options and mobilize a search for underlying organic causes.

As we have seen, this kind of thinking can be traced back to the early nineteenth century. It also contains elements of other philosophies. Like most good philosophical, medical and theological systems, its appeal involves incorporating commonsensical notions from earlier belief systems. In the eighteenth century also, the idea of a vital force became a popular notion. This was a secular force – not a soul in the religious sense – which was believed to inhabit living things. As Kant put it, a 'reaction of the living body means that there is a force but not necessarily a soul that is reacting to it' (Lohff 2001, p. 550). A life force, to some authors such as Medicus in the eighteenth century, was physically necessary because perpetual motion was impossible, yet motion occurred perpetually in nature. Therefore, a life force propelled these living things.

This tendency of the organism to propel itself towards health has been a mainstay of twentieth-century accounts of well-being. A good deal of theory in psychotherapy and counselling is formulated around the notion that human beings tend naturally towards health, growth and self-development (Rogers 1961; Maslow 1968). The idea of health care professionals providing the conditions under which their clients can heal themselves is one which derived from this vitalism, as is the idea that 'the core of personality is positive' (Rogers 1961, pp. 100–1).

Moreover, the idea that the stuff of our being that is desirable is ourselves, and is health, brings with it the notion that the stuff that is undesirable is somehow there as the result of disease or possibly the side-effects of the treatment. The sufferers of masturbatory insanity who consulted the late nineteenth-century psychiatrists and gynaecologists who we met in the previous chapter were convinced that this tendency was somehow the result or the symptom of a disease.

Looking at the kinds of concept formulations that are being used over time in the health care disciplines is important. It has some degree of anthropological interest in its own right, but more importantly, as Parker *et al.* (1995) remind us, the abstractions we talk about here are significant as forms of practice. They tell us what to do, give us tools for thinking and suggest means of dealing with whatever we decide is sickness. In Parker's view also, they are bound up with material structures of power and domination. The smorgasbord of different ideas we outline in this chapter is not something among which we can choose freely. In any period in history or in a particular culture, some ideas and practices will be more acceptable than others in the management of distress. Indeed, there will very likely be a complex web of governments, professional groups and bodies, large organizations such as drug companies, sectional interests, pressure groups and the general public as a whole, hard at work pressing forward the concept formulations they find acceptable and which interpret their world, however dire it is, in a more or less congenial way. It might even be possible to see family resemblances between concept formulations in the past and their contemporary equivalents. For example, the idea of vitalism, with its faith in vital forces and the ability of the body to repair itself under the right circumstances, can be detected in the current vogue for community treatment, shorter hospital stays and returning patients to their own homes as early as possible. The idea, then, is that convalescence is more readily accomplished by placing the patient in familiar surroundings. The practitioners who are involved in this kind of care do not necessarily speak explicitly about vital forces, yet it is possible to detect correspondences. One crucial difference, of course, is that in the present the concern is to save money and substitute home-based care for costly hospital stays. Yet this is made possible by means of all the vitalistic thinking which was done 200 or more years previously.

Now we have addressed the role of concepts and concept formulations about health and illness, it is worth showing how concepts work in diversity as well as coherence. Although concepts are part of our social currency and may be used in the processes of securing accord and consensus, it is equally apparent that concept formulations are important in dissent, diversity and in terms of specifying areas of schism, confusion or disagreement. There are many elementary examples. Our concepts, for example, of 'a good night out' will surely be different, and the levels of imaginative work to transform the symptoms of alcohol poisoning into a retrospective account of having had a good time will differ depending on the dedication of the speaker. Even our concepts of seductively simple phenomena such as chairs, tables and beds tend to differ. In health care, the roles of the people involved are subject to debate, dissent and historical change. Think, for example, about the concept of nursing. This has taken up a variety of different concept formulations, from obedience and duty through to interaction and nurse–patient relationship (Peplau 1988) and outcome approaches (Roy and Roberts 1981). Moreover, the notion of what nurses are supposed to be doing is one which is widely discussed and debated in the nursing literature and the status of nurses is subject to political and legislative change as some subgroups of the profession are granted new powers and responsibilities. Thus, even within cultures that might appear reasonably coherent, there is a great deal of diversity.

Cultures, concepts and communication: diverse conceptual literacies

To illustrate some of the possible diversity in contemporary ideas about health and illness and see how the concept formulations may differ, it is perhaps useful to consider how they might differ cross-culturally. Even when different cultures are living in the same geographical area, intriguing differences may persist. Jovchelovitch and Gervais (1999) found that among members of the Chinese community in England, thinking about health and illness was strongly informed by traditional Chinese concepts. Their Chinese informants deployed a highly structured system of knowledge so as to enable them to define health and illness, and to explain the causes of disease and to devise appropriate treatments. Their system of knowledge seemed to be rooted in the Confucian notion of maintaining balance and harmony between the universal complementary but opposite forces of yin and yang. Thus, in this view, the healthy working of the body is believed to depend on a harmonious balance between elements and forces within the body, and to sustain health this, in turn, must balance with the social, natural and supernatural environments. Illness may be caused by excesses and imbalance in any of these domains. Good health is believed to result from factors such as having a balanced diet, avoiding extreme weather conditions, having a good disposition, leading a disciplined lifestyle and respecting one's family members and ancestors. Illness, by contrast, is the symptom of an energy imbalance, perhaps caused by a hereditary predisposition, an inappropriate diet, old age, extreme emotions, exposure to overly hot/cold or humid/dry atmospheric conditions, or the displeasure of one's ancestors. This kind of social and spiritual embeddedness has not been seen in Western medicine since the Middle Ages, when the human condition was influenced by the ages of man, the winds and the signs of the zodiac. In Jovchelovitch and Gervais's study, Chinese people also partook of Western medicine, especially where it was believed to offer hope in the case of potentially lethal conditions. There seemed to be a complex system of translation at work to facilitate this bicultural medical literacy. This is in itself an important lesson in that it shows how different conceptual regimes can co-exist. The different healing practices are not incorporated randomly or unthinkingly, but different compartments or domains are carved out for each of them. It is as if the offerings of Western medicine were formulated as high-intensity interventions for otherwise fatal conditions. Thus, the concepts are formulated such that there are different spheres of competence for the different interventions.

Let us pause for a moment and try to made sense of what we are doing philosophically at his point. So far we have examined the concepts and concept formulations relating to health and illness by describing examples, some ancient and others contemporary. But we have not yet been able to define exhaustively what a concept is, or specify its role in research at this stage, a quarter of the way through the chapter. The interest we have in examining what sorts of concept formulations people use to make sense of what we now call health and illness is itself part of a philosophical tradition. We are not merely trying to pass off social science as philosophy here because the philosophical issue is too difficult – well, maybe it is – but we are also making use of a technique of twentieth-century philosophy. One of the enduring legacies of Wittgenstein on philosophy is to recommend that we redefine philosophical problems as empirical ones. That is, rather than worry about what concepts are in the abstract, we should take the role of the anthropologist and see how people are using the term or using concepts and begin our theorization from there. Within the social sciences we can see similar ideas at work in the promotion of techniques like grounded theory or analytic induction, which recommend that abstract and theoretical formulations be arrived at by studying the specifics of human interaction.

This study of concepts in their natural habitat as it were can throw up some interesting anomalies that are especially interesting from the point of view of philosophy. Perhaps on the face of it we might expect people to use concept formulations as a way of unifying or coordinating thought on an issue. Human enquiry might then be considered to proceed on the basis of shared meaning and shared practice.

The immune system: changing concepts and the choreography of metaphor

So far we have been discussing concepts as if they were somehow formulated before research and tended to drive research and lay thinking along. In this section, we consider the process in reverse. Sometimes as a result of especially close scientific scrutiny, the concepts at stake in a field of enquiry undergo transformation and reformulation. We shall illustrate this contention by considering some of the concepts that have been put to work in the description and presentation of the immune system. First, let us consider what it means to be immune to disease. Originally, the term had little to do with disease and was instead concerned with politics. Immune derives from the Latin *immunis*, which means to be exempted from a public service, burden or charge – in other words, taxes (Shipley 1965; Partridge 1966). Immunity was a political privilege, limited to an elite. It was only in the 1880s that Louis Pasteur and his associates started using it in connection with disease, inoculation and infection. Even then, connotations of privilege persisted in the term, because it was of course the masses who, in their filth and squalor, were more likely to have diseases anyway. In connection with our discussion of shifting conceptions of immunity, we shall be guided by Donna Haraway's notion that scientists create and recreate nature as a version of their own culture.

Scientific discourses, especially where these involve potentially contentious issues, topics and questions are, as Haraway describes them, 'lumpy'. That is, they 'contain and enact condensed contestations for meanings and practices' (Haraway 1992, p. 200). Extending this metaphor, we could perhaps see lumps in the otherwise epistemologically flat carpet under which controversies and socio-political disputes had been swept.

For example, there is, in the presentation of the story of the discovery of the immune system, a set of rather grand metaphors of exploration – a cross between Indiana Jones and Star Trek. As one of the textbook writers, Golub (1987) describes the work of pioneer immunologist Richard Gershon, who 'must have had what the earliest explorers had, an insatiable desire to be the first person to see something, to know that you are where no man has been before'. As he discovered the immune system, Gershon 'gloried in the layer upon layer of complexity. He thrilled at seeing a layer of that complexity which no one had seen before' (Golub 1987, pp. 531–2).

Through the 1980s as understandings of the immune system expanded by leaps and bounds, a number of popular pieces of artwork, books and journalism appeared. For example, a book complete with the triumphalist title 'The Body Victorious' (Nilsson and Lindberg 1987) and an article in *National Geographic* magazine (Jaret 1986) provide illustrations that make the whole process of immunity appear concrete, as if it is really there and really going on in front of the reader's eyes. For example, tendrils extrude from macrophages to ensnare a bacterium, flattened, distant hills of chromosomes lie on a blue-hued lunar landscape, and an infected cell sends off myriads of virus particles into the inner space of the organism, no doubt to infect others. Tumour cells are surrounded by lethal squads of killer T cells that eject chemical poisons at the body's traitorous malignant cancer cells in an evocation of biological warfare. The ravaged head of a femur from an autoimmune diseased patient glows in a kind of sunset against what appears to be another planet's landscape (Haraway 1992, pp. 208–9). This kind of imagery, says Haraway, reifies the space within that the immune system protects, and with these visual analogues makes it somehow similar to outer space and its exploration. The artistic motifs from science fiction art are hard at work creating a literal, believable landscape and moral economy of immunity where the body's defences root out and destroy the bad guys, typically depicted in darker colours. In a sense, the kinds of pictures of the body from within, depicting the activities of the immune system, are as revolutionary as the Renaissance illustrations from da Vinci or Vesalius in that they enable us to visualize an interior space that hitherto has only been imagined. They make the interior landscape visual. Warfare, inside the body and on the battlefield, is a spectacle which, as it creates reality, at once liberates itself from the concrete molecular realities it seeks to describe and creates spectacular landscapes with actors whose moral careers reinscribe peptide reactions as romantic fables.

Another analogue that is used when researchers describe the immune system is the idea of the immune system as somehow musical. It was a major theme of Gershon and Golub's account of the immune system that it was like an orchestra. The themes of cooperation and control in the many-celled organism have been common themes since the eighteenth century – around the same length of time as there have been large orchestras and large hospitals. There are diagrams, for example, of the Generator of Diversity (G.O.D.) from a vantage point in a lymph node conducting the orchestra of T and B cells and macrophages as they march around the body. In the later diagrams, from the 1980s, the G.O.D. is no longer the head of the orchestra, rather it is led by subsets of T cells. Later still, G.O.D. is torn between the conflicting advice of the angels of help and suppression, like the protagonist in some sort of Greek tragedy. The orchestra has not only a separate T cell conductor but two conflicting prompters. Yet the immune symphony plays on. The point here is not whether one or other of these metaphors is true. Rather, following Haraway, these illustrations help to shape and reformulate the kinds of concepts we have of bodily phenomena. If we can see the macrophages and the T and B cells, then this carries with it a great many connotations of how the system might work and how we might work upon it as health care practitioners.

To take a more mundane example, consider the fact that veins are blue and arteries are red in most illustrations of the circulatory system. This, of course, is something that depends on the availability of cheap colour printing for mass circula-tion textbooks. The earliest editions of *Gray's Anatomy* did indeed depict the body in shades of grey. The experience of practitioners investigating the actual fleshy body is a little different from the labelled diagrams, as the circulatory system does not come conveniently colour coded. A practitioner friend of one of the authors described an incident where a routine operation to remove a patient's varicose veins went tragically wrong when an artery was accidentally severed and stripped out. While the anaesthe-tized patient's bleeding was staunched with fumbling fingers, other members of the team frantically attempted to page a vascular surgeon to help repair the damage. Conceptual and schematic representations, then, can have devastating effects as health care procedures are implemented.

To pursue this question of the imagery of the body a little further, Haraway notes that in tandem with the imagery of the body's defences as a kind of orchestra, in the post-Second World War era the body is increasingly seen as some sort of communication system. One of the central notions in this idea of bodies as communication systems is that, in important respects, information flows one way. That is, information flows from DNA to RNA to protein and not the other way round. Information flow in this version of the body looks rather like the account presented in Claude Shannon's mid-twentieth-century theory of information. This was originally developed to help solve the problem of packaging the maximum amount of information down a phone line for the Bell Telephone Company and has subsequently been extended to cover communication acts in general. Information is the reduction of uncertainty. The original model of information as binary code has had some consequences for the way we think of communication outside and inside the body. Once communication has been specified and formulated as the flow of information, it doesn't have to look like anything in nature. That is, once upon a time communication was extremely mimetic. Communicative acts evoked other things in nature. Some systems of notation, such as that used in ancient Egypt, looked like stylized representations of the things the message was about. The twentieth century saw a very different approach to communication. At the beginning of the century, Ferdinand de Saussure proposed that there is no necessary connection between the signifier (the word) and the signified (the concept). Moreover, in Saussurean linguistics, the terms are defined crucially by where they come in the sequence of language; in other words, their syntagmatic relations. Any relationship between words and things in nature which they signify is, in this view, arbitrary. If this is true of natural languages, then it is even more true of the endless sequences of zeroes and ones that make up digitized communication. In Jerry Fodor's (1981) famous example, it might be a game of chess or it might be the Six Day War. There is no way of telling from the communicative sequence alone. Language, says Haraway, is no longer an echo of the *verbum Dei* or word of God.

Now, we have taken this detour into communication and language because this underlies some of the kind of imagery of the immune system that was important in much late twentieth-century thinking on the subject. One of the major concept formulations within immunology is that the fundamental process of immunity is the distinction between self and non-self. A binary distinction, in other words. Most interesting, from our point of view, is what the zeroes and ones in this system of information might represent. Is the self, as some propose, 'everything encoded by the genome' or 'everything under the skin'? Or, is it the set of antigens present in early life? Or could the self be only a certain subset of peptides found in the thymus gland, while all the other tissues of the body are merely ignored? (Matzinger 1994). Equally, the question of what is non-self is problematic. There are a great many non-self materials that do not provoke an immune response, such as silicone, bone, bacteria in the gut, foetuses, new antigens which appear at puberty, and most foodstuffs. So the model of self and non-self is curiously vague when it comes to referents in nature, despite its being precise in terms of the decision making and communicative process. Individuality, says Haraway, is a strategic defence problem.

This model of the immune system was itself challenged throughout the 1990s by alternative metaphors and formulations. One of the theories to gain a good deal of publicity is the model championed by Polly Matzinger (1994, 1998), who uses the 'innate sense of danger' metaphor. The immune system is 'turned on by danger' in this formulation. Public discourse, of course, is lurid with the discourse of danger at the turn of the millennium. The danger of unprotected sex, the dangerous classes, the danger of terrorism and the danger from 'mental patients', all are cornerstones of contemporary journalism and feature in the fabrication of our twenty-first-century 'scary world'. Cells expire within the body. They may do so in two major ways (another binary distinction). On the one hand, they may die a peaceful, natural 'programmed cell death' involving apoptosis, where the dying cells are shed to the outside of the body or scavenged by specialized cells. If, on the other hand, a cell dies suddenly, it might signal this to the dendritic cells in the surrounding tissues perhaps by shedding heat shock proteins or substances normally inside cells which leak out if the cell dies lytically, expiring violently and bursting open. This, then, in Matzinger's danger model, triggers an immune response. The crucial distinction is violence or peace, predestination or unruly rupture. All of a sudden a different set of social, legal and moral tropes appear in the immune system as a result of these new concept formulations. Matzinger can thus evoke new ways of making sense and map out new research programmes as a result of reconceptualizing the process.

Although these later ideas appeared after Haraway's germinal paper on the immune system, they nevertheless fit in with the overall drive of her thesis that:

> . . . the immune system is an elaborate icon for principal systems of symbolic and material 'difference' in late capitalism. Pre-eminently a twentieth-century object, the immune system is a map drawn to guide recognition and misrecognition of self and other in the dialectics of Western biopolitics . . . The immune system is a historically specific terrain, where global and local politics; Nobel Prize-winning research; heteroglossic cultural productions, from popular dietary practices, feminist science fiction, religious imagery, and children's games, to photographic techniques and military strategic theory; clinical medical practice; venture capital investment strategies; world-changing developments in business and technology; and the deepest personal and collective experiences of embodiment, vulnerability, power, and mortality interact with an intensity matched perhaps only in the biopolitics of sex and reproduction.
>
> (Haraway 1992: 200–1)

To illustrate this further, consider some of the primal myths of the science of immunity. Innocent bucolic scenes with cows, horses and milkmaids blushing as they offer their limbs to Edward Jenner like characters in a Constable landscape. Myths laced with heterosexual, patriarchal and class-privileged imagery that somehow is made to seem natural. To take another example, consider Bruno Latour's work on Louis Pasteur. In his essay, 'Give Me a Laboratory and I Will Raise the World', he shows how Pasteur's discoveries transformed the objects on which he was working, in this case the bacteria that caused anthrax in livestock. If Pasteur had not transformed nature by liberating the bacteria from other competition to enable them to multiply unhindered in the laboratory, it is unlikely that he would have been able to develop his vaccine. In Latour's work on the social relations of science, the microbes themselves become full-blown actors in the human drama of arresting the diseases they bring on. Pasteur, as a result of his experiments with anthrax and with chicken cholera, was able to develop an attenuated form of the diseases that could be used as vaccines, an approach also used successfully with rabies. Koch's work in isolating the bacillus responsible for tuberculosis was also proceeding apace at the same time. Indeed, in the late nineteenth century, exhibits of bacteria, busily proliferating in jars, were toured and displayed in Europe, making visible the hitherto invisible agents of disease (Brecht and Nikolow 2000).

We hope we have shown how scientific concept formulations, displays and illustrations are important in structuring the perceptual and discursive world of scientists, health care practitioners and the public. Moreover, the framework offered by these concepts has an effect on the kinds of work that are done, the order of scientific priorities and, if influential laypeople can be persuaded, it affects the kinds of research that get funded, find favour with the public and ultimately come to prevail. An unhelpful concept formulation can yield dead ends and frustration, yet the more helpful ones can transform, synthesize and educate, leaving their mark on our intellectual history.

Contexts of discovery and contexts of verification: concept validation and the 'strong programme'

To sum up so far, we have emphasized the relationship between scientific and practical healing activity in health care and the social context. Science is influenced by the concepts, ideologies and inferential frameworks at large in the societies where it is conducted and, in turn, through application, dissemination, journalism and even by travelling exhibitions, it transforms the culture in which it is embedded. But how deeply does this social construction go? Does it affect the very fabric of scientific knowledge, or does the truth of science have some independent existence aside from the individual researchers who originate it? Are the social influences just the wrapping paper for something more durable or truthful? Through the 1980s and 1990s in the UK, the presenters on the educational programmes from the Open University were often seen wearing the wide ties and lapels, the sideburns, moustaches and pageboy hairstyles of the early 1970s. While this was a source of amusement, it does not, presumably, affect the nature of the theories and findings they presented. The science is more durable than the fashions. At least it is in this case.

Traditionally, many scientists and philosophers of science draw a distinction between what is called the 'context of discovery', which involves the historical circumstances in which a discovery is first made and disseminated, and the 'context of justification', involving a more enduring and dispassionate epistemological assessment of the reasons we have for believing those results to be true or accurate. In this version of events, it follows that while the practice, concepts and cultural context of scientists may be interesting to the historian or sociologist, they are not directly relevant to the evaluation of current scientific theories and findings. Indeed, some philosophers, historians and sociologists of science steer away from the evaluation of findings as they consider themselves not to be expert enough to judge.

This, then, was the traditional position. We can, in this view, distinguish between the ephemeral fashions and the durable findings. From the 1970s, this approach to studying the social context of science was challenged by David Bloor (1976, 1981) and his colleagues at Edinburgh, who implemented what they called the 'strong programme' in the sociology of science. Most preceding work in the sociology of science had treated scientific knowledge as somehow categorically different from lay knowledge, or sociological knowledge, as if it had a privileged claim to truth. Thus, previously this knowledge was not susceptible to sociological analysis. Barnes (1974) and Bloor's 'strong programme' involved claiming that the sociology of knowledge can study not only the content of knowledge but its very nature. Here, they seemed to be annexing the theory of knowledge – epistemology itself – so that it becomes a branch of sociology. They had a 'naturalistic' conception of knowledge. That is, knowledge is whatever is collectively endorsed, and aimed to give a causal account of it in social terms. In this view, the theories and facts of science emerge for social reasons rather than because of what's 'out there' in nature. 'Out thereness' is just another rhetorical strategy and doesn't necessarily relate to what we can see down the microscope in any direct and simple sense.

In Bloor's original formulation, the strong programme of the sociology of scientific knowledge adhered to the following four tenets. In this way, he felt that the sociology of science could come to resemble the natural sciences themselves, and embody the same values that are taken for granted in other scientific disciplines. These are:

1. The sociology of science should be causal; that is, it should be concerned with the conditions that lead to beliefs or states of knowledge. There will be other causes apart from social ones that will combine to bring about beliefs and certainties, but social causes are accorded considerable significance.

2. The sociology of science should be impartial concerning truth or falsity, rationality or irrationality, and success or failure. Both sides of these dichotomies will require explanation; we cannot take it for granted that one side is real and the other unreal, because that involves 'going native' in the local community of scientists in question, and the student of science should remain disinterested.

3. The sociology of science should try to be 'symmetrical' in its style of explanation. The same type of cause would explain, say, true and false beliefs. Those beliefs that stood the test of time need explaining just as much as the ones that are rapidly dismissed as false.

4. Finally, the sociology of science should be reflexive. Its patterns of explanation would have to be applicable to sociology itself. As with the requirement of symmetry, this reflects Bloor's desire for general explanations. One reason why he needed this feature was so that the sociology of science would not refute itself. In other words, if knowledge is socially produced and caused, this means that this very sociological claim is invalid, because it must be socially caused itself. Reflexivity, Bloor believed, is a powerful way of navigating around this objection.

These four tenets – causality, impartiality, symmetry and reflexivity – defined the strong programme in the sociology of knowledge. The strong programme is sometimes referred to as a relativistic approach. In Barnes and Bloor's terms, it involves 'the observation that beliefs on a certain topic vary' and 'the conviction that which of these beliefs is found in a given context depends on, or is relative to, the circumstances of the user' (Barnes and Bloor 1982, p. 68). Moreover:

> Our equivalence postulate is that all beliefs are on par with one another with respect to the causes of their credibility. It is not that all beliefs are equally true or equally false, but that regardless of truth and falsity the fact of their credibility is to be seen as equally problematic.
>
> (Barnes and Bloor 1982, p. 69)

Having examined scientific knowledge in this way, and having argued that the concept formulations with which we interrogate and construct nature are embedded in human social affairs, some important questions about science remain unanswered. If scientific knowledge reflects social interests and processes and is not precisely about nature, how can scientific theories be coherent and predictive? How can experiments and, more importantly, their findings be replicated? Getting the same results reliably has been an important feature of scientific enquiry and lends confidence to knowledge, yet if knowledge depends on social processes rather than – or as well as – patterns in nature, how do scientists manage to replicate findings? Experimental results are reproducible because part of the craft of the scientist is to replicate the precise conditions of their production (Ravetz 1971). Whereas the method sections of empirical reports purport to be explicit, there is a good deal which is implicit too and which competent scientific practitioners can infer from the details given. In a sense, this idea that the results are reproducible because the conditions have been reproduced is an obvious platitude. The reproduction of experimental conditions enables the coherence and integrity of science. The fact that workers in contentious or cutting-edge fields try to replicate one another's findings provides a social check, and this ensures that the distributed production of scientific knowledge is a socially and discursively orderly, disciplined process. To some students of scientific knowledge, though, this reproducibility of research conditions does not mean that the resulting knowledge tells us anything about nature. To Latour (1987), this merely means that a particular negotiated reality is being reproduced under specified conditions.

Scientific knowledge looks the way it does, in Latour's view, because of the interpretive and procedural consensus among scientists. What does it mean when particular scientific facts leave the laboratory as it were, and produce successful results once they are transplanted into technological applications? Latour would argue that no-one has ever seen a laboratory fact move outside, or even from one lab to another, unless the original lab is first brought to bear on the 'outside' situation and the situation is transformed so that it fits the original laboratory prescriptions. Collins (2001) provides an example from the study of sapphires. The quality of the gem is related to how long it resonates after it is made to vibrate. In the early 1970s, scientists in Moscow were obtaining very long resonance times that were widely disbelieved in the West. However, one crucial feature unknown to Western scientists at the time was that the Moscow gems were suspended on Chinese silk thread coated with pig's grease. Eventually, in the late 1990s, when researchers in Moscow and Glasgow had visited one another's laboratories, it was possible to obtain concordant results from both sets of laboratories. Latour then makes a strong claim on the basis of events like this: 'scientific facts are like trains, they do not work off their rails' (Latour 1983, p. 155).

The example from Collins also highlights the importance of social networks in creating the right kind of conditions for scientific findings to become stable and reliable. In this case, it depends upon the end of the Cold War, the possibility of trust between different nations and the availability of funding for travel. This notion of a network to explain the development of scientific issues is one which we shall consider more explicitly in the next section. Modifying Clausewitz's famous maxim, Latour (1983) asserts 'science is politics pursued by other means' (p. 168).

Science, actors and networks: the 'web of deceit' and the construction of a scientific 'fraud'

The idea of a variety of interests, people and objects working together – or sometimes in opposition – to produce scientific knowledge has become known as Actor Network Theory (Callon 1986; Latour 1987; Law 1992; Law and Hassard 1999). This work is premised on the idea that materials are associated in 'networks' of relations. One of its key propositions is that technologies operate to open up certain obligatory ways of seeing the world.

These lines of sight become embedded in formal representations, such as maps or diagrams (Star 1989), or in artefacts, like computer imaging technologies, medical monitoring devices, graphics or exhibits, which ensure that the world appears in the same way wherever it is regarded. One foetal ultrasound scan looks pretty much like another, for example, and the same foetus looks similar when scanned by different machines in different clinics. Hence these technological artefacts are named 'immutable mobiles' (Latour 1990).

> This, then, is the core of the actor-network approach: a concern with how actors and organizations mobilise, juxtapose, and hold together the bits and pieces out of which they are composed; how they are sometimes able to prevent those bits and pieces from following their own inclinations and making off.
>
> (Law 1992, p. 386)

To try and illustrate some of these features, since the discussion of actor network theory has so far been rather abstract, let us consider a real case. We shall consider some events that took place in the world of obstetrics and gynaecology in the UK from 1993 to 1995 which were dubbed by some to be 'the scientific fraud of the century'. Indeed, for a few months in late 1994 and early 1995, it seemed to have eclipsed even Piltdown Man (a fake 'missing link' fabricated in 1912, allegedly by Martin Hinton, curator of the Natural History Museum). At St George's Hospital, Tooting, London, Malcolm Pearce, a consultant apparently with a flair for innovative surgery and research, published a revolutionary case report in the *British Journal of Obstetrics and Gynaecology* in August 1994 (Pearce *et al.* 1994). He claimed to have successfully transplanted a 5-week-old foetus growing ectopically in the fallopian tube of a 29-year-old African woman. The foetus had been removed from the fallopian tube and then been successfully introduced to the womb via the cervix, carried to term and delivered in a six and a half hour labour in March or April 1994. However, colleagues were sceptical as the mother and baby could not be found, and there was no record of such a person having been treated in the hospital. The person whom it might have been turned out to have been 25 not 29, and the baby was 3.7 kg not the 2.7 kg claimed by Dr Pearce in the article. It also turned out that the hospital's computer records had been tampered with and someone logging on to the system, with Dr Pearce's password or that of two midwives in his team, had substituted the case number of a dead patient who had been born in 1910 and was not likely to have been pregnant in 1994 anyway. In addition, he had published a paper in the same journal about the hormonal treatment of 191 women with a history of miscarriages and polycystic ovary disease, claiming to have allowed 132 of them to achieve a successful pregnancy (Pearce and Hamid 1994). It became clear that it was most unlikely that so many women could have been treated at St George's because patients meeting these criteria are relatively rare. The case, as one might imagine, resulted in Pearce losing his job and subsequently being struck off by the General Medical Council in June 1995.

It is not our intention to suggest that innovative treatments in general are tainted by fraud, or that Actor Network Theory is all about questioning the truth of medical or scientific claims. We have mentioned the case because it illustrates how the social bonds between colleagues are effective in creating medical research and medical work in a kind of ongoing 'liturgy of the clinic'.

Particularly obvious in this case were Pearce's efforts to retrospectively re-adjust the records so that the crucial actors in the piece, the mother and her baby, could be resurrected from the computer database. Alas, this was not done convincingly and unbeknownst to Pearce the computer system was capable of tracking the changes. What is interesting also in this case is the way Pearce was alleged to enlist others in his activities. His paper on the large-scale clinical trial was written up for journal submission by a colleague to whom he had passed some handwritten notes and invited to collaborate in the production of a journal article, which was eventually published as Pearce and Hamid (1994). The head of the department, Professor Geoffrey Chamberlain (who was also the journal's editor and the President of the Royal College of Obstetricians and Gynaecologists), had appeared as an author on the other paper (Pearce et al. 1994). This manoeuvre of including colleagues in research, even though they have not done the operations or collected the data, is a strategy for mutual career building in science. Also, from the point of view of the fraudster or someone with particularly tentative or controversial findings, it helps to authenticate the events whose veracity might otherwise be doubted by the audience. To question the integrity of such findings, then, involves questioning an array of actors, some of whom might be very senior indeed. In the play 'Julius Caesar', all of Caesar's attackers dipped their knives in the blood, so the task of indicting the guilty party is made all the more difficult. The network in the case of the Pearce scandal is even greater and incorporates rivals too. The paper included the comment: 'We freely admit that we stole the idea for uterine replacement of ectopic pregnancies from Professor J.D. Grudzinskas, who less freely admits that he stole it from Professor Ian Donald' (Hawkes 1995, p. 1). Thus, the apparently incredible operation is made more believable because it is identified as a concept that is being discussed as feasible in medical circles, and identifies the authors as being part of that network. Thus, the concept is formulated as 'uterine replacement of ectopic pregnancies' – a neat little phrase – and this is made to sound as if it is one being brought into the realm of possibility by others, thus heading off a reader's possible scepticism.

The networks in science, once established, are often also replete with strategies, courtesies and protocols that may have the effect of preventing problems coming to light. Indeed, one of the co-authors of the ectopic paper, Isaac Manyonda, became suspicious later in 1994 and challenged Pearce over the issue. He later described Pearce's response to his enquiries: 'He was very angry at me and expressed surprise that I had doubted his integrity. He was absolutely adamant that it had happened and said that the patient wanted anonymity. I felt rather silly that I had doubted his word' (Wilkins 1995, p. 1). Network building thus involves the deployment of a 'spectrum of methods that ranges from seduction to pure violence' (Callon 1986). Collectively these methods are referred to as strategies of *translation*. What is at stake is a way of convincing or simply forcing an actant to accept a given role and identity in a network, that is, the engineering of consent to *enrolment*. Of course, Manyonda may have been trying to distance himself from the scandal. In any event, his recollection to the inquiry conducted by the UK's General Medical Council is that he had a speculative discussion with Pearce about the possibility of such an operation, rather than actually doing one with him.

Thus, we hope these examples have shown how findings, processes and achieve-ments in science are made possible through the actions of people acting in concert embedded in a network. In this case, it is also apparent that entirely fictitious findings and procedures were not sustainable from the network alone. However, in Latour's account, it is possible for inanimate objects to take on a life of their own in the proceedings. Here we can see how inanimate objects such as the computer system on which records were kept, the passwords used to access the records and even the hastily fabricated confection of mother and infant are, in a sense, actors in the piece, brought into alignment with one side or another as the argument about the veracity of Pearce's claims progressed.

Scientific concepts, then, in Latour's formulation, exist by virtue of the network of actors within which they are embedded. It is as if concepts are suspended by the web of relationships between people, things, interests and values. Indeed, popular journalism at the time described Pearce as 'spinning a web of lies'.

This example also shows how the decommissioning of one part of a network, in the form of Pearce and his mysterious fictional patients, has implications for other actors' careers. Geoffrey Chamberlain, the professor who had supported him, enjoyed very little success afterwards. A possible knighthood had been mooted prior to the scandal, yet afterwards colleagues were keen to distance themselves: 'hardworking but ultimately naïve' said one. 'A real sweetie but intellectually past his best' said another (Jones 1995, p. 12). Geoffrey Chamberlain's disgrace was thus put down to human error – as they frantically sought to put distance between them-selves and their ex-colleague, other members of staff at St George's Hospital did the same as pilots do when one of them has an accident. They blamed the personal qualities of the person who has come a cropper. As if they would be too shrewd to be taken in themselves.

Hearts and minds: personalities, diseases and the discourse of stress

In the next section, we elaborate a little further on the role of concept formulations and ideas. To do this we examine the natural history of a concept, namely the idea of stress. In the health care sciences, this involves a curious intersection of themes from the physical sciences and biology with considerations of lifestyle, cognition, emotion and social context.

Within this field there are a great many issues that could be examined. There is a large literature on almost every part of stress that one might care to mention – occupational stress, post-traumatic stress disorder, life change and stress, and so on. To narrow down this discussion so as to illustrate some of the concepts at work, we consider the relationship between stress and heart disease, as this illustrates the social context of concepts and how there are traces of the vitalism we mentioned earlier still at large in contemporary health science. Let us emphasize that the aim here is not to challenge the truth or 'facticity' of this work. In the spirit of Barnes and Bloor, that would involve us claiming to be better physiologists than the authors we will discuss (see Barnes *et al.* 1996). Rather, we are interested in how facts are assembled, concepts are deployed and networks are created in the production of these concepts and findings, which nowadays have a very wide circulation.

There are a variety of possible origins of the notion of stress. One could point to the origins of psychological approaches to emotion in William James's work or the origins of Walter Cannon's 'fight or flight response'. The term stress was most famously applied to biological matters by Hans Selye (1976), who said 'Stress is the nonspecific response of the body to any demand' (p. 53). The relationship between stress and the cardiovascular system was being theorized rather earlier than this however. There have been a number of attempts historically to link heart disease to what later came to be known as 'styles of coping' and 'personality'. Sir William Osler (1849–1919) was reputed to have said in 1910 that the typical angina sufferer was 'vigorous in mind and body, and the keen and ambitious man, the indicator of whose engines is always set at full speed ahead' (cited in Chesney *et al.* 1980). As the twentieth century wore on, there were repeated attempts to relate circulatory disorders to the thought and behaviour patterns of the sufferer. The psychoanalytic theorist Franz Alexander was one of the first to try to explain the link between states of mind and states of the body. Here is his view of the causes of hypertension:

> The damming up of hostile impulses will continue and will consequently increase in intensity. This will induce the development of stronger defensive measures in order to keep pent up aggressions in check . . . Because of the marked degree of their inhibitions, these patients are less effective in their occupational activities and for that reason tend to fail in competition with others . . . envy is stimulated and . . . hostile feelings toward more successful, less inhibited competitors are further intensified.
>
> (Alexander 1950, p. 150)

Thus a good deal of the groundwork was laid outside the mainstream of psychology. Selye was a biologist, Osler was a physician and Alexander was a psychoanalyst.

These nodes in the network were given further impetus with the idea of a pattern of behaviour which predisposes persons to coronary heart disease (CHD) and elevates risk for myocardial infarction (MI). This arose from the interest in large-scale epidemiological studies of cardiovascular health in post-war North American medicine, which themselves emerged from the changing focus of medical research. Medicine included not just the consulting room or the hospital ward but the entire continent.

The now famous Framingham Study, commenced with 5209 participants in 1948, was pivotal in beginning the late twentieth-century concern with the demographics of disease. Unlike the squalor and deprivation catalogued in the nineteenth century, this latter initiative made visible a network of biochemical pathways between heart disease and the involvement of animal fats, cholesterol, being overweight and smoking (Kannel 1976; Inglis 1981). The progressive refinement of the causal pathways elaborated by the study has enabled the inclusion of factors such as blood triglyceride and high density lipoprotein. Stress was added to the list later as a result of Wolf's (1969) apparently inconsistent finding from Roseto, Pennsylvania. Here, obesity was correlated with lower mortality rates than those found in the surrounding area. Accordingly, Wolf brought the findings into line with the prevailing wisdom in the literature by describing Roseto as having a supportive community that protected the inhabitants from the stress of modern life. This manoeuvre was an important one, as it enabled stress to sit alongside the more obvious physiological factors in heart disease, as if there were a theorizable link waiting to be discovered. In doing this, Wolf also managed to reframe the long-standing narrative of the 'strains of modern life', previously centred on the notion of 'reserve force', around a different construct – the heart, as Brown (1997) notes.

There were other pieces of this puzzle waiting to fall into place to constitute additional anchoring nodes in the network. The concept of stress, in a sense, is made up as a mosaic from a variety of disciplines and research traditions. A further strand of thinking that has proved extremely fruitful as part of the modern conception of stress comes from the work of two cardiologists, Friedman and Rosenman (1959), who published a study purporting to link what they called an overt 'action–emotion complex', the now infamous 'type A behaviour pattern' (TABP) or even, significantly, the 'type A personality'. This involved aggressiveness, competitiveness and impatience and appeared to be correlated with the likelihood of developing CHD. In their formulation, it was characterized by 'muscle tenseness, alertness, rapid and emphatic vocal stylistics, and accelerated pace of activities' as well as 'emotional responses such as irritation, covert hostility, above-average potential for anger' (Rosenman 1993, p. 451).

Now what is interesting about the formulation of type A behaviour is the slippage it accomplishes between the meat and the morality, between cardiovascular health and the kind of life one leads and values one subscribes to. Friedman and Rosenman (1959) invoked the 'stresses of contemporary Western life' (p. 1286). They first hit upon the idea of TABP after noticing the wearing down of the front edges of the seats in their consulting rooms caused by a particular kind of irritable, hyperactive cardiac patient – the proverbial 'on the edge of their seats' stance – who came to serve as the model for the work-driven type As (Friedman and Ulmer 1985, p. 7). Thus, type A involves the enlistment of popular wisdom, the mobilization of popular stereotypes about heart disease from William Osler's era, and the intersection of this with contemporary notions of stress and personality. Moreover, a further component of the network, and one which again mobilizes established wisdom, is the finding of Matthews *et al.* (1977) that mothers of children who become type A continually stress the need for higher and higher achievement to obtain the same level of reward. This addition completes the circle, inasmuch as popular and psychological narratives of childhood, child-rearing and identifying mothers as being the responsible parties have been deployed to assist in the construction of a viable network to support the concept. It also fully individualizes the problem – as something that has its origins in early life and is presumably susceptible to individual solutions, of which more later.

In contrast to type A, Friedman and Rosenman also described a relatively low risk behaviour pattern, type B, characterized as a relaxed, unhurried, non-competitive interpersonal style. Recently – and we shall return to this point – type B's characteristics were redefined as involving less hostility (Rosenman *et al.* 1988). Evidence for the constructs came from a longitudinal study of Californian men, the Western Collaborative Group Study, where it was found that 'type As' were twice as likely as 'type Bs' to develop CHD, even controlling for other factors (Rosenman *et al.* 1976).

Once we consider the construct of stress, health and heart disease as a whole, and the various strands of evidence that go to make it up, the type A construct and the findings in Roseto serve as a powerful indictment of a society which literally made its members sick. It was as if type A was built into our culture just as much as it was built into our cardiac muscles. Moreover, type A pays off in the short run at least, in terms of increased productivity and accomplishment. Heart disease was thus associated with the Western way of life, an association underscored by Marmot's finding of higher rates of CHD among migrant Japanese in California who had become more 'westernized' than among those who maintained a 'traditional' lifestyle (Marmot and Symon 1976).

Overall, there is a curious relationship between the struggle to assume the 'American dream' way of life and the development of type A. Again, we see a curious interplay of the meat – the heart muscle itself – and morality in terms of what is considered desirable for the person. For example, insufficient social contact together with low income were strong predictors of death from heart disease (Williams *et al.* 1992). Increases in occupational changes and increases in job responsibility are associated with the development of CHD (Theorell *et al.* 1975; Karasek *et al.* 1982; Syme 1984). In the year after the death of their spouses, widows and widowers are more likely to develop and die from CHD. The problems associated with coronary artery disease have been demonstrated in the laboratory too. When Rozanski *et al.* (1988) got people with this syndrome to discuss their faults, the oxygen to their hearts fell dangerously low. Type A behaviour pattern is more prevalent in the African American community (Sprafka *et al.* 1990). Thus, people who are compromised in relation to the cultural ideals of affluence, leisure, sociability and togetherness are the ones at risk of CHD.

In their popular volume, *Type A Behaviour and Your Heart*, Friedman and Rosenman (1972) blame TABP on a society which commodifies time, justifies relentless toil by promises of future glory and values rationality as expressed in an obsession with quantification. This, then, was a story that fit very well with the spirit of the early

1970s. Persons expressing TABP embodied what was wrong with 'our flawed society' (Friedman and Ulmer 1985: 64). The solution was to foster alternative styles of life and work (Powell *et al.* 1984). Type As were encouraged to interest themselves in things 'that cannot be represented or contained by numbers' (Friedman and Ulmer 1985: p. 146), to ask themselves what 'should be the essence of my life' (p. 119). In a sense, the answer to this question is foreclosed, as the authors provide numerous pointers to the 'real' good life, for example: 'it is worth being cultured' (p. 151) and 'it is worth being aware of the transcendental' (p. 153). Here, we can see echoes of nine-teenth-century notions of vital energies. This can also be seen in Selye's work on the issue, where he engineers the shift from biology to society and to morality. From his deliberations on stress, for example, Selye (1973, 1975) offers a moral code for living that he called 'altruistic egoism', which was, he claimed, directly derived from the natural world. This pivots on the idea that people have a finite quantity of 'adaptive energy' to expend. Selye's ethics propose a way of living that optimizes the stockpile of adaptive energy. Thus, a sense of vitalism, the belief in a 'vital force' or 'natural energy' that animates the body, of a kind that would be familiar to any theorist of the eighteenth or nineteenth centuries, is, as they say, alive and well.

This picture of the relationship between stress, personality and the heart, while plausible, did not stay still for long. As the 1980s and 1990s progressed, new values came to prevail in European and American occupational life such that the advice to stop and smell the roses soon began to look outdated. All of a sudden the time scheduling, goal setting and the cult of long working hours were exonerated of blame for heart disease. The seeds of this redefinition were sown as early as 1977 when Matthews *et al.* discovered that of the cluster of characteristics of the original Type A pattern, the best predictors of heart disease were impatience, hostility and com-petitiveness. Moreover, aspects of people's speech style were associated with heart disease, such as 'explosiveness of speech'.

> Hostility consists of negative beliefs about and attitudes towards others, including cynicism, mistrust and denigration. Cynicism refers to the belief that others are motivated by selfish concerns, and mistrust is the often co-occurring expectation that others are likely to be provoking and hurtful.
>
> (Miller *et al.* 1996, p. 323)

Hearn (1989) identified hostility as the major predictor of heart disease. People high in hostility are more reactive to stress (Weidner *et al.* 1989) and are more likely to have higher levels of cholesterol (Weidner 1987). People who endorse items reflecting a cynical or hostile attitude on a psychometric measure, the Minnesota Multiphasic Personality Inventory, tend to have more artery blockage and a higher risk of coron-ary death (Barefoot *et al.* 1983; Williams *et al.* 1986). According to Houston and Vavak (1991), this cynical, hostile attitude is related to avoidance of social support, high levels of suppressed anger, greater consumption of alcohol and being overweight. Houston and Vavak (1991) suggest that hostility begins in childhood as feelings of insecurity and a negative attitude towards others. They argue that it is caused by parental behaviour that (i) lacks genuine acceptance, (ii) is overly strict, critical and demanding of conformity, and (iii) is inconsistent with regard to disciplinary treatment. This is believed to interact with parental behaviour that is related to the development of health-related attitudes and habits, like smoking, physical activity, drug and alcohol use.

Thus, the features that are bad for your heart turn out to be those that are bad for the organization or the economy. The worker under European or American capitalism is provided with a form of internal policing more vigilant than any manager. If negative feelings exist about one's work situation, the crippling commitments it extracts from the worker, then it is the worker's responsibility to police them out of existence. The everyday experience of fulminating about bosses with 'delusions of adequacy', poor pay, conditions or shortages of resources are, by this token, 'hostility and cynicism' and those who speak such treason do so at their own peril.

Instead, experts now advise an attitude of trust – the 'trusting heart' has been recommended by a number of authorities in the field (Williams 1989; Williams and Williams 1993). The trusting heart believes in the basic goodness of human beings and that most people will be fair and caring. Having these beliefs, the individual with such an attitude is slow to anger, and does not seek out negativity in others, nor does the trusting-hearted person expect the worst of them. He or she expects mainly good from others and, more often that not, finds it. The trusting heart treats others with sensitivity, kindness and love. Thus, individual adaptations are recommended – moreover, ones that leave the structure of hard work and long hours intact. Myocardial infarction, then, is the penalty for moral infraction. There is also much symbolism of the association of stress with the heart. As the seat of emotion and the engine that powers the body (Miller 1978), the heart seems to embody notions of personal efficacy (Brown 1997). In compromising the heart, hostility and cynicism threaten not only our power to work, but also seemingly everything about us that our heart holds in place. As Kott describes his own experience:

> After the infarct, the heart is constantly present . . . And only in saying so, did I realize that the heart really aches, and that I can feel in me everything language says about the heart. I have a heart. I am lighthearted or heavyhearted. My heart is in the right place. I pour out my heart. And what it means to break someone's heart.
>
> (Kott 1985, p. 83)

Also in the 1980s as the cult of business raged through Western economies, studies began to show that there were ways and means of surviving stress that more fully inscribed the commitment of the individual to the working organization. Maddi and Kobasa (1984) studied people who seemed to have many Type A traits and high stress. However, they did not have higher rates of illness and death. The authors therefore described these people as having 'hardy personalities'. The study examined 700 AT&T executives who were working during stressful changes in the company. The authors compared 200 executives who indicated high stress: 100 who stayed healthy and 100 who became ill. In contrast to their sick colleagues, hardy personalities seemed to have three viewpoints that contributed to better health: (1) They had a sense of personal commitment to self, work, family and other stabilizing values. (2) They had a sense of personal control over their lives and their work. (3) They had a tendency to see life changes as challenges to master rather than merely as threats or problems.

Thus, when workers are placed under stress by the organization for which they work, the responsibility for well-being rests with the individual worker. Type A itself has been rehabilitated as the villain of the piece and it is individual factors that are detrimental to the organization – hostility, cynicism and a sense of lack of commitment and personal control that are also hazardous to the individual. Indeed, with the right kind of attitude in this formulation, the experience of stress can be one of 'eustress' or good stress. This is a kind of mentalism or nominalism – the idea that the individual is somehow the captain of their own ship and their personality and attitudes are somehow psychologically prior to and causal of their circumstances.

Thus we have sought to show in this example how the concept formulations in the tradition of research and therapy concerned with stress, heart disease, morbidity and mortality are infused with political and moral values. It is difficult to separate the theorization of many issues in the health sciences away from the social and moral circumstances within which they are formulated. We are not suggesting that the 'proper' way to study stress is through a politically critical lens (though this might be a good idea). Nor are we saying that it would be 'better' to reformulate the story of what happens to people in organizations as something else, for example 'violence'. Nor are we suggesting that the stress researchers are ideologues for American corporate capitalism. These might be interesting arguments to pursue. What we have attempted to show is how concept formulations in this area are intimately connected with the climate of the times and with the interests and ideologies of the actors in the piece. They are embedded in research which may be eminently respectable and yield results which are reliable and more or less true. The therapeutic programmes to which they are linked may be considerably easier to implement than trying to convince sufferers that the employers to whom they have devoted the best years of their lives are evil exploiters who are trying to kill them. There might be, therefore, short-term pragmatic benefits for the individual, the corporation, the researcher and clinician.

Are we presenting a picture of researchers as somehow lacking integrity, as formulating concepts, selecting theories and generating findings as they are expedient? The answer is a qualified 'yes'. It is relatively rare to find successful researchers struggling against the mainstream for very long. Yet it is equally difficult to sustain a picture of greedy, avaricious researchers seeking to capitalize on what they see to be the most productive trends.

Conclusion: concepts, theories and the philosophy of science

It is perhaps fitting, now that we have addressed the idea of concepts and tried to show some of them at work in the production of scientific knowledge and health care practice, that we bring the discussion back to the philosophy of science and see where our deliberations fit within this canon. We have tried to describe the idea of a concept and discovered it to be a particularly slippery entity. The suspicion that concepts are created, refined and deployed to suit the circumstances of the debate in which they are embedded has led us to speak instead of 'concept formulations', an idea which highlights the contrived nature of the concept itself. Concepts inform research and open up slots for new lines of enquiry, while they may themselves be transformed as a result of new scientific endeavours. Concepts may, in some accounts of the scientific process, be like actors themselves.

Within the rubric of a theory, a variety of concepts may be brought together. Indeed, in the conventional view, a theory comprises a set of concepts, definitions, propositions or statements as part of a systematic view of the phenomenon in question, as well as a designation of specific interrelationships among concepts for the purposes of describing, explaining and predicting (Chinn and Jacobs 1987; Leddy and Pepper 1993). There are, according to Leddy and Pepper (1993), several important attributes of a theory. First, a theory involves building networks linking defined concepts together. Second, a theory should have a systematic structure and be goal-oriented. Finally, it will be tentative because it is often based on assumptions, values and judgements as well as on empirical observations. Theoretical frameworks pull concepts into an inter-relative whole. Theories comprise logically connected statements that will enable science to attempt to explain the world or predict what might happen in the future in the world. This, then, in theory is what theories might do. However, it is difficult to square this with the variety of activity that goes on in the form of theoretical development and practical research. Indeed, it is sometimes difficult to identify the difference between a concept and a theory. If we take the idea of stress, it is sometimes a theory, inasmuch as it proposes a particular kind of relationship between cognition, emotion and various indices of physiological arousal, yet in other instances it is a concept, a building block for some other theory about how our work can make us ill, for example. It is therefore sometimes difficult to separate out what the concepts are in human enquiry. In this respect, science is sometimes rather like everyday thinking, which needs to be studied using the techniques of social representations theory, discursive psychology or the sociology of science.

For interpretivists, scientific theories, or any theories for that matter, offer merely different, perhaps temporarily useful descriptions of the world, yet fail to achieve ultimate authority. There is, according to Quine, no neutrality in describing the world and furthermore there are no theory statements that cannot be removed and cast off if we so choose. In essence, adjudicating between competing concept formulations or competing theories is extremely difficult. There may well be no reliable or generally accepted way to accomplish this. As Williams *et al.* (1996) put it: 'Truth is not fixed or immutable, but is something that happens to an idea itself, not to the objects to which it refers' (p. 101). Here we can see echoes of the 'pragmatism' of Peirce, James, Dewey and Rorty – that the real issue is whether theories are 'useful' rather than true or false.

One of the messages that we hope is apparent from our discussion of the variety of concept formulations with which we have illustrated this chapter is that there is often a good deal of ongoing debate about the authority of concepts and theories to describe, explain or predict phenomena in the world. In Karl Popper's falsificationist model of scientific enquiry, the history of theories is often the 'history of wrong theories'. This could equally be applied to concepts, which are often purpose-built for particular experiments, arguments and findings and are rapidly abandoned once something more interesting comes along. Indeed, concept formulations, like paradigms in Kuhn's model of science, sometimes shift and change for reasons that may not appear to satisfy the standards of logic or rationality that their host disciplines often claim. In making sense of the value of theories and concept formulations, we need to be sensitive to their practical usefulness to the community which sustains them, rather than the issue of whether they are true or false in any absolute sense.

In examining the history of concepts in health care and the social sciences, a fitting end to our exposition can be found in the work of Karl Popper himself. In 1938, he began *The Poverty of Historicism*, a deliberation on social science methodology and history. In it he was critical of the 'approach to the social sciences which assumes that historical prediction is their principal aim and that this aim is attainable by discovering the "rhythms" or the "patterns", the "laws" or the "trends" that underlie the evolution of history' (Popper 1957, p. 55). Popper argued that it was not possible to reduce history to a set of laws. Here he was being critical of philosophies of history such as Marxism, which proposed an inevitable sequence of evolutionary stages in society. As there are no historical laws, it is very difficult to tell what will happen to concepts in health care or social science in the future. No theoretical science of history, or the history of ideas, is possible. Popper, in a sense, is preparing us for the even more radical indeterminacy of the philosophies that were to follow. History is made by the concepts, hopes and conduct of human beings. Historical development is informed by the growth of scientific knowledge, yet this process can never be predicted. There are historical trends, but these are most easily observed in retrospect and do not make predictions of the future possible. Even biological evolution to date is only a trend, and may be subject to change or even reversal. In the social or health care realm, conditional predictions may be possible. Indeed, this kind of prediction is the main business of the social scientist or the historian of ideas, but no historical prophecy about the concepts of tomorrow can claim a scientific status.

References

Alexander, F. (1950) *Psychosomatic Medicine*. New York: Norton.

Barefoot, J.C., Dahlstrom, G. and Williams, R.B. (1983) Hostility, CHD incidence and total mortality: a 25 year follow up study of 255 physicians, *Psychosomatic Medicine*, 45: 59–63.

Barnes, B. (1974) *Scientific Knowledge and Sociological Theory*. London: Routledge.

Barnes, B. and Bloor, D. (1982) *Rationality and Relativism*. Oxford: Blackwell.

Barnes, B., Bloor, D. and Henry, J. (1996) *Scientific Knowledge: A Sociological Approach*. London: Athlone Press.

Bloor, D. (1976) *Knowledge and Social Imagery*. London: Routledge & Kegan Paul.

Bloor, D. (1981) The strengths of the strong programme, *Philosophy of the Social Sciences*, 11: 199–213.

Brecht, C. and Nikolow, S. (2000) Displaying the invisible: *Volkskrankheiten* in exhibition in Imperial Germany, *Studies in the History and Philosophy of the Biological and Biomedical Sciences*, 31(4): 511–30.

Brown, S.J. (1997) The life of stress. Doctoral dissertation, Reading University.

Callon, M. (1986) The sociology of an actor-network: the case of the electric vehicle, in M. Callon, J. Law and A. Rip (eds) *Mapping the Dynamics of Science and Technology: Sociology of Science in the Real World*. London: Macmillan.

Chesney, M.A., Eagleston, J.R. and Rosenman, R.H. (1980) The type A structured interview: a behavioural assessment in the rough, *Journal of Behavioural Assessment*, 2: 255–72.

Chinn, C.L. and Jacobs, M.K. (1987) *Theory and Nursing: A Systematic Approach*, 2nd edn. St. Louis, MO: Mosby.

Collins, H.M. (2001) Tacit knowledge, trust, and the Q of sapphire, *Social Studies of Science*, 31(1): 71–85.

Edwards, D. (1995) Sacks and psychology, *Theory and Psychology*, 5: 579–96.

Edwards, D. (1997) *Discourse and Cognition*. Beverly Hills, CA: Sage.

Fodor, J.A. (1981) *Representations: Philosophical Essays on the Foundations of Cognitive Science*. Brighton: Harvester.

Friedman, M. and Rosenman, R. (1959) Association of specific, overt behaviour pattern with blood and cardiovascular findings, *Journal of the American Medical Association*, 169: 1286–96.

Friedman, M. and Rosenman, R.H. (1972) *Type A Behavior and Your Heart*. New York: Knopf.

Friedman, M. and Ulmer, D. (1985) *Treating Type 'A' Behaviour and Your Heart*. London: Guild.

Golub, E. (1987) *Immunology: A Synthesis*. Sunderland, MA: Sinauer Associates.

Haraway, D. (1992) The biopolitics of postmodern bodies: determinations of the self in immune system discourse, in L.S. Kaufman (ed.) *American Feminist Thought: At Century's End*. Oxford: Blackwell.

Hawkes, N. (1995) Lying your way to medicine's glittering prizes, *The Times*, 8 June, p. 1.

Hearn, M.D. (1989) Hostility, coronary heart disease and total mortality: a 33 year follow up study of university students. *Journal of Behavioural Medicine*, 12: 105–21.

Herzlich, C. and Pierret, J. (1987) *Illness and Self in Society*. Baltimore, MD: Johns Hopkins University Press.

Houston, B.K. and Vavak, C.R. (1991) Hostility: development factors, psychosocial correlates and health behaviours, *Health Psychology*, 10: 9–17.

Howells, J.G. (1975) *World History of Psychiatry*. New York: Bruner Mazel.

Hughes, J. and Sharrock, W. (1997) *The Philosophy of Social Research*, 3rd edn. London: Longman.

Inglis, B. (1981) *The Diseases of Civilization*. London: Paladin.

Jaret, P. (1986) Our immune system: the wars within, *National Geographic*, 169: 701–35.

Jones, J. (1995) Watching the researchers, *The Guardian*, 11 June, p. 12.

Jovchelovitch, S. and Gervais, M.C. (1999) Social representations of health and illness: the case of the Chinese community in England, *Journal of Community and Applied Social Psychology*, 9(4): 247–60.

Kannel, W.B. (1976) Some lessons in cardiovascular epidemiology from Framingham, *American Journal of Cardiology*, 37: 269–82.

Karasek, R.A., Russell, R.S. and Theorell, T. (1982) Physiology of stress and regeneration in job related cardiovascular illness, *Journal of Human Stress*, 8: 29–42.

Kitson, A. (1993) *Nursing: Art and Science*. London: Chapman & Hall.

Kott, J. (1985) The infarct, in M. Blonksy (ed.) *On Signs*. Baltimore, MD: Johns Hopkins University Press.

Latour, B. (1983) Give me a laboratory and I will raise the world, in K.D. Knorr-Cetina and M.J. Mulkay (eds) *Science Observed*. Beverly Hills, CA: Sage.

Latour, B. (1987) *Science in Action: How to Follow Scientists and Engineers Through Society*. Cambridge, MA: Harvard University Press.

Latour, B. (1990) Drawing things together, in M. Lynch and S. Woolgar (eds) *Representation in Scientific Practice*. Cambridge, MA: MIT Press.

Law, J. (1992) Notes on the theory of the actor-network: ordering, strategy, and heterogeneity, *Systems Practice*, 5(4): 379–93.

Law, J. and Hassard, J. (1999) *Actor Network Theory and After*. Oxford: Blackwell.

Leddy, S. and Pepper, J.M. (1993) *Conceptual Bases of Professional Nursing*, 3rd edn. Philadelphia, PA: J.B. Lippincott.

Lohff, B. (2001) Self healing forces and concepts of health and disease: a historical discourse, *Theoretical Medicine*, 22: 543–64.

Maddi, S.R. and Kobasa, S.C. (1984) *The Hardy Executive: Health Under Stress*. Homewood, IL: Dow-Jones-Irwin.

Marmot, M.G. and Symon, S.L. (1976) Acculturation and coronary heart disease in Japanese-Americans, *American Journal of Epidemiology*, 104: 225–47.

Maslow, A.R. (1968) *Towards a Psychology of Being*. New York: Van Nostrand Rinehold.

Matthews, K.A., Glass, D.C., Rosenman, R.H. and Bonner, R.W. (1977) Competitive drive, pattern A, and coronary heart disease: a further analysis of some data from the Western Collaborative Group Study, *Journal of Chronic Diseases*, 30: 489–98.

Matzinger, P. (1994) Tolerance, danger and the extended family, *Annual Review of Immunology*, 12: 991–1045.

Matzinger, P. (1998) An innate sense of danger, *Seminars in Immunology*, 10: 399–415.

Miller, J. (1978) *The Body in Question*. London: Jonathan Cape.

Miller, T.Q., Smith, T.W., Turner, C.W., Guijarro, M.L. and Hallet, A.J. (1996) A meta analytic review of research on hostility and physical health, *Psychological Bulletin*, 119(2): 322–48.

Nilsson, L. and Lindberg, J. (1987) *The Body Victorious: The Illustrated Story of Our Immune System and Other Defenses of the Human Body*. New York: Bantem Dell Publishing Group.

Padel, R. (1981) Madness in 5th century BC Athenian tragedy, in P. Heelas and A. Lock (eds) *Indigenous Psychologies: The Anthropology of the Self*. London: Academic Press.

Parker, I., Georgaca, E., Harper, D., McLaughlin, T. and Stowell-Smith, M. (1995) *Deconstructing Psychopathology*. London: Sage.

Partridge, E. (1966) *Origins: A Short Etymological Dictionary of Modern English*. New York: Macmillan.

Pearce, J.M., Manyonda, I.T. and Chamberlain, G.V. (1994) Term delivery after intrauterine relocation of an ectopic pregnancy, *British Journal of Obstetrics and Gynaecology*, 101(8): 716–17.

Pearce, J.M. and Hamid, R.I. (1994) Randomised controlled trial of the use of human chorionic gonadotrophin in recurrent miscarriage associated with polycystic ovaries, *British Journal of Obstetrics and Gynaecology*, 101(8): 685–8.

Peplau, H. (1988) *Interpersonal Relations in Nursing*. London: Macmillan.

Popper, K. (1957) *The Poverty of Historicism*. London: Routledge & Kegan Paul.

Potter, J. (2000) Post cognitive psychology, *Theory and Psychology*, 10(1): 31–8.

Powell, L.H., Friedman, M., Thoresen, C.E., Gill, J.J. and Ulmer, D.K. (1984) Can the Type A behavior pattern be altered after myocardial infarction? A second year report from the Recurrent Coronary Prevention Project, *Psychosomatic Medicine*, 46(4): 293–313.

Ravetz, J.R. (1971) *Scientific Knowledge and its Social Problems*. Oxford: Oxford University Press.

Rogers, C.R. (1961) *On Becoming a Person*. Boston, MA: Houghton Mifflin.

Rosenman, R.H. (1993) Relationships of the Type A behavior pattern with coronary heart disease, in L. Goldberger and S. Breznitz (eds) *Handbook of Stress: Theoretical and Clinical Aspects*, 2nd edn. New York: The Free Press.

Rosenman, R.H., Brand, R.J., Sholtz, R.I. and Friedman, M. (1976) Multivariate prediction of coronary heart disease during 8.5 year follow-up in the Western Collaborative Group Study, *American Journal of Cardiology*, 37: 903–10.

Rosenman, R.H., Swan, G.E. and Carmelli, D. (1988) Definition, assessment, and evolution of the Type A behavior pattern, in B.K. Houston and C.R. Synder (eds) *Type A Behavior Pattern: Research, Theory and Intervention*. New York: Wiley.

Roy, C. and Roberts, S.L. (1981) *Theory Construction in Nursing: An Adaptation Model.* Englewood Cliffs, NJ: Prentice-Hall.

Rozanski, A., Bairey, C.N., Krantz, D.S. *et al.* (1988) Mental stress and the induction of myocardial ischemia in patients with coronary artery disease, *New England Journal of Medicine*, 318: 1005–12.

Selye, H. (1973) The evolution of the stress concept, *American Scientist*, 61: 692–9.

Seyle, H. (1975) Confusion and controversy in the stress field, *Journal of Human Stress*, 1(2): 37–44.

Selye, H. (1976) Forty years of stress research: principal remaining problems and misconceptions, *Canadian Medical Association Journal*, 115: 53–6.

Shipley, J.T. (1965) *Dictionary of Word Origins.* New York: Philosophical Library.

Star, S.L. (1989) Layered space, formal representations and long-distance control: the politics of information, *Fundamenta Scientiae*, 10(2): 125–54.

Syme, S.L. (1984) Sociocultural factors and disease aetiology, in W.D. Gentry (ed.) *Handbook of Behavioural Medicine.* New York: Guilford Press.

Theorell, T., Lind, E. and Floderus, B. (1975) The relationship of disturbing life changes and emotions to the early development of myocardial infarction and other serious illnesses, *International Journal of Epidemiology*, 4: 281–93.

Weidner, G. (1987) The role of type A behaviour and hostility in an elevation of plasma lipids in adult women and men, *Psychosomatic Medicine*, 49: 136–46.

Weidner, G., Friend, R., Ficarroto, T.J. and Mendell, N.R. (1989) Hostility and cardiovascular reactivity to stress in women and men, *Psychosomatic Medicine*, 51: 36–45.

Wilkins, E. (1995) Consultant accused of inventing details of pioneering operation: Malcolm Pearce, *The Times*, 6 June, pp. 1–2.

Williams, M., May, T., Wiggins, R. and Bryman, A. (1996) *Introduction to the Philosophy of Social Research.* London: UCL Press.

Williams, R. (1989) *The Trusting Heart: Great News about Type A.* New York: Random House.

Williams, R. and Williams, V. (1993) *Anger Kills: Seventeen Strategies for Controlling the Hostility that can Harm Your Health.* New York: Times Books.

Williams, R.B., Barefoot, J.C., Haney, T.H. *et al.* (1986) Type A behaviour: angiographically documented coronary atherosclerosis in a sample of 2,289 patients, Paper presented to the *Annual Meeting of the Psychosomatic Society*, Boston, April 1986.

Williams, R.B., Barefoot, J.C., Califf, R. *et al.* (1992) Prognostic importance of social and economic resources among medically treated patients with angiographically documented coronary heart disease, *Journal of the American Medical Association*, 267:520–4.

Wolf, S.G. (1969) Psychosocial forces in myocardial infarction and sudden death, *Circulation*, 39/40 (suppl. 4): 74–83.

4

Concepts and theories II: operationalism and its legacy

> Whatever exists exists in some quantity and can be measured.
>
> (Thorndike 1904)

In this chapter, we consider the seductive but often problematic fusion between positivism and health care, highlight the difficulties of measuring health and disease and examine why researchers and clinicians have wished to measure people's experience of health and illness.

We cover concepts of measurement in the philosophy of science, including the idea of operationalism – the notion that concepts can be defined through the operations used to measure them. Generally, operationalism is associated with the belief that the meaning of scientific terms and concepts is wholly captured by a description of the process that determines their applicability in particular cases. On this view, theoretical entities are merely logical constructs. Such a view can be found in some of the early writings of Charles Peirce (Peirce 1998).

The idea of operationalism first gained strength in the early twentieth century, as scholars of physics struggled with the problems of knowledge that had sprung up in physics as a result of the Einsteinian revolution. The eminent physicist Percy Bridgman, later to receive the Nobel Prize, published *The Logic of Modern Physics* (Bridgman 1927). Here he proposed *operational analysis* to guard against the problems which, it seemed, had led to the end of Newtonian physics so soon after Lord Kelvin had confidently predicted that it would soon explain everything. Bridgman was thus lending his voice to a growing body of thought, which included other eminent scientists, such as Sir Arthur Eddington (1920), who had discussed similar notions. The basic thrust of Bridgman's argument was to eliminate all abstract concepts by defining them in terms of the specific operations by which they are measured. As he said, 'we mean by any concept nothing more than a set of operations; *the concept is synonymous with the corresponding set of operations*' (Bridgman 1927, p. 5; original emphasis). This vision of scientific concept formulation was taken up most enthusiastically not in physics, but in the human disciplines, notably psychology, but traces of it can be found just as easily in nursing and medicine.

Green describes his own experience in psychology but this could just as easily apply to the research methods taught to other trainee health professionals:

It is practically an article of faith among psychologists that in order to conduct empirical research each of the variables under study must first be operationally defined. The story usually goes something like this: You want to study some psychological variable – say anger. You have no way of measuring anger directly so you measure some purported behavioural or physiological symptoms of the variable – say loudness of voice or blood pressure – as an indirect measure of anger. These indirect measures are taken to be the operational definitions of anger. Ideally, one collects several different measures in an attempt to 'triangulate' the psychological variable itself. Those with a particularly behaviourist (or, in this example, Jamesian) bent might assert that anger *just* is those behavioural or physiological expressions.

(Green 1992, p. 291)

Even though psychologists might believe in the state of anger, or occupational therapists might believe that they are enabling clients to live independently and so on, they are befuddled by the difficulty of measuring these things. Thus, they might be likely to fall back on anger questionnaires or activities of daily living inventories.

This state of affairs has existed in psychology for some time and has come to prevail in other health care disciplines as well. This has led some sceptics to be particularly scathing about the possibility of finding out anything meaningful about psycho-social issues by means of this kind of operationalist approach. In the 1940s, Wittgenstein ([1953] 1958) argued that 'in psychology there are experimental methods and *conceptual confusion*' (p. 232). More recently, Jerry Fodor (1968) noted that 'many philosophers secretly harbour the view that there is something deeply (i.e. conceptually) wrong with psychology' (p. vii). This highlights the problem of using operational definitions and operational constructs to examine psychological issues. That is, if we can measure intelligence, say, with a test, does that mean that the test defines intelligence? According to Edward Boring (1923), one of the leading psychologists of the early twentieth century, this was pretty much the case. In the positivistic spirit of early twentieth-century psychology, this was, moreover, seen as a satisfactory state of affairs. Indeed, it was considered to be an improvement on the confusion and disagreement of the introspective and mentalistic psychology that this new scientific spirit was displacing.

Although the debate is brought into particularly sharp focus in the case of psychological issues, it might apply just as well to a great many other issues in health care. How can we examine internal states through the operationalization of their indicators? Constipation, fatigue, the progression of systemic lupus erythematosus ('lupus'), myalgic encephalomyelitis (ME) and many of the other disabling conditions of the twenty-first century involve considerable debate as to what the symptoms are and what the causal mechanisms might be. To what extent can these conditions be defined in terms of their measurable indicators?

These kinds of questions were asked very shortly after the idea of operational definitions was proposed. Although Bridgman's account of operationalism was generally applauded, a number of awkward questions remained. For example, L.J. Russell (1928) argued that if one were to take Bridgman's thesis literally, a variety of ways of measuring something would yield a number of different concepts. For example, argued Russell, instances where different operations give the same result would have no real significance. Measuring length with a ruler and by triangulation would yield different concepts rather than two stabs at the same underlying phenomenon. If operationalism were taken in a strong form, we would have no way of knowing it was the same underlying concept, any more than we could say the same construct was being measured if a thermometer and a ruler both read '37' when applied, respectively, to a person's mouth and chest. If operationalism were taken literally, we still wouldn't know whether the same thing was being measured if a person were to measure length with two different rulers, or two different people were to use the same ruler, and one person was to use the same ruler at different places or even at different times. Similarly, we should not worry if different operations traditionally thought to measure the same concept give utterly different results. The traditional understanding must be at fault. The idea of an underlying property being measured must be an unreliable piece of folklore and should have no place in science.

This tendency of operational analysis to turn each individual act of measurement into a separate concept came to be seen as a major limitation. Operationalism had a serious difficulty in that it went against the deeply ingrained common sense notion that objects have independent properties that people can record, usually with a number of different techniques. One ruler, commonsensically, yields pretty much the same results as another, unless one has a bit missing off the end. Operational analysis, taken literally, repudiates that belief.

Ironically, Bridgman himself, although he originated operationalism, did not appear to take it too seriously. He betrayed an underlying belief in abstract concepts by distinguishing between 'better' and 'worse' operations. Most people (including most scientists and philosophers) would agree that a micrometer yields a more accurate measure of length than a tape measure, even if they cannot explain why. Such a belief has no meaning, however, unless an abstract property of the object we are measuring, beyond its measurement by particular devices, is believed to underlie the various measurements.

In health care, although much research and practice centres on measurement, assessment and quantification, it relies on unobservable intervening variables and, just as important, much more complex morally and emotionally tinged speculative narratives about what these might mean. Blood pressure, for example, is relatively easily – if somewhat unreliably – measured, yet very often it is not merely blood pressure that is at stake when a health care professional straps the cuff onto a client. More often, there are a range of inferences at stake about the state of the person's cardiovascular system, their diet, their likelihood of having a stroke and their chances of perishing from heart disease.

As Green (1992) describes in his history of the concept of operationalism, following Russell's (1928) attack operational analysis underwent many transformations. Bridgman, as we have noted, softened his position about the admissibility of theoretical constructs (Bridgman 1938, 1961; Schlesinger 1967). However, another interesting point concerns the relationship between operationalism and positivism. The logical positivists endorsed many of Bridgman's ideas after Herbert Feigl, of the Vienna Circle, visited Bridgman in 1930. They later rejected Bridgman's analysis, however, as an ultimately unworkable oversimplification of the extremely intricate problem of meaning (Carnap 1936, 1939, [1936–37] 1953, 1956, 1966; Hempel, 1952, [1954] 1961, 1964, 1966). However, oblivious to these disputes, some authors have taken operationalism to be similar to, or even identical with, logical positivism (Pratt 1939; Langfeld 1945).

Despite this conflation between operationalism and positivism that one still occasionally finds in treatises on research methods and the philosophy of science, the schism between the two is worth noting because of what it reveals about the different ideas concerning science. The logical positivists split with Bridgman over two issues. One was the issue of the social or public nature of science. The logical positivists demanded that all scientific data must be available in the public sphere, whereas Bridgman (1940, 1945) argued that science is much more private, depending upon the individual's perceptions of phenomena. Furthermore, positivist thinkers broke with operationalism because of the difficulty in achieving explicit definitions of terms in science. By the mid-1930s, logical positivists were grappling with the difficulties involved in the definitions achieved through the operationalist strategy. First, they reluctantly came to the conclusion that scientific terms cannot be completely defined operationally, especially if there is a potentially infinite number of instances of whatever the term refers to. This concern led Carnap to replace the idea of complete definition with what he called 'partial reduction' of scientific terms (Carnap 1936, cited in Martin 1967) and 'verification' was moderated to the less inclusive notion of 'confirmation' (Carnap [1936–37] 1953). Second, the inherent incompleteness of these definitions, rather than being a drawback, is itself a compelling motive for scientific research. If terms did not have this 'openness of meaning', as Hempel (1952, p. 29) called it, there would be nothing left to discover, since all 'legitimate' scientific terms would merely be defined in terms of existing knowledge.

This emphasis on openness and lack of closure which the positivists asserted was very different from the turn which the philosophy of science was taking in the human science disciplines. As Green (1992) notes, this was a far cry from the positions being taken by leading behaviourists at the time who usually denied the importance, or even existence, of individual experiences. These individual, private experiences were, as we have seen, central to Bridgman's thinking.

Despite the popularity of operationalism in the human sciences – operational definitions are still touted in most research methods books that psychologists or trainee doctors and nurses are likely to see – it is widely regarded by many philosophers as having died out in the 1930s. Through the latter part of the twentieth century it was possible to see philosophers of science expressing views such as the following:

> Operational definition is a myth, a remnant of an obsolete philosophy of science, but a myth that commands the allegiance of most psychologists . . . But removed from its historical context and stripped of its philosophical justification, operationalism became a talisman and 'operational definition' a liturgical phrase. Continued use of the operational liturgy blinds psychologists to the nature of science as a pragmatic struggle of human minds against the facts of experience.
>
> (Leahey 1980, p. 141)

Therefore, in making sense of why operationalism has persisted, we will have to turn to factors beyond the scientist's laboratory or the philosopher's proverbial armchair.

Many writers put this continued popularity of operationalism down to social factors. Rosenwald puts it as follows:

> Social or cultural knowledge . . . which is shared by the members of the society and which guides our interpretation of everyday social experience despite being unsystematic and occasionally vague or self contradictory – such knowledge is not only more voluminous than that which we succeed in establishing scientific-ally, but enjoys *a normative privilege*.
>
> (Rosenwald 1986, p. 319; original emphasis)

The impact of these processes on science is that we press on with the process of operationalization because it is one thing over which the researcher has some mastery:

> because we wish urgently to gain mastery over pressing human perplexity, we are untiring in the pursuit of adequate operationalizations, and because we are rela-tively sophisticated about these perplexities [by virtue of our social knowledge], we tend to reject most of the attempted solutions as inadequate.
>
> (Rosenwald 1986, p. 321)

The message, then, coming strongly from people who have striven to make sense of the process of operationalization is that it persists because of the human processes of sense making and the human desire to establish order amidst complexity. It is ironic, then, that this aspect of scientific enquiry exists by virtue of the very processes it was designed to eliminate from human enquiry.

Perhaps, though, there is an important point to be salvaged from the idea of operationalism. Maybe Bridgman was right in one sense. The development of new measures leads to new ways of defining and constructing notions of the person. Equally, the development of new measures leads to new scientific theories. New measures could be argued to lead to new forms of consciousness. Following Foucault (1972) and Rose (1990), there is something to be said for the argument that new means of examining the human condition lead to new ways of conceiving of persons and perceiving ourselves. In the present day, some critics have alleged that the grow-ing popularity of folk diagnoses, such as shopping addiction, sex addiction and so on, is, arguably, fuelled by drug companies seeking to exploit new market niches for their products.

Despite the past 120 years being a time of great collapse for scientific edifices, and the way that philosophers have been able to thwart scientific attempts to know the world, this ambivalence and debate has existed at the same time as a burgeoning of faith in science itself. In the next section, therefore, we will examine some of the reasons why science has retained its credibility, prestige and intellectual hegemony despite such scepticism.

The very word 'science' has succeeded in retaining its connotations of credibility and truth. Indeed, it originates from the Latin *scientia* – knowledge. While 'science' has a very specific meaning in the current context, the word has been extensively popularized so that it adds prestige, cogency and plausibility to a whole host of assertions. For example, manufacturers, in an attempt to promote their products, lay claim to the fact that they have been scientifically proven or tested. At the time of writing, a quick flick through a leading woman's magazine had seven advertisements for beauty products that made reference to the scientific foundations on which they had been developed and tested, while there is currently a TV advert for a non-dairy spread that is claimed to 'be scientifically proven to lower cholesterol'. By including the magic word 'science', gravitas and weight are added to the claims of advertisers, presumably in the hope that more people will be persuaded to buy the product. But are these assumptions justified? Can we believe the claims of science? Are scientific findings beyond reproach? Science undoubtedly carries with it notions of kudos, prestige and veracity, thus transcending the intuition, irrational superstitions, hunch and time-honoured ritual that determine a lot of human behaviour, and which are not amenable to rigorous, formal investigation.

Perhaps, then, it is unfortunate that a considerable amount of health care provision has for centuries been based on unscientific irrationalities and assumptions. Walshe notes that:

> for far too long the patterns of clinical practice, and the way in which we organise and deliver health care have been too influenced by professional opinion, historical practice and precedent, clinical fashion, and organisational and social culture. As a result, we have often persisted in using health care interventions which are demonstrably ineffective, failed to take up other interventions which are known to be effective, and tolerated huge variations in practice which must mean that some patients receive ineffective care.
>
> (Walshe 1998, p. 270)

Widespread acknowledgement that treatment interventions and clinical decision making were very largely random, unfair and indefensible lay behind the inception of the new evidence-based health care (EBHC) culture, which has been theoretically (if not necessarily practically) accepted as the way forward by the NHS, government policy makers, health care professionals and other international health care systems. The brave new world of evidence-based care was a challenge to the historical precedents and clinician bias that had dominated health care for centuries. The aim of the EBHC agenda was to address the three core problems that Walshe outlined: the overuse of ineffective treatments (e.g. screening for prostate cancer), the underuse of effective treatments (e.g. drug treatment of essential hypertension in elderly patients) and the misuse of treatments for which too little is known about their effectiveness (e.g. selection of hip prostheses in hip replacement surgery) (Institute of Medicine 1999; examples taken from *Effective Health Care Bulletins* issued by the NHS York Centre for Reviews and Dissemination: http://www.york.ac.uk/inst/crd/). The examples provided above simply scratch the surface of the problems that pervaded health care delivery and which had resulted from a failure to use scientific evidence to guide clinical practice.

There are many other instances where the controlling forces of tradition and history have dictated clinical practice and which could be used to buttress the argument for a more scientific approach. Beyond the domain of medicine, the situation is hardly any better. For example, in nursing and midwifery, damage to the perineum was commonly managed by the use of salt water baths. Indeed, an early study by Austin (1988) found that the procedure was used for a range of conditions from incontinence to pressure sores and infected wounds. The same study also revealed that the amount of salt used varied from half a cup to three cups per (variable) quantity of bath water. Yet salt is not an antiseptic and, rather more worryingly, is used in 10 per cent solutions to culture *Staphylococcus aureus*, one of the most common causes of wound infection (Austin 1988). Patients were therefore being treated with a preparation that was more likely to exacerbate their infections rather than cure them.

Clearly, any policy development that aimed to eliminate pointless clinical practices, or even those that were downright dangerous, was to be welcomed. And hence the conception and incubation, though perhaps not yet the entire delivery, of the evidence-based health culture, a culture that was intended to replace unsystematic clinical practices with a more scientifically based approach to health care, a culture where clinical decision making could be founded more securely on rigorously derived evidence, rather than on personal preference and whim. The case for EBHC appears to be unassailable. Moreover, besides addressing the broad problem areas outlined by Walshe above, the new paradigm offered a range of additional advantages, as outlined below (taken from Rogers 2002):

- Improvements in clinical care and health outcomes
  - Efficacy
  - Consistency
- Transparency and accountability in medical decision making
- Accurate mapping of the limits of medical knowledge
- Informing research: targeting future research to areas of uncertainty or knowledge gaps
- Informing clinical practice: using up-to-date research findings
- Informing policy and health service provision: efficient use of resources
- Informing patients: empowering patients to make more informed choices about health care.

The claims for EBHC are so impressive that perhaps we should rest the case at this point. And yet the arguments in its favour are all founded on a set of assumptions about the validity, objectivity and veracity of the evidence and the best method of its collection – the scientific experiment and, more typically, the randomized controlled trial (RCT). It is with a challenge of these assumptions that this chapter will be concerned.

The idea of evidence-based health care was, of course, not new to medicine, since types of experimentation had been going on for centuries. It was, though, more clearly articulated by Archie Cochrane over 30 years ago, who noted to his alarm that many medical practices were at best ineffectual and, at worst, dangerous. He argued for clinical decision making to be based on proper scientific evidence, which he considered could really only be adequately derived from the randomized controlled trial (see next section). Cochrane's early idea was to develop a register of all randomized controlled trials, which would be analysed, systematically reviewed and then used to inform medical practice, although the idea has since been extended to other health professionals. His idea has been the driving force behind the centres for dissemination and systematic reviews, such as the Cochrane Collaboration in Oxford, the NHS Centre for Reviews and Dissemination in York and the Aggressive Research Intelligence Facility (ARIF) in Birmingham. However, implicit in this argument were two essentials: first, a considerable body of soundly conducted research was required, which could be analysed and synthesized; and, second, this then had to be disseminated through the publication process to inform clinical practice. Since it was decreed that the corpus of research had to be scientifically valid at least and a sound randomized controlled trial at best, it was hardly surprising that Cochrane's ideas would generate a tidal wave of published research of this kind. This is clearly reflected in the exponential rise in the number of randomized controlled trials reported in Medline, from 39 in the three year period from 1989 to 1992, to 485 in the single year period of 2000–2001. Furthermore, the higher education sector is responsible for conducting a significant amount of health research; since university funding is partly driven by research output, this has colluded with the EBHC ideology to buttress the near-obsession with scientific research. The result is a plethora of published information that often gathers dust on library shelves, or which rather than resolving confusion about appropriate clinical treatments, can often add to it. Together, then, the EBHC initiative and the revised funding model for higher education have provided the research and publication ingredients necessary to generate the research that could influence and enhance clinical provision. It would be reasonable to suppose, then, that the scene has been more than adequately set for ensuring cutting-edge treatments in all specialties and in all localities – a veritable Utopian health care system.

However, the quality of the information used to guide practice protocols depends very heavily on the research methods used to generate it and the skills of the individuals involved in the process. Cochrane and his successors all subscribed to the notion that it is primarily the scientific method, and in particular the randomized controlled trial, that have the necessary rigour to produce sound results. The randomized controlled trial has, in consequence, become the gold standard of health care research, the yardstick against which all other research and its methodologies are judged (Warlow 2002). Such is the commitment and devotion to the randomized controlled trial, that in true 'emperor's new clothes' fashion, it is now acknowledged as the only truly acceptable way of generating research of sufficient quality to inform clinical practice. But is this perspective a balanced one? Is the randomized controlled trial all it's cracked up to be? The monopoly of the experimental method in general and the randomized controlled trial in particular indicates quite clearly that the prevailing research paradigm is formal scientific, which will inevitably determine the sort of research question that can and will be addressed. Moreover, it generates numerical data, which in an era of almost obsessive target setting and bean counting by successive governments (e.g. Yates 2002), means that the randomized controlled trial is likely to win favour in the seats of power. The prevailing political ideology, then, coupled with the received wisdom about the superiority of randomized controlled trials and the university sector's part-dependence on published research output for its income, have further strengthened the stranglehold of the experimental method. Yet a closer inspection of what this means for health care research may raise questions as to whether it is time for a new paradigm. This chapter, then, aims to review the experimental protocol and to challenge the validity of the knowledge generated by this approach. In this way, it is hoped that the reader will be able to evaluate research conclusions dubbed as 'scientific' within a broader contextual framework. This chapter is not intended to tell the reader what to believe, but rather looks at how apparently rational beliefs emerge and how informed judgements are made. Underpinning these quests is the core question: How reliable and relevant are the evidence and information that are presented to us under the guise of science? The general proposition put forward by this chapter and Chapter 5 is that all research is value-laden, even the allegedly objective experimental method. Through widening experience of the complexity of health care provision, we have come to realize that the search for improved care doesn't begin and end with the randomized controlled trial, but must instead recognize the limitations of this approach and the value of alternatives. We should also point out, too, that the consideration of the experimental method in these two chapters raises questions about the objectivity and reliability of the findings that the method generates within the domain of health care research. However, the same limitations also apply to any subject discipline that uses the experimental method; the problems of the approach are not, therefore, confined to health research.

The randomized controlled trial and experimental design

The randomized controlled trial is a particularly stringent variant of the experimental design, intended to evaluate the effectiveness of intervention procedures and to establish reliable linear cause and effect relationships – for example, whether the administration of corticosteroids (cause) shrinks tumours in cancer patients (effect). The true experiment is designed in a sufficiently stringent way that conclusions about causality can confidently be drawn from the results. The randomized controlled trial, as the grand master of the experimental method, possesses the following characteristics:

- It is controlled, in that participants are randomly allocated to either an active intervention or no treatment (which may be a placebo). The intervention group is called the experimental group and the no-intervention group is called the control group. The application of different treatment/intervention protocols is called manipulating the variables.
- The groups are selected according to pre-specified inclusion and exclusion criteria, and because they are randomly assigned to either the experimental or control condition, the groups are considered to be comparable on all the characteristics that might influence the outcome of the study.

- The randomization process should ensure that all potential participants have an equal chance of taking part in the study and that, once selected, each participant should have an equal chance of being allocated either to the treatment group or the control group. The process has as its driving force the concept that there should be no bias in any of the selection procedures. It is carried out according to certain defined conventions (e.g. Jadad 1998).

- It adopts a double-blind procedure, in that neither the researcher nor the participants know to which group they have been allocated.

- Procedures are standardized, in that every participant is treated the same, with the obvious exception of whether or not they receive the intervention.

- A crossover design may be adopted, whereby participants are reassigned to the other treatment; their responses to each allocated treatment are then compared.

- Participants are analysed within their treatment group, which is called 'intention-to-treat' analysis.

- Data are analysed by comparing treatment with non-treatment outcomes, using effect size (the clinical importance of the findings) as a core element.

Less complex experimental designs do not always use a control group, but may instead compare two or more treatment groups; it may not be double-blind, use a crossover design or an intention to treat analysis. It should use randomly selected participants and identical procedures, but often it doesn't, simply because of the logistical problems and resource implications attaching to these requirements. Because they may be less rigorous than the randomized controlled trial and do not always follow the most stringent conditions demanded by the true scientific method, these approaches are often referred to as 'quasi-experiments'. Despite these variations, the philosophy underpinning all scientific methods is the same.

The principles and philosophy of the scientific method

The conduct of the scientific method conforms to certain principles and yet there is substantial disagreement as to the philosophical ideas that underpin the process. The traditional, conventional view of science demands that (Gross 1992):

1   There must be a defined subject for study.

2   Scientific observations must be explained by constructing an overarching theory; this theory will then generate a range of further hypotheses or predictions, which must be testable through the scientific process (and this is what typically forms the focus of research studies).

3   The scientific process must involve the collection of objective observations and measurements using sound empirical methods.

4   The results from the research studies are used to build general laws or principles about the world.

In other words, the traditional scientific process is inductive, in that it builds on observable facts to produce a broad theory, from the particular to the general. Many examples can be found in the history of medicine which confirm that many discoveries were predicated on an inductive scientific process, whereby specific observations led to theoretical frameworks. For example, Galvani's work, which reported that the legs of dead frogs positioned near a metal fence jerked when the metal wires came into contact with each other, led to the theoretical proposition that muscle movement is a product of electrical impulse. Similarly, Fleming's development of penicillin was based on a series of observations by bacteriologists and microbiologists describing the effect of moulds on bacterial growth. More recently, Harold Ridley's pioneering cataract operations, which have now saved the sight of an estimated 200 million people, had their foundations in observation. The ancient Greeks had simply moved the lens in the affected eye from its position, allowing unfocused light to penetrate the retina; more advanced approaches in the nineteenth century attempted to replace the lens with alternative materials. All were unsuccessful, because they were rejected by the body's immune system. Ridley, though, in his capacity as an ophthalmic surgeon during the Second World War, noticed that shards of Perspex embedded in the eyes of fighter pilots were not rejected and, in conjunction with an optical scientist, developed this material as a substitute lens. The rest, as they say, is history. Examples such as these abound within the literature, all of which demonstrate the process of building upon observations to construct theories. It is, therefore, unsurprising that the inductive approach has its advocates. But it also has its opponents, the most famous of whom was Karl Popper. His objections will be outlined later.

Continuing with the basic principles of the inductive method for the time being, if this is translated into a health care context, a researcher may be concerned with the issue of the barrier function of skin (defined subject for study); the researcher may have worked in a variety of clinical areas, such as care of the elderly, where pressure sores are common; surgical units, where the skin is injured via the surgical procedure; or in neonatal units, where premature babies have sticking tape on immature skins, to hold lines in place. In each situation, the researcher may have noticed that there was a raised incidence of hospital-acquired infection. These observations may give rise to the theory that if the barrier function of skin is compromised as a result of a surgical/treatment procedure, or of excoriation, then the individual will be more prone to certain sorts of infection (theory generation based on observation). This theory will spawn a number of hypotheses, for example, that patients on medical wards will have a lower incidence of hospital-acquired infection than patients on surgical wards, or that premature babies who did not require any adhesive tape to hold lines in place are less likely to develop such infections than those who had adhesive tape. These hypotheses would lead to the design of studies that compared patients on different interventions – patients on medical versus surgical wards or babies with and without adhesive tape. The researcher might then collect comparative data on infection rates in these two studies (objective data collection). If the relative risk is higher when the skin has been damaged in some way, the results will inform future clinical activities that involve some interruption to the skin's barrier function. This classical view of the scientific process will be familiar to most readers, although as Popper has pointed out, there are problems with this inductive approach to scientific discovery.

One of Popper's most critical objections related to the sequence of events in the inductive process – that is, that observation leads to theory (Popper 1968, 1972). He contested instead that all observations of scientific facts and data must be conducted within a framework of knowledge – how else would we make sense of what we see? How would the researcher know whether the skin in the above study is badly excoriated or just slightly so, without some prior knowledge of the subject area? I recall the first time I (CH) visited an intensive care unit and was appalled by what I perceived to be the very sick and frail state of an elderly woman who had just had bowel surgery. I asked the experienced nurse who was showing me round how long the patient was likely to last; my question was met with some surprise. The patient was, in fact, considered to be doing rather well and was scheduled to be moved to a high dependency unit within the next 24 hours. As a psychologist, I had no framework of knowledge or experience that would allow me to make a realistic observation of the patient in front of me. Popper would maintain that observations cannot be properly interpreted in the absence of theory or pre-existing information. Therefore, a critical requirement of the inductive approach to science – the truly objective observation and recording of facts – cannot be met because the researcher has to interpret the data within the context of his or her own experience, values and personal biography. These individual characteristics, together with the existing knowledge base, of necessity impact upon the interpretation of events. [It might be worth noting that the eminent philosopher Schopenhauer ([1851] 1974) believed that women were incapable of objectivity, so presumably they must be ruled out of all scientific research.] Observation (even that conducted by men) cannot therefore ever be unbiased and objective – it has to take place within a framework of prior knowledge. The point about objective evidence or observation, and the near impossibility of its acquisition, is a crucial one in scientific research, because research conclusions are predicated on the assumption that the data underpinning them are unbiased and neutral. This issue will be returned to later.

Popper's contradictory perspective challenges the traditional inductive notion that observation drives the theory, postulating instead that the process is deductive, with the theory driving the observation. Observation, in Popper's view, is used instead to justify a theoretical position and the theoretical position determines what sort of data are collected. Popper's argument has a logical appeal, yet it is easily embarrassed by many medical phenomena, such as the clinical effectiveness of aspirin, which while it has a range of well-established therapeutic benefits (based on observed evidence), had no satisfactory theoretical explanation for its mechanism until John Vane's work in the 1970s. In reality, then, the theory/observation process is interactive to a degree and is essential to progress science – one without the other takes us nowhere. The hiatus between Popper's perspective of the scientific process and the conventional inductive one is clearly demonstrated in Table 4.1.

From Table 4.1 it can be seen that the process followed in the traditional, induct-ive scientific method suggests that data from research are used to build theories, while Popper's deductive version claims that theory defines and dictates the research process. The contentious issue here, then, is one of sequence – which comes first, the data or the theory? Whichever conceptualization of the scientific process is accepted, researcher impartiality remains a stumbling block. The traditional approach relies heavily on the objectivity of the data collection process, while Popper's

Table 4.1 A comparison of the traditional inductive scientific method with Popper's deductive approach

Inductive method	Popper's version
1. Observation and method	1. Problem (usually a challenge of an existing theory or prediction)
2. Inductive generalization	2. Proposed solution or new theory
3. Hypothesis	3. Deduction of testable statements from the new theory (i.e. hypothesis)
4. Attempted verification of hypothesis	4. Tests to refute by methods including observation and experiment
5. Proof or disproof	5. Establishing a preference between competing theories
6. Knowledge	

Source: Gross (1992, p. 25).

conceptualization makes objectivity impossible, because all observation must be interpreted and recorded within a context of prior experience. If Popper's line is accepted (as, indeed, logic would instruct), then the possibility of achieving an impartial database from which to make clinical recommendations is almost non-existent. Since data cannot be collected in a vacuum, the scientific evidence base on which clinical practice must be founded will, by definition, be biased by the personal biographies of the researchers involved in evidence-generation. Whatever else is accepted from Popper's theorizing, the impossibility of value-free data is almost a given. This point of disagreement notwithstanding, both processes seek to use theory in the search for scientific truth. And the better the theory, the better the research.

Characteristics of a good theory

Verification versus falsification

The logical positivists (see Chapter 2) worked on the principle that the observed facts should be used to verify the hypothesis: that was the original starting point for the research. In other words, a prediction was made and the researcher set out to collect data that would verify it; data that would not act as a source of verification were presumably not collected. This means that the focus of the research in the logical positivist view, is a search for confirmation of the researcher's assumptions and predictions, an investigation that will potentially corroborate the original hypothesis. Thus it is conceivable that there is always a degree of selectivity in terms of what research is conducted and which data are collected. If we accept that there is inherent bias in the interpretation of any event (because interpretation is governed by the value system and knowledge of the researcher and the context in which the study is conducted), then it follows that there is considerable potential to report selectively only that information which supports rather than rejects an idea. Numerous examples of selective information processing can be found in everyday life. For example, there is a huge social psychology on how first impressions impact upon on our subsequent opinions of other people. Known as the 'primacy effect', in essence, it would seem that the first information we receive has more impact than subsequent information, simply because once an opinion or judgement has been formed, we selectively look for evidence that supports and confirms this; evidence that contradicts this perspective is given short shrift. An early study by Jones *et al.* (1968) found that observers who were asked to rate the intellectual ability of a student solving some maths problems over-rated the IQ if the student solved the problems at the beginning of the observation period. When the student solved exactly the same number of problems, but at the end of the observation period, ability was underestimated. In other words, the observers made a preliminary judgement of the student's ability and then sought evidence to support that judgement. It is easy to see how the primacy effect could lead to some very distorted conclusions about events and people. The same potential for distortion must exist if the scientific process relies on the verification of hypotheses through the selective collection of confirmatory data.

Popper, unsurprisingly, challenged the validity of this approach, and replaced verification with falsification, on the grounds that it is more conclusive (though more difficult) to falsify a theory than to verify it. A recent quote by a former MP, Joe Ashton, who apparently announced that 'there are no lesbians in Barnsley' (cited by Liddle 2002), illustrates this concept perfectly. This hypothesis would be easy to support or verify by a quick glance at the marriage register in the Town Hall, or at the activities at a local nightclub. However, this ready source of evidence tells us nothing about the existence of any other sexual proclivity or contradictory data, and while it might support Ashton's contention, it is far from conclusive. A single example of lesbian activity would instantly refute the original hypothesis. A more classic and commonly quoted example that 'all swans are white' is similarly easy to verify by focusing on the numerous white swans that are around. This tells us only that there are a lot of white swans, but nothing about the existence of swans of any other colour. Consequently, a search for data that verify either of these propositions may undoubtedly be easier, but could be misleading and certainly inconclusive, whereas the location of a swan of any other colour, or a single lesbian in Barnsley, instantly refutes or falsifies the hypothesis and is therefore self-evidently conclusive. The search for a not-white swan, though, may be a longer-term project, since the evidence is not so easy to find; and until the rogue swan is found, the original hypothesis may hold firm, even though it has not been definitively and conclusively supported. Consequently, knowledge is only provisional and lasts until better evidence comes along.

The research on peptic ulcers is an example of the falsification process (Marshall 2002). Peptic ulcers were widely held to be the product of excess gastric acids. The research undertaken in this area had been concerned with demonstrating such an excess of acids, thereby adding confirmation to the hypothesis. Marshall, though, in the face of enormous opposition, demonstrated instead that peptic ulcers were the product of infection by the *Helicobacter* bacterium, thus instantly and conclusively falsifying the original hypothesis (Marshall 2002). Marshall, like many before him, faced enormous opposition from the medical community, because he challenged their belief system, the theory–knowledge *status quo*. Implicit within this example is the concept that medical knowledge about the gastric acid cause of peptic ulcers was temporary and could only be sustained until better evidence was provided.

Schopenhauer again: 'all truth passes through three stages: first it is ridiculed . . . second it is violently opposed . . . Thirdly, it is accepted as being self-evident'.

How relevant this is to the evolution of medical knowledge, but how worrying. The acceptance and acceptability of evidence that contradicts the current received wisdom and theory may be ignored or criticized to the detriment of the health and safety of the patient. John Snow's revolutionary work in the nineteenth century on the mechanism of cholera transmission challenged medical opinion of the time. Snow's proposition and evidence clearly pointed to a water-borne infection, whereas the existing theorizing favoured a miasmatic mode. It was over 30 years before Snow's work was accepted, with catastrophic results for many inhabitants of sewage-strewn London (Longmate 1966; Eyler 2001). Falsification of knowledge is clearly more uncomfortable than verification and may require of the researcher almost superhuman levels of dogged determination, self-belief and commitment to pursue alternative lines of enquiry.

Published health research similarly often appears wedded to the inductive, logical positivist view, in that reports of findings that are significant and support the hypothesis are more likely to be published. Conversely, the relative number of studies that are published which report negative results that do not support the hypothesis is low (Warlow 2002). This, of course, may reflect what is submitted for publication, in that researchers may believe that only significant results will be considered worthy of dissemination or, alternatively, it may reflect what is selected for publication. Either way, the message is clear – verification of hypotheses, which provides no conclusive evidence, may be the name of the research and dissemination game.

This premise generates its own source of further bias. The fact that the prevailing paradigm in health care research is formal experimental, and derives from the world of science, both reflects and defines the value system in which it is embedded. Because it is seen as superior and of high quality, it is also the case that grants and research sponsorship are more likely to be awarded to research that employs scientific methodologies rather than qualitative approaches. Similarly, research papers are more likely to be published if they report findings from experimental research that abounds with statistical analysis, compared with the softer, qualitative methods (Ingram 1996; Hicks and Hennessy 1997). Implicitly this announces to the research world that the experimental method is king, that it is superior, preferred and more valuable. An inevitable corollary of the domination of the experiment and randomized controlled trial in health care research is a surge in research that employs this paradigm. Since the investigative approach determines what is researched and how, it means that research topics are favoured if they can be studied using these methods, thereby leaving a considerable amount of clinical activity on the sidelines (Ingram 1996). The result of this is that much of the holistic clinical care conducted routinely as part of any therapeutic process will not come under randomized controlled trial scrutiny, simply because it doesn't lend itself to this sort of methodology, although it is fair to say that attempts have been made to force it to fit into this paradigm. There are a number of issues that emerge from this that demonstrate quite clearly that the inevitable selection that takes place of what is researched (and indeed published) must of itself impose bias. Consequently, the findings that are presented to the world, by virtue of their origins, will also be but a limited, unrepresentative and hence biased view of the world of health care research. The appropriateness of the scientific method for health care research will be discussed in the next chapter. These comments notwithstanding, it would appear that the prevailing value system attaching to science and its processes precludes objectivity and impartiality – what we read and what we see is not the whole picture or even an accurate picture.

Such adherence to the conventional scientific paradigm is concerning when the consequences are applied to health care. The selectivity of data that support preconceived ideas will inevitably lead to error and bias and may be one reason for many of the litigations that are lodged for wrong diagnosis of conditions. An example close to home illustrates this perfectly – the presenting symptom of breathlessness in a close relative was initially ascribed to the ageing process and indeed a check of the case notes confirmed that the patient was 85 years old. Thus the general practitioner (GP) hypothesized that the cause of the problem was age and sought confirmation of this hypothesis from the biodata. The verification process provided no information about alternative explanations. When the breathlessness got worse, further advice was sought from another GP. This GP worked on the alternative paradigm of falsification; he provisionally offered three hypotheses to account for the symptoms – that they were caused by heart trouble, lung problems or a blood disorder – and then set out, by a process of elimination of the alternatives, to establish which explanation was correct. The investigations he initiated, in essence, ruled out, or falsified, each hypothesis in turn, finally arriving at the conclusion that a blood disorder was the cause. Through the alternative process of systematic falsification – that is, the generation of diagnostic possibilities and the search for evidence that would refute them – the correct explanation and treatment were conclusively identified. A good theory, then, must be potentially falsifiable and the more it withstands attempts at falsification, the more robust the theory.

Predictive power

A second essential quality of a good theory relates to how well it predicts future events. A theory built upon a small set of data and which only explains that data set is clearly of limited value – the theory should be able to make predictions about what will happen in other similar circumstances. For example, in his early work, Sir Richard Doll theorized that there is a link between smoking and lung cancer; observations of a group of patients confirmed a relationship. Doll's proposition that toxins contained in cigarette smoke caused lung cancer led to the prediction that other smokers would have an enhanced chance of developing the disease. His predictions turned out to be accurate. The ramifications of his work are so huge, well known and all-pervasive that they need no further discussion here. Doll's theory would have been of restricted use had his theory only applied to the relatively small sample of smokers that he originally observed. One useful facet of Doll's work is the degree of predictive value it had, for all smokers as well as for any individual smoker, in other words, the general law that there is a relationship between smoking and lung cancer has probabilistic relevance for every individual smoker, even though it cannot predict precisely whether a given person will get the disease.

This point illustrates an important concept inherent in the experimental work carried out within health care – the distinction between the idiographic and the nomothetic. The former relates to the individual and the latter to the group, which in methodological terms represents the difference between the case study approach on the one hand and the randomized controlled trial and other experimental methods that attempt to find general laws of human response, behaviour, reactions and the like on the other. The case study, by definition, makes the use of conventional inferential statistical analysis irrelevant (see below), telling us instead only about the individual being studied and making no predictions at all about other people. This approach, therefore, does not enable generalizations to be made about anyone else (although it can spawn hypotheses which may be tested using experimental methods). It might be useful for recording the passage of disease of a particular patient suffering from essential hypertension, but can make no statement about other sufferers from the condition. Indeed, it is worth pointing out that the predictive capabilities of the case study may be limited even for a well-studied individual – after all, a problem-free first pregnancy and birth have no real power to prophesy what will happen in subsequent pregnancies. Likewise, early school reports on Einstein, which predicted that he would never amount to much, demonstrate perfectly the limits of the case study even in individual forecasting. The generalizability of the single case approach, then, is zero, which means that it is rarely the method of choice in medical research.

The experimental approach, in contrast, relies heavily on inferential statistics, which allow the assumption that the data which derived from the group being studied would also apply or generalize to other similar groups. If the results can be confirmed through repeated replication, then the germs of a universal law may be evident. The predictive capacity afforded by the experimental method is clearly an essential feature of medical research – a drug or intervention must be comparably effective for the majority of similar patients as for the sample on which the drug was tested, or there would be neither a moral nor logical justification for developing or prescribing it. Treatments that are only effective for random individuals are unreliable, generally useless and potentially dangerous. It should be pointed out though, that even robust universal laws about the efficacy of treatment interventions cannot accurately predict the reaction of any given individual; all they can do is to make general statements about probable effectiveness. Translated into health care terms, a drug may be useful in the treatment of the majority of patients with atrial fibrillation, but it cannot guarantee that it will be successful with a specific sufferer. The frequently quoted statistics on treatment success for various types of cancer may appear convincing and comforting, until someone points out that such figures are meaningless because any given cancer sufferer cannot know whether or not he or she belongs to the 'survival at five years' group.

The more negative and alarming side of this issue relates not to non-effectiveness of a treatment intervention, but to adverse side-effects of an intervention (e.g. Andrews 2001). The current debate on the safety of the MMR vaccine and its relationship to autism provides an example of this. While the vast majority of children suffer no ill-effects from the triple vaccine, there appears to be evidence that for a very small minority, gastric problems, inflammatory bowel disorders and autism may be adverse outcomes (Fombonne and Chakrabarti 2001). The government continues to promote its use, while public pressure groups contest its safety. Even in the face of the overwhelming statistical data, which suggest negative side-effects are a comparative rarity, how could any parent evaluate whether their child would be one of the minority? The data and research still fail to provide a foolproof means of assessing individual risk. Moreover, none of this helps the clinician, who needs to know what to do with any given patient. All the results from a randomized controlled trial or true experiment can do is to provide an 'average' result, in that if a trial demonstrates that a given drug has a positive impact on a medical condition, then the majority of patients with that condition will improve – the old utilitarian principle of the greatest good for the greatest number.

Because of the importance and high stakes placed on the predictive capacity of the experimental method, the relative value placed on the methodologies that generate the universal laws is also very high. The research approaches derived from the natural sciences have the power to reduce (though not eliminate) the uncertainty or random effectiveness of health treatments, to maximize the chances of their effectiveness, to guide the practitioner's clinical decision making, to reduce the use of inappropriate and useless interventions and to optimize the patient's recovery. Small wonder that these methods are so revered by clinicians and policy makers alike. By contrast, the non-experimental, non-statistical qualitative methods, which focus on the uniqueness of the individual and not the sameness of the group, cannot offer the same advantages. Unsurprisingly, then, the qualitative methods do not have the same kudos or the same pulling power in terms of grants and publication opportunities (Ingram 1996; Meerabeau 1997). It is sad, therefore, that it is with these methodologies that nursing has allied itself, while medicine has typically conducted experimental research (e.g. Roe 1994; Bonell 1999). By a simple process of deduction, this means that the associated worth of nursing research is often considered to be lower than that of medical research, a point illustrated by a study conducted by Hicks (1992) and which is discussed in the next chapter. The net result of such value-laden assumptions about the relative quality of the different research paradigms will inevitably mean that the formal scientific methodologies, whether they follow inductive or deductive protocols, will continue to dominate health research, marginalizing both the topics that might be fruitfully researched by alternative methodologies and the health care professionals most likely to research them. The insidious forces that result in research bias through selectivity of the topic, the process, the outcome and who conducts the research, are many, various and powerful. What we see is not necessarily what we get, what there is to get or we want to get.

Economy, fertility and problem solving

There are three other criteria that define a good theory. First, a good theory should be economical in its explanation and should be based on as few unsupported assumptions as possible. This principle is known as Occam's Razor, or the law of parsimony (Thorburn 1918). Based on the writings of the fifteenth-century William of Ockham [sic], the theory simply states that if there are two or more theories that can explain the observed data, then the simplest one should be used, until it is proved wrong. The razor says nothing about the veracity of the theory, but merely tells the researcher which theory to test first, on the grounds that the simpler the theory, the easier it is to falsify. It appears, for instance, to govern the diagnoses provided by many GPs, as exemplified above by the elderly patient with breathlessness – the most economical explanation is adopted for the presenting symptoms. If this diagnosis is incorrect, and the patient returns uncured, then in the absence of any additional information or symptoms, a diagnosis is sought from the next layer of complexity.

A good theory should also generate new hypotheses and research. Despite the appalling tragedy of thalidomide, the theoretical understanding of the drug's action and impact has enabled its (safe) application to a variety of other clinical conditions, including leprosy, AIDS and cancer. It is, though, undoubtedly the case that many treatments work without a prior or even concomitant theoretical understanding of the hows and whys. The example of aspirin given above demonstrates this, as does a new approach for the treatment of Parkinson's – deep brain stimulation – which miraculously seems to stop the uncontrollable tremors, yet no-one really knows how it works. And, finally, a good theory should offer solutions for everyday problems. Epidemiological studies that provided a route for explaining clusters of diseases, such as leukaemia in residents near nuclear power plants and among people who worked with benzene and its derivatives, or the raised incidence of glaucoma among African-Caribbean men, are examples of the explanatory application of a theory.

Scientific research and the philosophies of power

The principle on which the EBHC culture was originally founded had huge merit, in that it sought to overcome the quixotic clinical decision making that often made health care little more than a lottery. However, the narrow focus of what was (and still is) considered to be acceptable evidence and how this might best be obtained, has meant that there has been an over-reliance on the experimental method, largely to the exclusion of other data. Moreover, a further consequence of the domination of the randomized controlled trial has been an emphasis on medical research, because much of it can be reduced to component parts that easily lend themselves to scrutiny by experimentation. Those areas of health care which often form the heart of patient/ professional contact and service delivery, such as nursing and allied health care activities, have been largely excluded simply because the essence of these jobs cannot be similarly distilled to their constituent parts. The therapeutic relationship between patient and carer, based on a mixture of trust, experience and 'tacit knowledge' (Meerabeau 1992), cannot be mechanistically investigated by science or applied through rigid protocols – a point cogently made by Dixon and Sweeney (2000).

It takes no great leap of the imagination, then, to conclude that in research terms, some of the most critical aspects of health care provision have been left out in the cold, because they couldn't be readily moulded to fit the preferred and prevailing research paradigm. Add to this the proposition that the randomized controlled trial may not be the sole answer to the problems that result from capricious and unsystematic care, and a new problem emerges – one of terrier-like adherence to a methodology of limited application and flawed by cumulative bias at each stage of the research process. Such unwavering commitment to and belief in a single solution for a multifactorial problem smacks of over-simplicity and naivety. But more than this it reflects a governing value system that favours science and medicine, and disadvantages allied health care and alternative evidence.

Rogers (2002) cogently supports this position by suggesting that the series of decisions that is made when deciding the focus of a randomized controlled trial, its design, its conduct, the selection of measurements to be collected and their interpretation, all restrict the topic and its value. Similarly, at the next level – that is, that of systematically reviewing the available research on a given area prior to disseminating the findings to clinicians – more decisions are made about which studies to include, which outcomes are relevant, which quality criteria to adopt and how to conduct and interpret the systematic review, all of which add another layer of restrictive decisions. The effect of this decision-funnelling is that a lot of health care practices are left unresearched and unassessed. Therefore, to conduct a rigorous systematic review means that only a limited pool of studies is eligible for review, because only when like with like is being compared can valid conclusions be drawn. Thus the more general or complex the topic, the less amenable it is to systematic review. The inevitable outcome is that a sound systematic review of the sort that Cochrane had envisaged and which is conducted at the major dissemination centres, might generate a valid conclusion about the value of one particular treatment over a placebo, but would have more difficulty arriving at such definitive conclusions if multiple comparisons were being made about the whole range of alternative treatments versus the placebo. The methodologically valid reviews can only focus on small aspects of treatment interventions, making them less valuable in clinical practice, because they only enable patients to make a choice from a very restricted range of options. Moreover, as Rogers (2002) points out, patient perspectives on treatments are rarely a focus of interest of systematic reviews and randomized controlled trials, because the data are considered to be too subjective. Thus the production of evidence for use in informing clinical care is the outcome of value-laden decisions at every level, which limits patient choice and which cannot be considered to be objective in any sense of the word.

In practice, there is further restriction of patient choice and further evidence of value-driven control within the EBHC arena. The application of EBHC via organizations such as the National Institute for Clinical Excellence (NICE), National Service Frameworks (NSF) and Local Protocol Developments, involves the production of a set of clinical guidelines on a particular medical condition, based on research evidence. The selection of the medical condition is made by government agencies, which means, by default, that these agencies also commission the research in this area and the development of the guidelines. Thus EBHC will support government agendas and priorities and will not necessarily reflect areas of concern identified by patients (Rogers 2002). Clinical guidelines also include recommended interventions, which to be manageable must also be simple, and to be evidence-based must have a significant corpus of research underpinning them. Consequently, most of this evidence comes from pharmaceutical research, because it more easily complies with the randomized controlled trial paradigm, yields fairly objective data, can be more rigorously systematically reviewed and typically comes with generous funding. Non-pharmaceutical treatments do not meet these criteria and so are less likely to be presented as viable options in the clinical guidelines. While patients are represented in guideline development groups, the dynamics of such forums make equality of input and discussion difficult (Rogers 2002). Taken together, the whole process from topic selection through to guideline recommendations do little to enhance patient choice and much to ensure Hobson's Choice. A very basic driver of the EBHC culture – that of empowering patients through informed choice – may have succeeded only in doing the reverse.

Health care professionals have been similarly disempowered by the rise of research-based guidelines. While many advocates of the evidence-based health care culture would regard clinical judgement as a euphemism for prejudice, hunch and tradition, many doctors have resisted not only the instruction to base their clinical practice on empirical research evidence, but also taking part in trials. Prescott *et al.* (2002) found that loss of clinical autonomy constituted a significant deterrent to clinician participation in randomized controlled trials. One outcome of clinician opposition can be found in a report by the Kings Fund in 1993 which suggested that only 15–20 per cent of medical interventions had any scientifically demonstrated effectiveness (Kings Fund 1993), while Walshe and Ham (1997) found from a survey of all health authorities and trusts that there was widespread inertia when it came to implementing research-based clinical effectiveness strategies.

One explanation for the research/practice gap may be that research evidence is only deemed to be relevant and acceptable if it reinforces the values and existing ideology of the professional groups involved (Stewart 2001). In other words, not only is the research process influenced by value-laden decisions, but its uptake in practice may consolidate these values in an ever-perpetuating cycle of bias and belief. The assumptions and prejudice that characterized care before the inception of the EBHC culture may have been replaced by another set of assumptions and prejudices that define the concept of evidence and how it is obtained. As Stewart points out:

> Definitions of evidence may be framed or constrained by the culture of the health service. The organisation, in turn, appears to embrace evidence which promotes and maintains its own mores and ideologies, reinforcing the impression that some types of knowledge are more legitimate than others ... Until and unless the influence of the cultural beliefs is acknowledged, evidence-based practice may simply be used as a means of legitimising and reinforcing current ideologies of authoritative knowledge
>
> (Stewart 2001, p. 287)

The resistance of many health care professionals, then, to alter their practice in accordance with available evidence may relate to the fact that many scientifically supported interventions may not resonate with the dominant cultural ideology in a given profession or specialty and in this way adds another layer of bias in the EBHC system. The contention that research is value-laden grows in strength.

That the evidence-based health care culture was originally supported in part by a government-driven need to increase individual professional accountability is widely accepted (Rogers 2002). It is almost certainly not a coincidence that its inception occurred at a time when the then Prime Minister, Margaret Thatcher, was deter- mined to free the NHS of its medical stranglehold, while simultaneously harnessing the powers of the professions. By taking away health professionals' authority to make independent clinical judgements and replacing this instead with research-based protocols, professional autonomy was effectively undermined, while accountability was at the same time increased. A sub-text of these policies may have been an imperative to reduce litigation claims – if best-evidence protocols were followed during a care episode, this would presumably reduce the number of successful claims against the NHS. Heightened professional accountability was further encouraged by the introduction of various charters that spelled out the rights of several consumer groups, including patients. In a marketplace ideology whereby the government attempted to deliver public services as though they were a private supermarket – witness the purchaser/provider divide following the Griffiths Report (DHSS 1983) – the notion of consumer rights and redress gathered momentum. The result was not a reduction in litigation, but a rise. Claims settled in the year 2000–2001 represented a seven-fold increase over the three years up until 2000 (National Audit Office 2001), with claims against GPs rising from 38 in 1989 to 500 in 1998. The size of settlements also increased, with the highest settlement in 1989 being £777,000, but that in 1999 being £3.9 million. The evidence-based health care culture curbed the freedom of health care professionals, and replaced it instead with rule-governed research-based protocols, which, although providing patients with the most up-to-date care, also removed the goodwill between the patient and doctor. It offered benchmarks and definable criteria against which performance could be assessed. Thus while evidence-based health care should have offered some theoretical protection from litigation because it gave health professionals an official guiding hand in clinical decision making, instead it may have compromised the therapeutic relationship and given patients some direct, hardline evidence that could be used in the rising compensation culture. The prevailing ideology in the current health service is often not so much one of research, but one of fear, a fear that prompts the collection of numbers and statistics to demonstrate improvements in care outcomes and delivery, and which provides the government and viewing public with hard, objective, numerical evidence that should have offset further claims of incompetence, negligence and inappropriate practice, yet may, conversely, have fuelled litigious action. While it was widely accepted that clinical care should be removed from the realms of whim and chance, it is also conceivable that the (less quantifiable) trust and faith in the authority of the doctor may have been the price paid, simply because individualized care was replaced with rule-governed mechanistic decision making. This inherent and essential aspect of clinical care may have been eroded and with it the belief in the value of the treatment and the psychological investment in getting better. Perhaps randomized controlled trials are a challenge to the grand narrative of medicine.

Other forms of distortion, though not necessarily intentional distortion, are also possible in scientific research. Where the research is being sponsored by a commercial company or even a government agency, results that run counter to requirements or profit margins may be suppressed. While it is now widely acknowledged that poverty and ill health go hand in hand, when Sir Douglas Black first reported the connection in 1980, the Conservative government rejected his findings. Black's 37 recommendations included rises in benefits, a campaign against child poverty, free school meals and phasing out the tobacco industry, all of which would have cost the exchequer billions of pounds and, furthermore, flew in the face of conservative ideology.

Consequently, his report was never formally published, with only 260 copies being made available, and those on August Bank Holiday weekend (*Health Service Journal* 2002).

The thalidomide scandal of the 1960s is another example of top-down suppression of economically and politically sensitive data. Despite a growing body of worldwide evidence that thalidomide caused birth defects in animals, and that it was teratogenic in humans because of its highly toxic effects on the nervous system, the manufacturers, Chemie Grunenthal, and its licensees suppressed the findings for years (Sjostrom and Nilsson 1972). Numerous other examples exist within the literature and news – for instance, in 1998, Dr Arpad Pusztai completed a £1.6 million research project on the effects of genetically modified foods on rats, and concluded that on a short-term diet of genetically modified potatoes, some critical organs shrank or did not develop properly. In addition, he reported that the rats' immune systems were compromised (Ewan and Pusztai 1999). The results were clearly neither economically nor politically acceptable and he was summarily sacked and professionally discredited. In the process, Pusztai was publicly humiliated by his employers who claimed he had misinterpreted his results. Prime Minister Tony Blair and Cabinet Office Minister Jack Cunningham both rejected his conclusions and the *Lancet* was heavily criticized by one of the leading governmental sponsors of research, the Biotechnology and Biological Sciences Research Council, for their irresponsibility in publishing Pusztai's findings. Subsequently, Pusztai was exonerated by an independent, multidisciplinary international team of experts, who re-examined the data and found the results and conclusions to be valid. It may be coincidental, but the research was sponsored by the Scottish Office: Agriculture, Environment and Fisheries Department (http://news.bbc.co.uk/1/hi/sci/tech/278354.stm).

Despite the notorious frauds of the Piltdown Man and the elaborate botanical hoax committed by Professor John Heslop Harrison (Sabbagh 2000), cases of deliberate fabrication are still rare (as far as we know). But the enormous international and national prestige that accrues from conducting high-quality research means that the possibility of intentional distortion must remain. Certainly, the recent expose of Jan Hendrik Schon's falsification of his data not only brings the academic community into disrepute, but also demonstrates clearly that the kudos attaching to scientific findings, and the pressure to achieve these, may be sufficient incentive to some scientists to fabricate potentially publishable and commercially valuable findings (http://www.cbsnews.com/stories/2002/09/26/tech/main523335.shtml). Perhaps more fundamentally, it also challenges the objectivity and integrity implicit within the scientific process. Hendrik, a physicist who had been tipped to win the next Nobel Prize, worked on microscopic nanocomputers the size of a molecule and his 'findings', had they been true, would have heralded the end of further miniaturization of computers because of the limits of matter itself. The implications of his research were far-reaching and would have had an important application to medicine, in that these microscopic computers could have been embedded in a patient's body to control and monitor the release of drugs. However, despite having published extensively in two of the most scientifically renowned journals (*Nature* and *Science*), it was found that identical data and charts were reproduced in several articles, even though the experiments were different in each case. Moreover, other scientists failed to replicate his findings. Sufficient suspicion was aroused to have Schon's work investigated by an independent review committee, which found that he either made up or altered data at least 16 times between 1998 and 2001. It is likely that the shock waves will continue to impact upon the academic community for some time, not least because of the credibility that was afforded Schon's work by its publication in such prestigious peer-reviewed journals – normally assumed to be some sort of safeguard against error. This point will be taken up later.

Indeed, the impact of the socio-political climate and the desire for personal kudos was implicated in one of the biggest frauds in research history – that committed by the eminent psychologist, Sir Cyril Burt. This was indeed a triumph of self-aggrandisement over truth, but had far-reaching effects on the social and educational structure of the UK, especially through the introduction of the 11+ examination, which was one of the longer-term outcomes of Burt's work. Burt was concerned with demonstrating the extent to which intelligence is either inherited or created by environmental circumstances – the old nature/nurture controversy that continues to be the focus of heated debate (e.g. Steve Pinker *versus* Oliver James 2002). To this end, Burt devised an elegantly simple study, which involved assessing the IQs of identical twins who had been reared apart from each other and away from the family home, a fairly unusual and numerically limited subject sample. He reasoned that any degree of similarity in IQ scores between the twins would be attributable entirely to genetics (or nature) because, as they had been reared apart in different homes, the only thing the twins would have in common would be their genetic inheritance. Any dissimilarity in IQ scores would, therefore, be attributable to environmental factors (or nurture). The study was an important one in its time, because it would inform educational policy and provision, in that if IQ was mainly genetically determined, then very little could be done to alter performance. In this case, remedial provision would be largely pointless and there would be a strong case for providing education appropriate to the inherent ability of the child (an argument that supported the thinking on selective education at the age of 11). If, on the other hand, IQ was determined by environmental factors, then additional educational input was likely to be effective and essential (if expensive). The issue was both educational and political. Burt found that in 53 sets of twins reared apart in this way, there was around 0.77 similarity in IQ scores between the twins and concluded that it was, for the most part, genetically determined. However, shortly after Burt's death, Kamin (1974) reported a number of flaws in Burt's research and queried the veracity of his data. Further investigative journalism by a *Sunday Times* correspondent (Gillie 1976) ultimately found that Burt had not only falsified the data (unsurprising given the rarity value of the sample), but also the research assistants that had apparently worked with him. While such an example of deception is relatively rare, it does illustrate the point that what appears to be objective scientific evidence may be quite corrupted, in this case by a wider political agenda.

Nor is such fraud unknown to the medical profession. Audits in the USA have suggested that an estimated 5 per cent of published medical research includes falsified data and that dozens of doctors have been struck off for such deceptions (Ayres 2002). Coulter (1991) focused on randomized controlled trials conducted between

1977 and 1978 and found serious methodological deficiencies in 11 per cent of them, the four most frequent being:

- deliberate falsification and misrepresentation of results for personal and academic promotion;
- deliberate deceit for economic gain;
- inadequate application of a good randomized controlled trial protocol;
- unintentional errors resulting from incompetence and lack of experience.

In an era when the economic gains from publishing high-quality research are enormous, it is hardly surprising that such problems occur.

Coulter's work identified the individual and academic benefits that could be achieved from published research. This gain may also apply at the level of the institution, through the four-yearly system of evaluating the research output of British universities (where a significant proportion of health research is conducted, either solely or in conjunction with other organizations). The Research Assessment Exercise is used as a basis for measuring the quality of university research activity and thence for allocating government research funds. The higher the unit of assessment's rating, the more money is allocated, with units scoring low marks receiving nothing. Once a researcher or an organization attains five-star status, further research opportunities and funding almost inevitably follow. Since there is an established correlation between the rating given to an organization and the relationship of the panel members to it (www.medicine.man.ac.uk/epidem/biostats/raepanel.rtf), it becomes painfully obvious that high marks in the Research Assessment Exercise may not exclusively reflect high-quality research activity, but a form of academic patronage. It also becomes hard to see quite how any low-ranked unit might actually move into the funded research arena, which inevitably means that research funds may not be awarded on any meritocratic basis, but rather on hype, halos and reputation. In short, research is not necessarily being carried out by the best researchers.

Likewise, the case of Jan Hendrik Schon, outlined above, adds support to the contention that the halo effect operates in research. Schon had nine publications in the prestigious journals *Nature* and *Science*, both of which use rigorous peer review to ensure the high quality of any research published in these journals. Clearly, the quality control mechanism failed in Schon's case, and it may have failed because the reviewers were influenced by the fact that Schon was employed at the renowned Bell Laboratories. Karl Ziemelis, the physical science editor of *Nature*, believed that Schon's results might have been treated with more scepticism had he come from a more obscure organization. He is quoted as saying that 'There may be a higher degree of trust with known quantities than with unknown ones' (quoted in Ayres 2002). Similarly, Donald Kennedy, editor-in-chief of *Science*, said in the same paper, that 'I think there is no question that distinguished institutions and famous authors carry a little prestige and an advantage'. In other words, the identity of the researcher and institution, rather than the quality of the study, may enhance the chances of getting research findings into the public domain and hence ultimately into clinical protocols. While many journals operate the expedient of blind reviewing, from personal experience it is relatively easy to identify the authors from the myriad clues that pepper the article.

This point was reported some years ago by Peters and Ceci (1982). In an elegant and somewhat risky study, these researchers selected 20 articles published in top-ranking psychology journals. The authors of all the research papers were well known in their field and the institutions from which they came were all top of the league. For each article, Peters and Ceci replaced both the author's name and affiliation with an alias; they then re-submitted the articles to the journals in which they had been published within the previous 12 months. All but two of the journals rejected the articles and none recognized that the article had not only been submitted before, but that it had also been published. Peters and Ceci concluded that the influence of name and place precluded the possibility of a totally impartial reviewing and publishing process. The authors also nearly lost their jobs and were virtually excommunicated from their academic disciplines.

External sponsorship of research has contributed a further huge source of potential bias. Academic freedom used to mean that research findings could be published without fear of reprisal, job loss or other adverse consequence. Researchers were answerable to no-one in their pursuit of truth. But that was in the days when the freedom to conduct research was an expected part of the job and when external sponsorship for research was almost unheard of, and would anyway have been seen to compromise the freedom of the academic. The situation has shifted so dramatically now that it is incumbent upon academics to find external monies for their research activities, usually through competition, from government departments and commercial organizations. Such funding carries with it great prestige – higher Research Assessment Exercise ratings for the university, with consequent enhanced government funding, personal promotion and power, and national and international research esteem. The stakes, then, are high.

The logic behind the pressure to obtain external funding stems in part from the growth of the marketplace approach to public services, which had its genesis in the 1980s, and which was intended to provide better value for fiscal budgets. It was also a way of subsidizing a core activity of higher education without having to fork out more from the public purse. But the outcome has been another raiment from the emperor's outfit of new clothes. Spurgeon and Hicks (2003) in a ball-park cost analysis of the tendering process, suggested that the development and submission of a bid for a grant would, in real terms, cost an additional £10,000 to £20,000 per institution, per bid – a cost rarely built into the accounts. Given that several organizations are likely to tender for sponsorship, this additional cost can be multiplied several times. For example, in response to a call for bids for £4 million of NHS Research and Development money, 407 initial proposals were received for the first stage of a three-stage submission process. From the above figures alone, this first stage would incur overall additional costs to the interested institutions of between £814,000 and £1,628,000 or 20.4–40.7 per cent of the total amount to be distributed. If to this is added the costs to the sponsor of advertising, selecting and monitoring the successful projects, Spurgeon and Hicks suggest that to allocate a small budget of £50,000 for a two-year project would cost an additional £100,000 to £200,000 – that is, between twice and four times the award. From these figures, it can be seen that the financial investment in research is extremely high to all parties and, where investment is high, so are the stakes. It would be unlikely that even the most committed entrepreneur would agree that external sponsorship either represents value for money or promotes the same degree of impartiality that the previous system afforded. In other words, the potential for corruption may have risen in direct relation to the amount of research that is outside-funded.

Indeed, evidence from both sides of the Atlantic suggest that the influence imposed by external sponsors, especially by the large pharmaceutical companies, generates huge potential for fraud. Morin *et al.* (2002) noted that in the USA, pharmaceutical companies will need to generate more than US$25 billion in increased sales if they are to maintain current profit levels, which in effect means the launching of between 24 and 34 new drugs per year. It would not be unreasonable to suppose that the pressure to generate acceptable results from pharmacology trials would increase in proportion to the pressure to produce new drugs – a sure-fire breeding ground for sins of omission and commission in the research process (Morin *et al.* 2002). In addition, the payment of patients and doctors to participate in trials has also been a cause for concern. Morin *et al.* (2002) note that many companies allow for between US$2000 and US$5000 per recruit for drug trials, while Foy *et al.* (1998) also found that, in the UK, pharmaceutical companies offered GPs substantial sums of money for each patient recruited. Non-monetary incentives are also frequently used. The sample representativeness demanded by the defining criteria of the randomized controlled trial is unlikely to be achieved under such circumstances. When resources are short and public sector pay is relatively low, the likelihood of impartial, objective research activity would appear to be receding all the time. The economic pressure existing within this sector, coupled with the kudos attached to successful drug development, may lay the foundations of impropriety.

Of course, allied to this is the control that the external sponsors impose upon publication of results. Government agencies, such as the Department of Health, often demand that recipients of their grants sign the Official Secrets Act, effectively precluding the publication of results that conflict with the current political agenda. Many examples of top-down publishing restrictions litter the annals of research history, but the case of Dr Arpad Pusztai outlined earlier demonstrates the pressures and implicit threats that may be imposed on the publication of research findings. More direct control may also be imposed by drug companies. Publishing favourable results about a drug will expand its usage and also is likely to influence formal approval decisions by the Food and Drug Administration, whereas unfavourable results may end the development of a drug or at least limit its use (Morin *et al.* 2002). Consequently, sponsors may seek to prevent or delay the dissemination of unfavourable results. This widespread control over the publication process may have negative consequences, both in the short and long term, for human subjects and for the integrity of the research and the researchers (Office of the Inspector General 2000).

A rather depressing possibility emerges from all this: the personnel and organizations involved in any stage of the research process add further potential for partiality. Cumulatively, this may add up to a considerable deviation from a pure scientific truth.

While safeguards could theoretically be put in place to reduce some of the biasing influences, the fact remains – research cannot ever be value-free. Whatever sense is made of a set of research findings must be mediated by the knowledge that these do not represent immutable truths.

Conclusion

The scientific method is the prevailing research paradigm in health care. The objectivity, generalizability and incontrovertible integrity that were assumed to be its core qualities meant that the evidence generated by rigorous randomized controlled trials was considered to be the 'gold standard', the way forward in improving health provision. The clear preference for experimentation, though, has led to an over-focus on medical activities, especially those that can be reduced to component parts small enough and controllable enough to be amenable to investigation via a randomized controlled trial. While these studies may have provided an invaluable source of evidence, especially in the area of pharmaceutical research, they have simultaneously ensured that much of the core business of health care – that of the patient–carer interface – has been eliminated from scientific study, simply because it cannot be controlled and managed according of the principles of sound scientific conduct. Moreover, the pressures that macro- and micro-level socio-political contexts bring to bear upon research, its sponsorship, publication and uptake, have together conspired to ensure that only that research which conforms to and reinforces the dominant ideology is conducted and adopted. In other words, there is a significant selection bias in experimental research – exactly the sort of selection bias that the randomized controlled trial was designed to overcome. Add to this the fact that the objective observation and recording of data that is the cornerstone on which scientific research is founded is virtually impossible to achieve, due to the bias of the personal biographies of the researchers. This means that the value of the experiment may be more limited than was previously thought. The point here is not to condemn the randomized controlled trial as unworthy, or to promote the superiority of other methods; instead, the aim has been to illustrate how a single method cannot be accepted as the sole route to establishing facts in a highly complex area, where the outcomes must of necessity be multifactorially determined. The chapter has also tried to bring a degree of questioning acceptance and scepticism to an area where scientific facts and figures have traditionally held a position of supremacy and indomitability. It should be acknowledged, though, that while this chapter has outlined and challenged some of the major principles that are central to the scientific method and to its claims of objectivity, the case for the prosecution has rested heavily on evidence (deliberately) derived from a range of sources. This evidence may have been susceptible to the same value-driven distortions. What claims can ever be made, then, about scientific truth?

References

Andrews, N.J. (2001) Statistical assessment of the association between vaccination and rare adverse events post-licensure, *Vaccine*, 20 (suppl. 1): S49–S53.
Austin, L. (1988) The salt water bath myth, *Nursing Times*, 84: 79–83.

Ayres, C. (2002) World's tiniest computer vanishes without trace, *The Times*, 28 September.

Bonell, C. (1999) Evidence-based nursing: a stereotyped view of quantitative and experimental research could work against professional autonomy and authority, *Journal of Advanced Nursing*, 30(1): 18–23.

Boring, E.G. (1923) Intelligence as the tests test it, *New Republic*, 35: 35–7.

Bridgman, P.W. (1927) *The Logic of Modern Physics*. New York: Macmillan.

Bridgman, P.W. (1938) Operational analysis, *Philosophy of Science*, 5: 114–31.

Bridgman, P.W. (1940) Science: public or private, *Philosophy of Science*, 7: 36–48.

Bridgman, P.W. (1945) Some general principles of operational analysis, *Psychological Review*, 52: 246–9.

Bridgman, P.W. (1961) The present state of operationalism, in P. Frank (ed.) *The Validation of Scientific Theories*. New York: Collier.

Carnap, R. (1936) *Über die Einheitssprache der Wissenschaft [The Unity Language of Science]*. Actes du Congrès International de Philosophie scientifique, Fasc. II, Paris.

Carnap. R. (1939) *Foundations of Logic and Mathematics*. Chicago, IL: University of Chicago Press.

Carnap. R. ([1936–37] 1953) Testability and meaning, in H. Feigl (ed.) *Readings in the Philosophy of Science*. New York: Appleton-Century-Crofts.

Carnap, R. (1956) The methodological character of theoretical concepts, in H. Feigl and M. Scriven (eds) *Minnesota Studies in the Philosophy of Science*, Vol. 1. Minneapolis, MN: University of Minnesota Press.

Carnap, R. (1966) *An Introduction to the Philosophy of Science*. New York: Basic Books.

Coulter, H.L. (1991) *The Controlled Clinical Trial: An Analysis*. Washington, DC: Centre for Empirical Medicine.

Department of Health and Social Security (1983) *NHS Management Inquiry: The Griffiths Report*. London: DHSS.

Dixon, M. and Sweeney, K. (2000) *The Human Effect in Medicine: Theory, Research and Practice*. Abingdon, Oxon: Radcliffe Medical Press.

Eddington, A. (1920) *Space, Time and Gravitation*. Cambridge: Cambridge University Press.

Ewan, S.W. and Pusztai, A. (1999) Effects of diet containing genetically modified potatoes expressing *Galanthus nivalis* lectin on rat small intestine, *Lancet*, 354 (9187): 1353–4.

Eyler, J.M. (2001) The changing assessments of John Snow's and William Farr's cholera studies, *Soz.-Praventivmed*, 46: 225–32.

Fodor, J.A. (1968) *Psychological Explanation: An Introduction to the Philosophy of Psychology*. New York: Random House.

Fombonne, E. and Chakrabarti, S. (2001) No evidence for a new variant of measles-mumps-rubella-induced autism. *Paediatrics*, 108(4): E58.

Foucault, M. (1972) *The Archaeology of Knowledge*. Harmondsworth: Penguin.

Foy, R., Parry, J. and McAvoy, B. (1998) Clinical trials in primary care, *British Medical Journal*, 317: 1168.

Gillie, O. (1976) Crucial data was faked by eminent psychologist, *London Sunday Times*, 24 October.

Green, C.D. (1992) Of immortal mythological beasts: operationism in psychology, *Theory and Psychology*, 2: 291–320.

Gross, R.D. (1992) *Psychology: The Science of Mind and Behaviour*, 2nd edn. London: Hodder & Stoughton.

Health Service Journal (2002) Obituary: Professor Sir Douglas Black, *Health Service Journal*, 112(5823), 19 September, p. 5.

Hempel, C.G. (1952) *Fundamentals of Concept Formation in Empirical Science*. Chicago, IL: University of Chicago Press.

Hempel, C.G. ([1954] 1961) A logical appraisal of operationism, in P. Frank (ed.) *The Validation of Scientific Theories*. New York: Collier.

Hempel, C.G. (1964) Aspects of scientific explanation, in *Aspects of Scientific Explanation and Other Essays in the Philosophy of Science*. New York: Free Press.

Hempel, C.G. (1966) *Philosophy of Natural Science*. Englewood Cliffs, NJ: Prentice-Hall.

Hicks, C. (1992) Of sex and status: a study of the effects of gender and occupation on nurses' evaluations of nursing research, *Journal of Advanced Nursing*, 17: 1343–9.

Hicks, C. and Hennessy, D. (1997) Mixed messages in nursing research: their contribution to the persisting hiatus between evidence and practice, *Journal of Advanced Nursing*, 25: 595–601.

Ingram, N. (1996) The research basis of health care decision making, *Journal of Advanced Nursing*, 23: 692–6.

Institute of Medicine (1999) *To Err is Human: Building a Safer Health System*. Washington, DC: National Academy Press.

Jadad, A.R. (1998) *Randomised Controlled Trials: A User's Guide*. London: BMJ Books.

James, O. (2002) *They F*** You Up*. London: Bloomsbury.

Jones, E.E., Rock, L., Shaver, K.G., Goethals, G.R. and Ward, L.M. (1968) Pattern of perform-ance and ability attribution: an unexpected primacy effect, *Journal of Personality and Social Psychology*, 9: 317–40.

Kamin, L.J. (1974) *The Science and Politics of IQ*. Potomac, MD: Lawrence Erlbaum Associates.

King's Fund (1993) *Annual Report: Strengthening the Knowledge Base of Clinical Practice*. London: King Edward's Hospital Fund.

Langfeld, H.S. (1945) Introduction to symposium on operationism, *Psychological Review*, 52: 241–8.

Leahey, T.H. (1980) The myth of operationism, *Journal of Mind and Behaviour*, 1: 127–43.

Liddle, R. (2002) And no lesbians in Barnsley, *The Guardian*, 21 August.

Longmate, N. (1966) Victory in sight, in *King Cholera: The Biography of a Disease*. London: Hamish Hamilton.

Marshall, B. (ed.) (2002) *Helicobacter Pioneers*. Oxford: Blackwell Scientific.

Martin, N.M. (1967) Rudolf Carnap, in P. Edwards (ed.) *The Encyclopedia of Philosophy*, Vol. 2. New York: Macmillan/Free Press.

Meerabeau, L. (1992) Tacit nursing knowledge: an untapped resource or a methodological headache?, *Journal of Advanced Nursing*, 17: 108–12.

Meerabeau, L. (1997) Why are our grant applications continually rejected?, *Nurse Researcher*, 5(1): 5–13.

Morin, K., Rakatansky, H., Riddock, F. *et al.* (2002) Managing conflicts of interest in the conduct of clinical trials. *Journal of the American Medical Association*, 287(1): 78–84.

National Audit Office (2001) *Handling Clinical Negligence Claims in England*, HC 403. London: NAO.

Office of the Inspector General, Department of Health and Human Services (2000). *Recruiting Human Subjects: Pressures in Industry-sponsored Clinical Research*. Washington, DC: Office of the Inspector General, Department of Health and Human Services.

Peirce, C.S. (1998) *The Essential Writings* (edited by C. Edward, E.C. Moore and R. Robin). New York: Prometheus Books.

Peters, D. and Ceci, S. (1982) Peer review practices of psychological journals – the fate of accepted, published articles submitted again, *Behavioural and Brain Sciences*, 5(2): 187–95.

Pinker, S. (2002) *The Blank Slate: Denying Human Nature in Modern Life*. Harmondsworth: Penguin.

Popper, K. (1968) *Conjecture and Refutations: The Growth of Scientific Knowledge*. New York: Harper & Row.

Popper, K. (1972) *The Logic of Scientific Discovery*. London: Hutchinson.

Pratt, C.C. (1939) *The Logic of Modern Psychology*. New York: Macmillan.

Prescott, R.J., Counsell, C.E., Gillespie, W.J. *et al.* (2002) Improving the quality, number and progress of randomised controlled trials, in L. Duley and B. Farrell (eds) *Clinical Trials*. London: BMJ Books.

Roe, B. (1994) Is there a place for the experiment in nursing research?, *Nurse Researcher*, 1(4): 4–12.

Rogers, W.A. (2002) Evidence-based medicine in practice: limiting or facilitating patient choice?, *Health Expectations*, 5: 95–103.

Rose, N. (1990) *Governing the Soul: The Shaping of the Private Self*. London: Free Association Books.

Rosenwald, G.C. (1986) Why operationism won't go away: extra-scientific incentives of social-psychological research, *Philosophy of the Social Sciences*, 16: 303–30.

Russell, L.J. (1928) Review of the logic of modern physics, *Mind*, 42: 355–61.

Sabbagh, K. (2000) *A Rum Affair: A True Story of Botanical Fraud*. Gordonsville, VA: Farrar, Strauss & Giroux.

Schlesinger, G. (1967) Operationalism, in *The Encyclopaedia of Philosophy*, Vol. 5. New York: Macmillan/Free Press.

Schopenhauer, A. ([1851] 1974) *Parerga and Paralipomena: Short Philosophical Essays* (translated by E.F.J. Payne). Oxford: Clarendon Press.

Sjostrom, H. and Nilsson, R. (1972) *Thalidomide and the Power of the Drug Companies*. Harmondsworth: Penguin.

Spurgeon, P. and Hicks, C. (2003) The tendering process: flaws and all, *Health Services Management Research*, 16(3): 188–93.

Stewart, M. (2001) Whose evidence counts? An exploration of health professionals' perceptions of evidence-based practice, focusing on the maternity services, *Midwifery*, 17: 279–88.

Thorburn, W.M. (1918) The myth of Occam's razor, *Mind*, 27: 345–53.

Thorndike, E.L. (1904) *An Introduction to the Theory of Mental and Social Measurements*. New York: Teacher's College Press.

Walshe, K. (1998) Evidence-based practice: a new era in health care?, in P. Spurgeon (ed.) *The New Face of the NHS*. London: Royal Society of Medicine Press.

Walshe, K. and Ham, C. (1997) *Acting on the Evidence: Progress in the NHS*. Birmingham: University of Birmingham Services Management Service, The NHS Confederation.

Warlow, C. (2002) Comparing like with like and the development of randomisation – goodbye anecdotes, in L. Duley and B. Farrell (eds) *Clinical Trials*. London: BMJ Books.

Wittgenstein, L. ([1953] 1958) *Philosophical Investigations*, Oxford: Blackwell.

Yates, J. (2002) Mixed message, *Health Service Journal*, 112(5823), 19 September, p. 21.

5

The philosophy of experimentation

Why think when you can experiment.

(Bernard 1885)

In this chapter, we will introduce the philosophical rationale behind experimental design, induction and inference to enable the reader to gain a critical appreciation of the explanatory power of experiments in social and scientific discourse. The rise of positivism has been intimately connected with the development of experimental methods and their growing prestige in human sciences, such as medicine and psychology. Therefore, to introduce this chapter, let us remind ourselves of some of the key features of these approaches because it was on account of these intellectual movements that contemporary science looks the way it does.

The rise of medical science as we now know it through the nineteenth century went hand in hand with a number of developments in the philosophy of science which privileged the 'hard nosed' end of the scientific spectrum. Mill's canons of induction established a logical rationale for experimental designs and nineteenth-century positivism was given a new lease of life through the efforts of the Vienna Circle, whose thinkers sought to define with increasing rigour the kinds of knowledge that would pass muster as real science. These philosophical developments eventually led to Karl Popper's attempts to identify what was so special about experiments in science, which led him to describe the hypothetico-deductive approach in which the major part of science involves testing hypotheses. There is a special status attached to the falsification of hypotheses in this view. Yet even in the mid-twentieth century, leading scientists such as Sir Peter Medawar felt that the hypothetico-deductive stance that most scientific papers portrayed was deceptive and that sometimes the hypotheses were made up after the scientist had performed the experiment rather than before.

The hypothetico-deductive process in science is often described in the following terms: Scientific knowledge comes from testing theories by logically deducing predictions or hypotheses from them, using experiment and careful observation to test the hypotheses, and revising theories that lead to incorrect predictions. It is worth pausing over because it is such an important part of the process of science. Popper's account of scientific discovery makes a great deal of this. Earlier variants of positivism had stressed the verification of ideas. Popper (1968) stressed instead the development of hypotheses and the systematic attempt to falsify them. To go back to the example of the swans (which Popper used as well), the statement 'all swans are white' can never be fully verified by observing additional white swans. However, we can establish the truth of the statement much more effectively if we go out looking for a swan that isn't white. In this way we can establish knowledge that is empirical, logical, objective and universal. If the hypothesis fails in one instance, then it fails completely.

Karl Popper's claim that it is the 'falsifiability' of scientific theories that demarcates true science from pseudo-science gave a sense of the historical and sociological aspect of science – that is, the falsification process reveals the change and development at the heart of science. Popper was also able in this way to define science so as to exclude Marxism and psychoanalysis. They did not in his view generate testable predictions and so could not be considered scientific. What was left of science, however, by diligent application of this hypothetico-deductive method might achieve successive approximations to the 'truth' in an evolutionary way.

The impact of hypothetico-deductive models of science has left its mark, not so much on the process of enquiry and theory building itself, but on the narrative form of science. Journal articles – one of the principal forms of narrative communication in science – have existed in a recognizably contemporary form for about a century and a half. Overwhelmingly, when empirical research is presented, it is written so as to make it look like theory or prior research has suggested the topic and the hypotheses and the data collection exercise has been conducted apparently untouched by human hand. Just looking at the language can be instructive: 'The theory predicts . . .', 'The data suggest . . .' imply that this is happening all by itself without the intervention of humans to manipulate the theory and construct the data. Indeed, it could be argued that to enable one's ideas to appear compelling to the scientific establishment it is necessary, because of the reverence for hypothetico-deductivism, that the ideas be expressed as theory-generated hypotheses that have undergone the 'ordeal' of experiment.

This viewpoint has been strengthened by the claim that the certainty of empirical inductions comes from employing deductive logic in the form of the 'hypothetico-deductive' model, whereby a set of statements connected by logical rules express the following: 'whenever A, then B'. This, of course, is subject to the same 'initial conditions' or empirical circumstances to which the law is applied being met, for example exactly the same water temperature, and so on. Then a hypothesis can be deduced that can be tested against empirical observation. The statement 'whenever A, then B' cannot be conclusively proved but can be falsified by one instance that A is not followed by B. It is this falsificationist approach to scientific laws that was championed by Karl Popper. Popper stressed the provisional nature of scientific discovery and saw the rigour of science as part and parcel of its striving to falsify its own laws. The history of science, of course, has been of scientific laws being replaced by more effective ones. On this thinking, science is a succession of wrong theories! The sense of approximation going on here gave positivistic and hypothetico-deductive approaches in social science a bit of a let-off. Since social phenomena were arguably more complex than natural objects, it was not surprising that exact, precise laws were difficult to obtain. This gave an impetus to those social scientists with a positivistic bent to try to construct more rigorous research methods – if you like, to increase the probability that their explanations have validity. Such an approach might appear like the search for the Holy Grail. After all, how can you exclude all the variables impinging on social cause and effect? Correlations between variables such as, for example, socio-economic status and educational attainment, or stress and illness, are always imperfect. Social research often has a non-experimental nature and relies on this kind of correlation of variables. Such correlations cannot provide laws so much as 'empirical generalizations' that are restricted to time and place. As Hughes and Sharrock (1997, p.65) conclude, 'no empirical generalisation can ever logically entail a law'. This scepticism sits oddly with the ambition of many scientists, such as Lewis Wolpert (1992), to discover the lawful regularities which they believe to be immanent in nature, or like Jaques Monod (1972), who believe that science should or could commit itself to objectivity.

Science is concerned not simply with producing theories of empirical connections in the positivist sense of the relationship between one observable and another observable, but also with providing a convincing rationale as to why such a relationship exists. It often attempts a logical explanation in terms of rational, lawful, regular processes. It abstracts from the properties of empirical objects to laws such as the law of motion. As such, laws are not causal empirical generalizations but rationally connected statements.

The social sciences and the health care disciplines, however, must often be content with less formidable explanations than those chased down through the hypothetico-deductive model. The health care disciplines are in a most interesting position in this respect. Here, the 'social' and 'natural' sciences both operate and co-exist, occasionally with some friction, but often very comfortably. Traditionally, within the philosophy of science, scientific laws are causal statements describing events in nature and are capable of being true or false, their truth or falsity being determined by observation. But whether this happens is another matter. Scientists are perhaps less critical than we might hope, holding onto pet theories for dear life. Popper was sceptical about social science and felt that much of it did not articulate theories which would expose themselves to the possibility of refutation. Yet this indeterminacy and theoretical slipperiness did not appear to handicap the social sciences in their rise through the twentieth century. Neither does it appear to have prevented them finding their way into health care, both to study it and to attempt contributions to human welfare more directly.

Like his predecessor Comte, Popper gave a sense of the historical and sociological aspect of science, in terms of how the disciplines, theories and methods change and develop. The emphasis was placed on successive approximations, but in an evolutionary, hierarchical kind of way so that a sense is given that science was going somewhere in a progressive fashion.

Thomas Kuhn (1996) had other ideas. Kuhn saw scientists as holding onto general frameworks and theories – paradigms or models – chugging along in a normal, cautious, conservative manner, until another paradigm insisted on taking its place, usually involving the death of the old science, and the ascendancy of a new breed of scientists working under a different paradigm. Over time, scientists become aware of an accumulation of problems that do not fit the orthodox paradigm or model and a new paradigm condenses around these problems as new theories and explanations for phenomena are constructed. Kuhn did not see this process as necessarily being rational in the sense that Popper insisted upon. In Kuhn's view, science does not move ever closer to 'truth'. Kuhn highlights the way that the choice of theory may be the outcome of non-rational, extra-scientific considerations and factors, such as social power or reputation and the wider cultural and political context.

Positivistic approaches in social science led to a great deal of reductionism in the explanation of human activity. In the early stages of social science, Auguste Comte and Emile Durkheim took this deterministic view, and developed theories of human society where the culture and social behaviour were seen as the result of converging forces. Durkheim in particular was concerned with how one could adhere to the scientific demands of 'positivism' yet still attain an understanding of such human phenomena as morality, beliefs, opinions and so on, in the same way as if they were material, physical objects. In this sense, empirical observations only skim the surface of the behaviour or activity being studied. Durkheim tried to make social, human phenomena look as if they were a kind of material factuality. In positivistic style, he sought 'social facts' as if they were 'things', real objects in their own right, like the social fact of suicide (Durkheim 1953). That is, social 'facts,' which are external to the observer, resist distortion or contamination through our will and constrain our behaviour or activity. For Durkheim, the sociologist should 'describe the essential characteristics of social facts, explain how they come into being, enter into relationships with one another, act on each other, and function together to form social wholes'. As such, social 'facts' are observed from 'outside' as objectively, it is claimed, as if one were examining physical facts. To sustain this point of view, the definition of the social 'fact' is of paramount importance. Originally, in the nineteenth century, the scientific search for the causes of social 'facts' such as suicide was done not through experiment but by linking or correlating social 'facts', so as to explain one social fact by another. Strong social bonds, for example, led to more 'altruistic' suicides, whereas the lack of these bonds might lead to anomic suicides. Like Comte, Durkheim hoped that a stronger knowledge of social 'facts' would lead to social improvement. Both aimed to reveal objectively the laws of society by a properly constituted science of the social. But this positivistic view of social science – with its stress on laws, causal explanation, objectivity and rigorous method – has attracted much criticism. It is seen to reify or spuriously treat social affairs as if they were material objects, and reduce complex human phenomena to 'social facts' in such a way that they lose their richness, meaning and political, moral and ethical qualities with which they are imbued in the human world.

To toughen up a positivist status, social science introduced the neutral sounding language of variables. These are general attributes or properties which can be compared in relation to supposed causes. Positivistic social science turned to look at patterns between various indicators of a social phenomenon such as, say, 'suicide' or 'adultery' – finding links and variations between these and building up empirical descriptions and then theories. What can follow is a quantification of variables, perhaps even just their presence or absence. But the indicators only stood in for the actual phenomena and were not the 'things' themselves. The problem posed here is whether we can capture reality in language – in definitions, propositions and the protocol statements of the positivists – to the point where we can speak with scientific certainty of any correlations made. They are by this time, after all, a long way from the actual social phenomena they purport to describe.

Critics of this method of social research have objected to the way in which the reality of social phenomena and processes is concealed behind a descriptive apparatus whose character owed more to the technical requirements of developing the meas- urement instruments and of manipulating the statistics than it did to capturing the underlying connections between the phenomena it attempted to describe (Hughes and Sharrock 1997). Part of the problem of this approach is the way it derives vari- ables from social wholes or collectivities rather than individuals. Paradoxically, such social wholes cannot be reduced to the individuals that compose them and that have provided the empirical evidence through their individual behaviours out of which the social whole is built. Many of the ideas we have about social wholes, for example those of hierarchy, class, privilege or economically based differentials in health, may there- fore be difficult to justify in concrete terms. Yet the statistical significance of their impact on health is difficult to deny (Townsend *et al.* 1990; Acheson 1998). Even so, the notions of inequality as they are used by the social scientist or epidemiologist are little more than theoretical entities, despite their explanatory usefulness. By the time they enter the statistical process, they are far removed from the subjective sense of hunger, for example.

There are further concerns with 'positivistic' science in attempting to produce laws or generalizations which state the causal relationships that hold between phe- nomena, since causal generalizations result from sensory experience and cannot be guaranteed because they only apply to events so far. Therefore, knowledge of em- pirical causes and effects can never be certain, merely probable. Even if, like Mill, we appeal to the uniformity of nature, the inductive process of reasoning at the heart of empiricism is only promoted by yet more induction of the uniformities and stability of nature. Monod's (1972) exhortation to moral disengagement and objectivity is itself a profoundly moral statement.

As we hope the reader will appreciate, the issue of what is true and not true is a complex one. What you experience and claim as objective, someone else may argue against, as in a court case. The question becomes even more complex when we are dealing with events that are beyond the speakers' and hearers' experience. For example, some people, such as David Irving (1983) and Richard Harwood (1978), claim, perversely to our thinking, that the Holocaust – the murder of the Jews in the 1930s and throughout the Second World War – never happened and that, perhaps, this was an elaborate hoax (Guttenplan 2001). As part of this, others argue that since the true witnesses are all dead, the facts can't be fully established. Others liken the Holocaust to an earthquake that destroys the instruments set to measure it. The loss of the instruments does not take away the 'fact' that people feel the seismic shock (Lyotard 1988). The issue of what stands as knowledge and what does not is full of difficulty, especially when we are somewhat distant from the events in question. So what is it that people do to strengthen their claim that what they observe in the world is accurate?

The usual suspects are evidence, measurement and proof, used repeatedly to justify claims to factuality. These are powerful rhetorical devices that serve to anchor the statements we are making and enable the hearers to suspend their disbelief. If whatever you are claiming has been tested; if you can claim by means of certain kinds of anecdotes that the theories you have about phenomena have stood up to experiment, then the claim is correspondingly more powerful. Of course, we have to have the right kind of anecdotes. In health care, the systematic review of several 'methodologically sound' randomized controlled trials is an especially persuasive anecdote. In everyday conversation, appeals to reality may take different forms. One popular style of argument is the 'death and furniture' approach (Edwards *et al.* 1995), where people resort to the 'hit the table' approach when faced with the notion that something is illusory. Look, this is 'real', nothing 'socially constructed' about that. Alternatively, people say things like 'step outside and get run over by a bus' and claim a warrant to have accessed the same sort of ultimate reality. It is a kind of 'facts will speak for themselves' common sense approach. But what is 'real' and 'not real' is not simply dealt with; nor, according to post-positivist philosophies, can our findings or knowledge of the world through research be anything other than cloudy, temporary and replaceable. Ultimately, of course, we want this book to have a destabilizing effect on the reader's notions of certainty. This is partly motivated by our subversive tendencies, but more importantly to encourage the reader to ask 'how do we know that?' when confronted with the conclusions of research and statements of fact. We must come to terms with the philosophical debate that runs through the work of research, its validity, the level of evidence it provides, and the politics behind accepting one form of knowledge over another. The knowledge of the world provided through observation and research is debated, which might seem odd if one were to accept a strict positivist point of view. This becomes a little easier to understand if we see scientific life as being more like a courtroom, where the defenders of particular theories try to use evidence to make the best kind of argument for their case. In a courtroom the audience might be the magistrate, jury or judge, but in everyday life it is less clear who the audience is. It might be other members of the scientific community, health care practitioners or the public. In presenting arguments about phenomena, it may even be that scientists are trying to convince themselves.

In the traditional account of knowledge contained in most positivist and falsificationist accounts, knowledge itself is fairly sensible stuff. Unlike metaphysics, knowledge is empirical, logical, objective and universal – allegedly. If we test a hypothesis and it fails in one instance, then it fails completely and should be ruthlessly rejected, in Popper's [1935] (1959) account.

However, a great many theoretical systems are not rejected even when confirmations are not forthcoming. For example, most Western intellectuals believe in the theory of evolution. However, as it was originally formulated, based on Darwin's study of finches in the Galapagos Islands, it stressed gradual change and adaptation based on relatively small individual differences. However, as palaeontologists try to piece together the fossil record, it is clear that there are a great many gaps and missing links. Rather than reject evolutionary theory and the specific hypotheses it leads to, scientists have instead searched for the intervening species even more diligently. Finding the remains of species that might have evolved into modern humans has exercised a great many scientists and has led to some spectacular mistakes and possible frauds. Neanderthal man was believed to walk in a stooped posture because the original specimen from the Neander valley suffered from arthritis, Peking man was probably a monkey and Piltdown man was a fake. These disappointments have not resulted in the theory's abandonment, but have instead led to some revisions. Perhaps the fossil record contains not a continuous record but merely snapshots from occasional periods of rapid extinction and rapid sedimentary rock formation. Or, alternatively, maybe evolution itself proceeds as a sequence of punctuated equilibria where periods of rapid change occur interspersed with periods of relative stability. The point is that a real life scientific theory is often not simply discarded, especially if it is a popular one. The data or the theory itself are reinterpreted so as to come into alignment.

A focus on the hypothetico-deductive method as a way of explaining science has also been considered to be somewhat misleading because it underemphasizes the role that observation and description play in establishing exactly what there is to invent hypotheses about. Archaeology, astronomy, botany and health care itself rely on the observation of the phenomena in question, even when this is not obviously theory led in any way. Observations are important even when they are not used to test theories and important discoveries have originated this way. For example, before 1803, scientists did not believe that rocks could fall from the sky, but the observation of a large number of stones falling in the village of L'Aigle in France in August of that year, after a display of shooting stars, finally convinced most of the scientific community and probably constituted what we would now call a meteorite shower. Observations, then, help invent theories.

Theories are not necessarily built on new evidence. Theoretical development can sometimes be largely conceptual, logical or mathematical, and allow a better understanding of existing evidence.

A good deal of observation and exploration is based on things that are not necessarily formal theories from which hypotheses derive. Scientists may be exploring their world out of curiosity, or following hunches.

Standardized experiments are very difficult to perform – indeed, might even be a myth, at least in social science, and possibly the health care disciplines too. Phenomena are not facts in the sense of being sensory data or the protocol statements beloved of logical positivism. Rather, the observations may be better thought of as interpretations constantly under review as events unfold. Hypotheses relate to situations, and what is true in one situation may be false in others. The values and agendas of the researcher are embedded in the survey instruments or experimental designs. This is sometimes called imposition. For example, consider the situation of patients who have had an operation. They may be in considerably more pain and feeling worse than when they first came into hospital. However, if we focus on other things about them and their situation, such as the wounds healing or the number of days until discharge, it is a lot easier to make it look like the operation was a success. Indeed, this is exactly what the surgeons did in Nicholas Fox's (1993) study of ward rounds. Positivism, and its relative, hypothetico-deductive science, leave us with very few tools to make sense of this process.

Many scholars of a humanist or interpretivist bent would argue that human behaviour is meaningful and that people actively interpret and make sense of their circumstances and social behaviour, according to this point of view, cannot be explained easily in terms of external stimuli. The methods which purportedly allow us to measure objectively the phenomena in question yield results which reify a dynamic social process and give rise to an overly mechanistic way of making sense of people. Moreover, the statistical methods which often accompany these data collection strategies tend to misrepresent the phenomena because they tend to average out diversity. The forces at work in human affairs are not the same as gravitational forces or the forces at work in the movement of elementary particles. A good deal of interpretivist enquiry in the human sciences can be summed up in the 'Thomas Maxim' that 'If men define situations as real they are real in their consequences' (Thomas and Thomas 1928, p. 572). Thus, what is important for understanding human behaviour is not what is objectively real, but what people think is real. Put another way, a positivist might say that 'seeing is believing', whereas an interpretivist might argue that 'believing is seeing'.

Scientists learn things from events that confirm theories as well as refute theories. The first atomic bomb, even though it exploded as predicted, still enabled physicists to learn something. Indeed, once we look at the published literature of science, the overwhelming majority of papers reporting empirical studies contain results that support rather than refute the theory. Arguably, then, science is in theory deductive but in practice inductive, or in theory falsificationist but in practice verificationist.

Sometimes events or observations are surprising. For example, *Ustilago maydis* or corn smut is a fungus that affects corn plants. One might initially be surprised to learn that one variety of this fungus has hundreds of different sexes. However, once we know this, discovering a variety that has a few more isn't so surprising.

Thus, we have hoped to show that despite appeals to an external reality, many of the more scientific aspects of science remain controversial. What we can observe, what it means and what theories it might not support are issues which are argued about a great deal. Even objects apparently as incontrovertible as lumps of rock – fossils or meteorites – are part of some of the most controversial areas of enquiry of all, in the form of evolutionary theory. The problem of knowing gets even more complex when we start looking at human affairs. Not only that, but the protagonists sometimes seem unwilling or powerless to examine the descriptions, categories and typifications which helped to consolidate that particular view of the world and understand why other groups of people find them objectionable. In a sense, the appeals to evidence and fact inherent in nineteenth-century science facilitated some kinds of value-blindness. The drive to make things visible led researchers away from scrutiny of the moral and ontological frameworks and inferential structures which helped to constitute their objects of enquiry. Thomas Huxley, the friend and supporter of Charles Darwin, hatched a scheme to have the 'aboriginal peoples' of the world photographed because, of course, since they were more primitive people they would soon be extinct, according to the predictions of evolutionary theory. This caused offence when his collaborators attempted to put this into practice in Australia, for reasons which Huxley was at a loss to comprehend.

Returning to the scientific method itself, and the implications of the foregoing arguments for how we might characterize it, we are left in a state of some confusion. Paul Feyerabend (1924–1994), the noted philosopher, added to this when he proposed an especially anarchical model of science. It is his contention that we cannot describe what scientists do – verification, hypothetico-deductive enquiry or whatever – because, whatever we say, there are examples of 'good science' that don't follow these rules. In Feyerabend's (1999) view there are a plurality of co-existing and sometimes competing theories and methods which he calls 'epistemological anarchism'. In this view, there is, as with postmodernism, nothing fundamentally superior about scientific knowledge. Feyerabend has suggested that there is nothing to allow us objectively to distinguish science from voodoo. By the same token, perhaps, there is little to distinguish phrenology from neurology or the nineteenth-century epidemic of nymphomania from the early twenty-first-century epidemic of 'sex addiction'. Indeed, in Feyerabend's view, examining voodoo might well enrich or humanize our understanding of physiology. Nevertheless, as a number of scholars of science as a social process have pointed out (e.g. Mulkay 1979), the ethos of science, including its hypothetico-deductive mantle, has done a great deal to enable scientists to justify their own behaviour and characterize that of others as improper.

Hacohen (1998) reminds us that Karl Popper himself felt that there was nothing special about science. Indeed, he challenged philosophers' and scientists' claims of expertise. Moreover, for him, there was no single pre-eminent philosophical method. Every person can be a problem solver and, by extension, in Popper's philosophy, every person is a philosopher: 'Science is nothing but enlightened and responsible common sense – common sense broadened by imaginative critical thinking' (Popper 1983, p. 260). Popper was concerned to demystify science, yet he felt there was something hopeful about the growth of knowledge. He thought science at its best was an interminable quest for uncertain but expanding and more effective knowledge. Despite his stringency about what could and could not constitute science, Popper was also one of the early anti-foundationalists, he insisted that objectivity meant intersubjectivity – the agreement of observers – rather than reflecting an incontrovertible state of some external reality. Rationality was thus a product of informed critical debate, bringing Popper into line with thinkers such as Habermas. As Popper put it:

> Science does not rest upon solid bedrock. The bold structure of its theories rise, as it were, above a swamp. It is like a building erected on piles. The piles are driven down from above into the swamp, but not down to any natural or 'given' base; and if we stop driving the piles deeper, it is not because we have reached firm ground. We simply stop when we are satisfied that the piles are firm enough to carry the structure, at least for the time being.
>
> (Popper [1935] 1959, p. 111)

Although Popper describes science as a kind of contrived edifice that draws on common sense, there are still elements of his philosophy which a good deal of science would find it hard to live up to. There is a problem with Popper's demand for predictive theories – that is, theories that can be tested to show that they, provisionally, predict in a precise manner – since this assumes that strenuous testing is taking place all the time and that scientists are deeply critical of established theories. But this is simply not the case. A good deal of material, once it has passed through the hoop of controversy, is taken for granted.

In Chapter 4, we dealt with some of the underlying issues attached to the scientific method. We sought to challenge the idea that science and its findings are above reproach, by visiting some of the principles on which the scientific method is founded. This chapter looks at the conduct of the experimental method, with the same aim – to what extent does the scientific process provide results in which we can place our faith and confidence, and how far are they inherently distorted by the values and beliefs that operate at national, local and individual levels? In the UK, the national level may be thought of as having to do with the government and at a local level the influence of health authorities and health care trusts will be apparent, and all this may itself influence what goes on in individual health care encounters.

Objective observation

Enshrined within any philosophy of scientific method is the need for objective observation. Medawar (1963) describes the scientific process as involving the simple, impartial, objective observation of events, usually in the form of numbers, recordings and so on, which can be analysed statistically and from which conclusions are drawn and theories generated. It has already been noted that Popper (1968) challenged this claim, contending instead that there is no such thing as objective observation – rather, all observation takes place within the context of a set of theoretical assumptions. This grandiose position also operates in a simpler form, in that the experience, values and knowledge of the person making the observations will influence what is recorded. Therefore, the recording of a 'fact' in the course of an experiment (for example, the quality of life of a multiple sclerosis patient, or a blood pressure reading) is as heavily dependent on who is doing the recording as it is on who is participating in the study and what is being recorded. Indeed, even Gregor Mendel's work on the laws of inheritance may be suspect because the assessments of whether or not a pea was wrinkled were not made 'blind' but were vulnerable to experimenter bias, in that Mendel did the observations and knew which seeds each pea crop had come from.

One good example of observational unreliability that will be familiar to most people is the visual illusion, in which two identical silhouetted profiles face each other. One observer may record this as two profiles, while another may interpret it as a white vase against a black background. Thus, a piece of static objective evidence can be easily interpreted in two quite different ways by two observers, but even more than this, a single observer may see the image repeatedly alternate between both interpretations within a short space of time. Not only can evidence be interpreted differently by different individuals, it can also be interpreted differently by the same individual. What reliance can be placed, then, on the objective recording of events?

While plausible neurological explanations have been put forward to explain this particular figure/ground phenomenon (Gregory 1977), they don't eliminate the unreliability of the interpretation or guarantee objectivity in the scientific process. Although the individual may be aware of alternative images in figure/ground illusions, the potential for, or existence of, bias in research studies is not always as readily acknowledged by the researchers. Other influences on the observation process are less easy to harness and interpret than the profile/vase example above, with the consequence that their biasing impact is harder to recognize and assess. It is known that numerous other individual differences, such as the personality of the observer or the appearance of the participant, may affect judgements and observation. The literature is replete with interesting examples. An early seminal study by Else Frenkel-Brunswick (1949) classified children as being racially prejudiced or not, using a well-tested, psychometrically reliable ethnocentrism scale. She then showed each child a picture of a dog, followed by an identical sequence of pictures in which the drawing of the dog gradually changed into a drawing of a cat. For each picture the children had to record what they saw. She found that the prejudiced children tended to hold on for longer to the idea that the drawing represented a dog, while the unprejudiced children altered their interpretation earlier. The prejudiced children were more rigid in their interpretations than the non-prejudiced. The point here is that the value-system of the observer influenced what was seen, even though both groups had seen exactly the same image at each stage of the study.

Other studies have demonstrated fairly clearly, if rather undemocratically, that the degree of facial attractiveness can distort the way in which other attributes are perceived – the much researched 'beautiful equals good' hypothesis. Darbyshire (1986), in a succinct review of some relevant studies within health care, found that there was abundant evidence in health care that attractive patients are assumed to have a whole range of positive qualities irrespective of whether they actually possess them. Bordieri *et al.* (1983), for instance, found that attractive victims of paralysis were assumed to have significantly better prognoses than less attractive but comparably paralysed patients, while Corter (1978) found that experienced nurses assumed that attractive premature babies would have better intellectual attainment than unattractive babies, all other things being equal. What is even more depressing is that Stephan and Langlois (1984) also found that these differential assumptions about prognosis led to differential treatment by health care staff. In an era of health care rationing, it requires just a small stretch of the imagination to see what effect such attributions may have – if the above findings can be legitimately extrapolated, it is conceivable that in a cash-strapped NHS, attractive patients may get a better health care deal, simply because they are assumed to be a better investment. Whatever the outcome, the evidence challenges the assumption that observations and judgements can be truly objective in the sense desired by some scientists and philosophers. Therefore, it will never be unhampered by the biases and intuition that science and the evidence-based health care culture have tried so hard to avoid.

Even the recording of apparently value-free data may be unreliable. A classic example is blood pressure monitoring. While this procedure can be an invaluable screening technique for potential cardiovascular problems, its routine use on an average 30-bed ward can consume as much as 14–21 hours of a nurse's time per week – in other words, 0.5 of a Whole Time Equivalent (WTE) (Walsh and Ford 1994). This investment of time would be easily justified if the readings were reliable (and hence useful), but there is considerable evidence to demonstrate that a minimal raising or lowering of the arm away from the heart can affect the blood pressure reading by 5–6 mmHg. Similarly, taking the reading from an unsupported arm can raise blood pressure by 8 mmHg, while supporting the patient's back can reduce it by the same amount (Webb 1980). Even the choice of arm can alter the readings by 10 mmHg (Kristensen and Kornerup 1982). Given that the way in which blood pressure readings are taken varies within and between health care professionals, these errors of unreliability may have serious clinical significance for certain categories of patients, as well as being hugely wasteful of resources. Even relatively objective measures may be vulnerable to bias.

Other sources of bias in research

The question of who does the research is intricately bound up with the values and evaluations that attach to the findings. In this sense, the nature of the researcher imposes another potential source of bias. There are numerous anecdotal and formal accounts from the non-medical professions of how their research proposals are over-looked in funding applications, in favour of those submitted by the doctors, particularly if a non-experimental paradigm is proposed (e.g. Meerabeau 1997), which will inevitably add further weight to the assumption that only medical and scientific research is worthy of consideration. The influence of the professional status of the researcher on how research is assessed has been demonstrated in a series of studies carried out by one of the co-authors (C-H.).

Hicks looked at how nurses evaluated research and researchers. In one study (Hicks 1992), one group of nurses was given a journal article on a piece of experimental research apparently conducted by a nurse, while a second group was given the identical article, but apparently conducted by a consultant. The task was to rate the paper on each of six criteria. The results clearly demonstrated that the overall quality of the research, the author's grasp of statistics and understanding of research methodology were rated significantly higher for the article believed to be authored by a doctor. No difference was observed in terms of clarity of expression and level of expertise on the research topic. Not only did these results suggest that nurses in the study perceived doctors to have more credibility as researchers but, furthermore, that the doctors were attributed with greater expertise on the essential competences of the scientific process – in simplest terms, they were considered to be better at experimental research, which may of course explain the relative paucity of experimental research that emerges from non-medical health care professionals. At the least, the study suggests that the prestigious experimental research methodologies are seen by nurses to be located fairly and squarely within the expertise of the medical profession. The logical upshot of this is that the high-status research is likely to be dominated by the medical professions, who may conceivably focus primarily on issues of medical interest, thereby abandoning many highly relevant health care interventions to the mercies of unresearched ritual and tradition. Not only does this appear to be a sure-fire recipe for relegating non-medical research to the second division, it also introduces a further element of selection bias to health care research.

Hicks's results gained further corroboration from a follow-up study, in which two groups of nurses were asked to rate a hypothetical candidate for a nursing post along 15 criteria. To provide the participants with some information about the applicant, they were all given a description that included six adjectives (Hicks 1996). Of these, five were identical for each group, but the sixth descriptor varied, in that one group of nurses was told that the applicant was a good clinician, while the other was informed that the applicant was a good researcher. The task was to evaluate the candidate according to 15 personal qualities, which had not been specifically referred to in the description. The evaluations were therefore simply based on assumptions and inferences generated from the six descriptors – a variant of Asch's Central Trait Theory. The findings showed that the applicant described as a good researcher was rated significantly higher on those personal qualities that were associated with the conduct of conventional research (e.g. logical, rational, analytical, more controlled) and lower on those qualities traditionally associated with nursing (e.g. kindness, compassion, intuition) and which go back as far as Florence Nightingale. It would appear, then, that the attributes required of a good researcher may be fundamentally incompatible with those traditionally required of the good nurse. Again, this seems to confirm that nursing and scientific/experimental research are not considered to be natural bedfellows, a position which may leave nursing research out in the cold when it comes to credibility ratings, impact and kudos.

But underpinning these sets of results may be the additional factor of gender differences. The qualities attributed to high-quality research and high-quality researchers are manifestly male – in other words, the traditional association of maleness with logic, rationality, emotional control and the like are also the qualities associated with experimental research as it is construed within the health care community (Davies 1998). This proposition enjoys considerable support from a large corpus of educational research, which demonstrates that despite the supremacy of girls in overall achievement, the subject disciplines remain heavily gendered, with boys assumed to be better at science and maths and girls better at the arts and humanities (Archer 1992). Schopenhauer's ([1851] 1974) sexism (quoted in the previous chapter) would be vindicated, no doubt, as would Florence Nightingale's, whose assertion that to be a good nurse, you must first be a good woman, has influenced much of the thinking and developments in the nursing profession (Gamarnikov 1978; Shepherd *et al.* 1996; Davies 1998). For example, even the original role titles, such as 'sister' and 'matron', are inherently feminized. Similarly, Cleverly (1998) notes that in academic nursing departments, female lecturers were more likely to prioritize student welfare while back-burnering research, while for their male counterparts the reverse was true. If there is, as would seem, a gender bias in the research process, then it is conceivable that this would further influence the topics chosen for research and the methods selected to undertake it, a contention reinforced by the fact that feminist research typically follows a qualitative paradigm. Whatever the explanation, though, it is clear that evidence is not absolute and that it is defined within a cultural, value-laden framework and belief system (Walsh 1998; Stewart 2001).

The better evaluation given to the putative consultant's grasp of scientific method and statistical understanding in Hicks's (1992) study may be explained by the male domination of the consultant tier of the medical profession (at the time of writing, women occupy less than 7 per cent of the consultant surgeon posts in the UK; *Health Service Journal* 2002). The implications of these findings are that research in general, and experimental research in particular, are male gendered, while nursing (and qualitative research) are female gendered. Thus the emphasis on experimental research may be antipathetic to nursing, which might in part explain the relatively low profile of nursing research in the new randomized controlled trial-based, evidence-based health care (EBHC) culture. Indeed, the most recent Research Assessment Exercise which evaluated universities' research output (www.herp.ac.uk/rae/overview/docs/UoA10.doc) noted in its assessment of the nursing submission, under the sub-title 'Issues of concern', that the 'majority of research [submitted] used social science methods . . . a large amount of descriptive work . . . There was an almost complete absence of laboratory work' (4.2.3). Such a verdict makes quite clear that the reviewers perceive methods other than the formal scientific ones to be an 'issue for concern', substandard substitutes for real research. And given, too, that bureaucracies are inherently patriarchal and male dominant/female subordinate (Witz 1992; Davies 1998) and that the NHS is a huge bureaucracy, the environment in which the female-dominated non-medical professions work may also conspire to ensure that the research methodologies more suited to their areas of activity and interests are confined to the low-status ranks. Thus the values and the associations embedded in the prevailing research paradigm may have ensured that some health care topics, in particular holistic nursing ones, are effectively consigned to the wayside. The inevitable selection procedure of topics capable of being researched by experimental protocols, therefore, introduces its own bias.

Control groups

The randomized controlled trial and the true experiment depend heavily on the use of the non-intervention, or control, group. The reasoning behind this is as follows: if one group is given active treatment and the other a non-active placebo (all other factors being the same), then any differences in outcomes between the groups must be attributable to the effects of the treatment. In other words, the use of the control group contributes to the capacity of the experiment to establish linear cause–effect relationships. The principle is simple, logical and unassailable, at least in theory, but it is not without its ethical and practical problems.

Because of the importance of the control group concept to the randomized controlled trial, it may be worth illustrating it with a health-related example. If a researcher is concerned with evaluating a new analgesic drug for patients with pancreatic cancer, two groups of very similar patients might be selected, with one group being given the new drug and the other group a placebo. The data on pain levels would be collected and compared; if the patients on the new drug had lower pain levels, then providing the design of the study had been sound, this intervention would be deemed to be more effective than the placebo. Thus in an ideal scientific study, a control group is used, one which receives no active intervention or treatment. If the only difference between the groups is the use of some form of active treatment, then any disparity in outcomes must be the result of the intervention. But while the use of control groups provides a methodological ideal, it raises serious ethical issues that relate to the non-treatment or placebo-only treatment of some patients.

The concept of the placebo not only demonstrates an important feature of sound research design, but also reflects the old mind/body problem, and the relationship between them. Rapidly growing interest in the mind/body relationship or psycho-neuroimmunology (PNI) is a testament to the widening acceptance that within health there is a reciprocal impact of the body and the mind. Consider, for example, research that has demonstrated that the effectiveness of a placebo is about half that of the actual drug, that two placebo tablets are more effective than one, that big pills are more effective than small pills, and that red ones are better than white ones (Dixon and Sweeney 2000; 'Placebo: Cracking the Code', *Discovery Channel*, 26 October 2002). How else is this to be explained except by mind over matter, a belief in the power of the treatment, however useless it may be? Or take the evidence on hysterical conversion symptoms, whereby physical problems are manifest, with no corresponding aetiology. Numerous accounts exist throughout the centuries, ranging from demonically possessed nuns demonstrating extreme psychomotor agitation, to pupils in strict religious schools who suffered a range of symptoms including palsy, and uncontrollable tremors and the appearance of chemical burns during the anthrax scare in 2001, when a number of individuals opened letters thought to contain a suspect powder when there was no trace of any (Bartholomew and Wessely 2002). The mounting corpus of evidence on the impact of stress on the immune system (e.g. Burns *et al.* 2002; Kiecolt-Glaser *et al.* 2002; Sepa *et al.* 2002; Thomas *et al.* 2002) adds weight to the fact that the mind and the body do not have parallel existences, but rather they are part of an interactive system. The point here though is quite simple: the randomized controlled trial can try to pin down the effects of a drug on cancer or coronary heart disease, but it can never evaluate or control the impact of the human mind. Interestingly, as Evans (2003) notes, placebo effects work partly because not only patients but doctors also believe they work. A group of men and women who have been trained in (and for the most part believe in) a material, cause and effect universe might be expected to be sceptical of quasi-mystical notions concerning the mind affecting the body. Yet in the case of the placebo effect, most of them are true believers and this, Evans argues, affects the success of placebo medication too. The human mind, then, is clearly critical in health care outcomes, so the value of the randomized controlled trial in making statements about best treatment options must be questionable.

This point notwithstanding, the concept of the control group had an early genesis in medical research, and was increasingly seen as a critical aspect of treatment evaluations. For instance, in 1545 Paré dressed parts of wounds with crushed onions, while leaving other parts untouched; the onions appeared to be more effective. Likewise, during an epidemic of scarlet fever, Balfour (quoted in West 1854) selected two groups of boys, one of which was prescribed belladonna prophylactically, to see if it would prevent the development of the disease. And Fibiger (1898) administered anti-diphtheria serum to alternate patients and monitored its effect. While such studies were undoubtedly informative, they had serious ethical flaws in that some patients were left without any treatment. Moreover, while there was a primitive understanding of the need both for comparability of groups and for reducing selection bias, early techniques of simple alternation of treatment with control failed to address the potential for experimenter and subject bias, in that both parties were aware of whether or not they were receiving active treatment and thus had the potential to distort the results (see section on 'Random allocation' below). The fundamental issue here, though, is the comparability of the participating groups; if this cannot be assured, the outcome cannot be conclusively attributed to the intervention – a serious consideration when the multiplicity of human variation is taken into account. While many known and quantifiable factors (gender, age, previous medical history, existing co-morbidities, etc.) can be taken into account when trying to establish comparability, there are numerous unknown, random factors, such as the psychological profile of the participants, their moods, temperament and the like, which can neither be assessed nor balanced out. This inevitably means that any attempt at claiming group comparability in experimental studies must be treated with an element of healthy scepticism.

Despite the obvious need for similarity between groups, many studies have carelessly overlooked its importance, often with potentially adverse consequences. One striking example of the distorting effects of non-comparability is the study conducted on the efficacy of the Bristol Cancer Help Centre (Bagenal *et al.* 1990). The study compared the outcomes of women with breast cancer who were attending the Bristol centre, with those attending standard oncology departments in the NHS. The authors concluded definitively that the Bristol Cancer Help Centre was no more effective than conventional treatments and, in some cases, it was worse. The findings, sensationally represented in the press (e.g. Richards' 1990 article entitled 'Death from complementary medicine') had a devastating effect on donations to the Centre, which has charitable status; at one point, it came close to closing. However, closer scrutiny of the results demonstrated that the people who attended the Bristol Centre were doing so because, for many, it was a last resort – they were terminally ill and had a very poor prognosis; conversely, those attending the NHS clinics typically had a better prognosis, because they were not as seriously ill (Hayes *et al.* 1990; Sheard 1990). While there was no deliberate intention to distort the results, the fact that the two comparison groups were quite dissimilar from each other meant that the results and conclusions were flawed. The random allocation of patients to treatment groups that is demanded by the randomized controlled trial is designed to minimize such discrepancies between participating groups; nonetheless, even with the best matching in the world, individual differences are bound to exist between the groups.

Comparability of groups requires the identification of inclusion and exclusion criteria for patients taking part in any study. In essence, this means that certain parameters are defined and all patients who meet these requirements (and who consent to take part) are included in the sample pool and then randomized to a treatment group. For example, a report in the *British Medical Journal* (de Fine Olivarius *et al.* 2001) concluded from a multicentre randomized controlled trial that a structured personal programme in primary care does not improve mortality and morbidity for Type 2 diabetes. The patients were excluded from participating if they had any serious somatic disease, doubtful diagnosis, mental illness or non-white ethnicity. Yet diabetes is a particular problem for the Asian population, who were presumably excluded from this study and for whom the recommendations may not apply. Consequently, the conclusions that can be drawn from randomized controlled trials using inclusion/exclusion criteria must, of necessity, be limited to a population with the same characteristics as the sample. Since in the above example not all people with diabetes are white, devoid of somatic disease and mental illness, and have a clear diagnosis, the generalizability of this study and every other that applies stringent inclusion and exclusion criteria must be limited. Yet it is on the basis of findings from research such as this that systematic reviews are conducted and the results disseminated to practitioners in the form of clinical guidelines.

Ethics

The control group, as a non-treatment or placebo group, is an important feature, by definition, of the randomized controlled trial and the experimental method. Such a feature claims to ensure that linear cause and effect relationships can be established. While non-intervention for some participants is a reasonable option in many subject disciplines, such as botany, within health care serious ethical issues arise (Campbell *et al.* 2001). The classic abhorrent use of the control group is the Tuskegee Syphilis Study (e.g. Gamble 1997; Brawley 1999). Treatment was deliberately withheld for 399 black men from low socio-economic backgrounds who had syphilis, so that the course of the disease could be monitored. Apart from the self-evident immorality of this study, it also serves to illustrate the role of values in conducting research. Beyond the brutality of the indefensible decision to withhold a treatment known to be effective, the participants were black and poor – minority, disadvantaged groups. Undoubtedly the value of a non-treatment group is unassailable in methodological terms, especially where the participants are delphinium plants or leeks, but in human terms it is highly questionable. Scientific research must be very careful to ensure that it doesn't unquestioningly adopt sound and logical methodological principles in a search for the truth, while simultaneously abdicating responsibility for the participants. Yet if no control group is used, what confidence can be placed in the findings? It is also true that unless the effects of treatment can be compared rigorously with those of non-treatment, it is possible that interventions may be used that are unnecessary, providing no discernible benefits to the participants. Without a control group to validate the findings, people may be subjected to unnecessary treatment. A classic example of this is the current debate over the value of routine breast screening. Despite the received wisdom that mass screening has a positive effect on mortality and morbidity of women (e.g. Blanks *et al.* 2000), a number of meta-analyses of the available evidence have found that breast screening is not necessarily useful and, in some cases, is positively harmful, because it leads to a range of invasive and disfiguring surgical procedures that are sometimes unnecessary (Olsen and Goetzsche 2000, 2001a,b). The only way to resolve this issue would be to randomly assign women with suspect lumps to either treatment or no treatment – hardly a proposal that would enchant an ethics committee or entice potential participants. Meanwhile, this challenge to the current political grand narrative goes unheeded in government quarters.

Ethical considerations apply as much to treatment groups as to control groups. The testing of new procedures requires the use of human volunteers, which could potentially place them at risk of unknown side-effects. Classic examples of particularly morally bankrupt studies include injecting live cancer cells into elderly patients at the Jewish Chronic Disease Hospital in Brooklyn, without the patients knowing what was being done (quoted in Polit-O'Hara and Hungler 1995), and the human radiation experiments sponsored by US federal agencies, many with elderly people, pregnant women, children and prisoners (for a discussion of these studies, see Samei and Kearfott 1995; Kass and Sugarman 1996; Roff 2000). While these studies have been deliberately selected to illustrate the adverse side-effects that medical research may have, they also demonstrate the importance of providing information to potential participants before recruitment to experimental trials. Yet a critical feature of the randomization process in randomized controlled trials is the concealment of the treatment option at the point of allocation (see next section). In other words, neither patients nor researchers know which intervention will be used with whom (double-blind procedures), or who is on the placebo. Duplicity of this sort, while essential to the sound conduct of the study, contravenes the basic principles of right to full disclosure and right to self-determination, even where informed consent has been obtained. The near perfect scientific principles of the randomized controlled trial may take priority over decent human behaviour. The question of when this is appropriate is one for ethics committees, whose decision will be governed to some extent by the beliefs and values of the constituent members. Scientific endeavour cannot escape subjectivity.

Random allocation

A key feature of the randomized controlled trial and true experiment is the random allocation of participants to either the treatment or control groups, based on the assumption that selection bias will be eliminated as a result. Unbiased allocation of participants is not a new idea. Silverman and Chalmers (2002) cite numerous interesting examples from various historical documents that suggest that the casting of lots in order to allocate goods has been deemed for centuries to be the fairest way to eliminate preferential treatment and bias. For instance, despite the Church's opposition to such games of chance (even though the Bible is replete with references to them, e.g. Book of Judges 20:10), the body of St Leger, claimed in A.D. 782 by three different bishops, was awarded to the Bishop of Poitiers via the casting of lots. David (1962) even noted that the very serious business of choosing a wife was decided by John Wesley through the casting of lots. Clearly, lotteries addressed the issue of selection bias through their recourse to chance, but offended the Church because of its connotations of demonic activity, gambling and the challenge to the ultimate authority of God. It was indeed an affront to the grand narrative and was therefore sacrilegious. Interestingly, Darwin, some time later, while writing *The Origin of the Species*, succumbed to a range of psychosomatic illnesses (Pasnau 1990; Barloon and Noyes 1997). Since his theories could have been seen as an insurrection against the authority of the Church, the resultant anxiety which induced the neurotic disorder from which Darwin suffered may be attributable to a fundamental and heretical challenge to contemporary teachings. Silverman and Chalmers (2002) also quote a number of instances in military history (even as recently as the Vietnam War) when recruitment into the militia and the allocation of tasks was decided by a simple lottery.

However, these authors note that the casting of lots to ensure even-handed delivery of health care has a relatively recent history, quoting an example of an argument in 1662 between the Flemish physician, Van Helmont, and the Galenists. The latter favoured indiscriminate use of bloodletting and purging for a variety of illnesses, while Van Helmont opposed the practice. To settle the dispute, he recommended that a number of patients suffering from fevers should be divided into two groups and lots cast to see which group would be treated by Galen's bloodletting intervention, or by

Van Helmont's non-intervention (the ultimate control group). The outcome measure was to be the number of funerals recorded for each group.

These early studies used alternation as the primary means of allocation and it is fair to say that despite the availability of more sophisticated randomization techniques, a healthy debate still continues over whether alternation methods constitute randomization (Cox 2002). Alternating the allocation of patients remained the main method of eradicating selection bias, until Bradford Hill's seminal work on the use of streptomycin for pulmonary tuberculosis patients. In this he allocated patients to either the treatment or control group using random numbers and sealed envelopes which were centrally controlled. The drive for this more complex, reliable and sophisticated approach to allocation of patients was partly determined by logic and partly by social and political pressures (Yoshioka 1998).

However random allocation is achieved in practice, in theory it means that a particular treatment group is not selected by the researcher or the participant, but rather that any participant has an equal chance of being allocated to any group – preference or choice do not come into it. In reality, this means that if participants are to be allocated to one of two groups, tossing a coin can be used to determine which treatment is used. If participants are to be allocated to one of more than two groups, a dice can be rolled. As long as the allocation rules are identified at the outset (e.g. heads = treatment A; tails = treatment B; 1 or 2 on the dice means treatment 1; 3 or 4 means treatment 2; 5 or 6 means treatment 3) and that the allocation is conducted by someone who is independent of the research study, these processes should be free of bias (Jadad 1998). Alternatively, random number tables or computer-generated sequences can be used. The essential rule of allocation must be decided in advance, it must be adhered to throughout the allocation procedure and the allocation must not be known either to the researcher or patient (Prescott *et al.* 2002). Indeed, many researchers consider that the most critical requirement of randomization is concealment of the treatment to both the participant and the researcher, until the point of allocation (e.g. Berge and Sandercock 2002; Prescott *et al.* 2002). Only if this is assured can selection bias be truly eliminated. Yet there is evidence that many randomized controlled trials do not employ sufficiently stringent randomization processes (Prescott *et al.* 2002), and that the interpretation of random allocation remains variable. In consequence, then, the randomization processes used may not always eliminate selection bias or produce accurate results (Schultz *et al.* 1995). Indeed, many studies described (often in eminent journals) as randomized trials often do not conform to conventional randomization protocols (Altman and Dore 1990; Moher *et al.* 1996; Jadad 1998), thereby calling into question the reliability of their findings and conclusions.

The concealment imperative has a logical and obvious appeal, since it clearly minimizes the biasing effects of autosuggestion and expectation. Its application, though, is rather more complex. Blinding patients in drug trials is easy enough – short of expert chemical analysis, how would any participant know whether the little white pill was an active or inactive treatment? But what if the treatment is surgery? No placebo equivalent is ethically truly acceptable in such studies (although it's fair to point out that placebo arthroscopy has been carried out successfully in America; 'Placebo: Cracking the Code', *Discovery Channel*, 26 October 2002), so the patient may well know to which group they've been assigned. Furthermore, patient preference for one treatment over another is an insurmountable barrier to recruitment for randomized controlled trials; if patient participation is reduced because expressed treatment preferences prohibit participation in the trial, then so too must sample representativeness be compromised through low recruitment.

Yet whether or not a patient consents to take part in clinical trials may be determined to some extent by a range of personal attributes and these have the potential to impact upon the results. Early studies in psychology (Rosenthal and Rosnow 1975; Cowles and Davis 1987) highlighted the individual differences that were evidenced in participants recruited for studies by a variety of methods. Not only did participants react differently compared with non-participants, but in addition the demands of the experiment together with a range of biographical factors, such as the participant's gender, also impacted upon the outcomes. Individual patient tendencies towards compliance and non-compliance with treatment regimes also have the potential to influence reactions in randomized controlled trials, especially when this is a fundamental feature of the trial. It is a reasonable assumption that patients prepared to take part in a trial may be generally more compliant, with a desire to respond appropriately. But even this assumption must be tempered by the fact that total compliance is not guaranteed by the patient's agreement to participate. Indeed, Prescott *et al.* (2002) report that disposing of unused medicines before a clinic visit, or only taking the medication before a clinic visit, are common practices that cannot be adequately monitored – the so-called 'white coat compliance'. Since non-compliance reduces the power of a trial and yet is rarely assessed, it has the potential to distort the effects of the treatment and the conclusions that can be drawn in consequence (Prescott *et al.* 2002). Thus, the differences in psycho-social variables between participants and non-participants in research studies may mean that the samples are not representative and the conclusions limited in their generalizability.

Low recruitment remains a major problem for the sound conduct of randomized controlled trials. Where knowledge about treatments is suspected to be a reason for non-participation, some doctors omit to advise their patients that they are in fact taking part in a randomized controlled trial. In a survey of European clinicians, Williams and Zwitter (1994) found that a concerning 12 per cent did not inform their patients that they were involved in a research study. Similarly, the UK Breast Cancer Coalition (1997) has raised concerns that research is still being undertaken without prior consent. The ethical issues surrounding this expedient are considerable and highlight the conflict of adequate recruitment versus informed choice and ethical practice. Unfortunately, recruitment problems and their associated dilemmas are further compounded by the pressure to conduct large sample trials, because of their enhanced power to detect clinical effects (Duley and Villar 2002). Therefore, small trials that operate on the basis of full consent/low recruitment may be less valuable and informative than large-scale trials, in that the results may have less relevance for the wider population; yet to conduct larger trials may involve a breach of medical ethics.

Moreover, while random allocation theoretically satisfies the needs of sound research principles, it challenges the rights of patients to choose their treatment and usurps the ultimate authority of the doctor, who by precedent has prescribed those interventions assumed to be appropriate based on what is usually referred to as clinical judgement (Downie and Macnaughton 2000). Taking account of patients' treatment preferences not only acknowledges their moral status, but also their power of self-determination and their right of autonomy. To ignore this fundamental principle is to disregard the essence of medical ethics, and yet this is precisely what the random allocation process involves. Where there is a potential treatment choice, the blind allocation of patients to intervention inevitably contravenes these issues. Thus another Catch 22 prevails: to establish a good scientific base of research on which the EBHC culture depends requires random allocation of patients to treatment, yet this disempowers the participating patients from making informed choices about their care – one of the governing principles of the new NHS culture. Thus while the generation of sound research evidence provides the information on which future patients can (at least in theory) select their treatment, the participants in those research studies may have been deprived of choice and information.

Statistics

The experimental method involves the collection of objective, numerical data, which have to be interpreted to establish whether or not they support the hypothesis under investigation. The interpretation process involves describing the data, in terms of their interesting features, as well as testing their significance, using inferential tests. The results of these tests permit the researcher to ascertain whether or not the results are due to chance factors or whether they support the hypothesis. In health research terms, the concept can be illustrated by a randomized controlled trial carried out by Steen *et al.* (2000) on childbirth-induced perineal trauma. Many women experience oedema, bruising and pain as a result of instrumental deliveries. Standard treatment procedures at the hospital involved in the study employ the local application of ice packs and Epifoam. The researchers compared these standard treatments with an alternative cooling device (maternity gel pads), for women's experience of pain, bruising, oedema and perceived effectiveness. The results were analysed using techniques of inferential statistics and demonstrated that the innovative gel pads were significantly better on each of the measures ($p = 0.048$, $p = 0.021$, $p = 0.01$, $p < 0.0005$, respectively). These probability values led the authors to conclude that the results were not due to chance factors operating at the time, but rather to the method of perineal treatment. The findings, then, would also permit the inference that the results obtained from this study would also apply to other women suffering perineal damage following instrumental deliveries and, in this way, would become recommended practice. On the basis of these results, a large clinical trial was commissioned to extend the study by examining the impact of the maternity gel pad on women who had not had instrumental deliveries and who were being cared for in the community. This study also embodies many of the features of a good theory, in that it's simple, falsifiable, makes predictions, generates other research and addresses a practical problem.

The findings obtained in this study (as with any that uses inferential statistics and probability values) provided information about the probability that the results were due to chance factors; they demonstrated evidence of a relationship between the method of treatment of the perineum and a range of clinical outcomes. But as with all inferential statistics, Steen and co-workers' findings could not claim that this relationship was invariable and constant, that it would always happen. This is a critical concept underpinning experimental research – however good the results, however strong the apparent support for the hypothesis, however many times the results are replicated, there is no absolute certainty that the same results will always be achieved (see section on 'Control groups' above). All that can ever be said is that there is support for the hypothesis, support which, of course, will grow each time a study replicates the findings. Such a notion drives systematic reviews, which are a corner-stone in the evidence-based health care culture. In these, reviewers assess a large number of studies to establish whether the studies are sound and whether the results accord with each other. If the studies sing from the same song sheet, then the findings are circulated with a view to modifying clinical practice.

Implicit within this idea of collecting together a large number of studies on the same topic and assessing the quality of their results, is the assumption that the studies are replications of each other. If they are and the findings are the same each time, then a mounting body of evidence is built up to suggest a link between the intervention and the outcome. But to what extent can a study ever be a true replica of any other? Where human participants are concerned, there will always be individual differences – in personality, medical condition, unknown idiopathic biochemical reactions, compli-ance with treatment, influence of other extraneous factors and the like that will make one sample of participants subtly different from another. In this respect, no study can ever replicate exactly any other, but if the samples of participants used in each study are typical or representative of the groups from which they're drawn, then the studies will bear greater similarity to each other than if the samples are not representative.

The use of statistics, then, goes some way towards informing the researcher as to how far the results of any given study may be due to random factors, such as indi-vidual differences. Moreover, despite the fact that most people are familiar with Disraeli's saying that 'there are lies, damned lies and statistics', they add credence and an air of objectivity to the findings. Most people, though, having listened to party political debates would accept that statistics can be used creatively to illustrate a point and bolster arguments. Even when there is no intention to deceive, statistics can still be hugely misleading. A Sunday broadsheet carried a very interesting and useful interpretation of breast cancer statistics that demonstrates just this point (*Independent on Sunday* 1997). The author of this article, Markie Robson-Scott, notes that women are told that they have a 1 in 12 chance of getting breast cancer, and that it is the most common cause of death for women aged 35–54 years. Robson-Scott deconstructs these statistics in a comforting manner and in a way that makes more sense. For instance, he points out that the 1 in 12 statistic applies to women who live to the age of 85 and that breast cancer is a disease of the older woman, with a third of all breast cancers being diagnosed in the 70–85 year age group. The 1 in 12 figure, then, is a cumulative risk and not a figure that applies to all women irrespective of their age. The incidence for the 35–50 year group is 1 in 1000, and for the 50–65 age group it is 1 in 500. The same argument can be applied to some of the risk factors associated with breast cancer. For instance, an early puberty is associated with a 33 per cent increased risk, which, for a woman aged 45, means that her chances of developing breast cancer are 1.3 in 1000. The statistics that should lend objectivity and credibility to this sort of epidemiological research cannot only mislead but alarm.

Suitability of the randomized controlled trial for health care research

While there are numerous problems attaching to the conduct and interpretation of any research, the theoretical appeal of the randomized controlled trial remains self-evident, because it at least attempts to minimize sources of potential bias to isolate the effect of the treatment. It should be science at its most logical, objective and accurate. But is it? Like other health care research, the randomized controlled trial involves the allocation of people to different interventions, with the assumption that providing due process has been followed, the groups will be more or less the same and that any differences in outcome between them will be the result of the treatment. But an intervention can be any treatment, from the administration of an anti-inflammatory drug to rheumatoid arthritis patients, to open-ended psychodynamic counselling for anorexic adolescents. While the randomized controlled trial may lend itself easily to the study of limited, definable treatment interventions, it is less valuable when it comes to holistic therapies, such as mental health care. For example, supposing an eating disorders unit sets up a randomized controlled trial to compare the effectiveness of a token economy system, psychodynamic counselling and rational emotive therapy in the treatment of anorexic patients. The study allocates the patients randomly and conforms to all the other requirements of the trial. The groups may look comparable, in that they don't differ significantly in age, gender, admission weight, weight loss, length of time anorexic, and so on – in other words, all the easily quantifiable characteristics. But what of the personality, both morbid and pre-morbid, the original cause(s) of the anorexia, the social factors and family influences, the extent of the peer group pressure, the susceptibility of each patient to media influences? How are these to be measured? How can we be sure that the groups are comparable on these more intangible, less quantifiable features? And what of the treatment processes? Psychodynamic counselling and rational emotive therapy are especially heavily dependent on the therapeutic relationship between therapist and patient for their success, and this relationship is, of necessity, a dynamic fluid one, governed to some extent by the personalities of the participants. How can the effect of this be isolated from the actual nature of the therapy itself? One intervention may indeed be revealed to be more effective than another, but maybe the patients and the therapists in that group simply liked each other more and hit it off better. Such uncertainties mean that the randomized controlled trial is less suitable for investigating complex interactive therapies, yet a great deal of health care activity is based on a total care package of treatment, which involves the relationship between health professional and patient. Where attempts have been made within the mental health arena, for instance, to use the randomized controlled trial paradigm to evaluate clinical interventions, the resulting problems have highlighted clearly the lack of universal relevance of this methodology. Adams (2002), in a survey of randomized controlled trials conducted on treatments for schizophrenia over the past 50 years, found that 86 per cent of the reported studies focused on pharmacological interventions, rather than the talking therapies. Moreover, Adams also found that 25 per cent of the studies did not use rating scales to measure outcomes (in other words, the results were not quantified, as properly befits the scientific process) and, of those that used numerical outcome measures, a third of these scales were unpublished and were therefore of doubtful

psychometric value. He also points out that as scales are rarely used in clinical practice, their value is clinically irrelevant.

Likewise, the nursing process, founded on the care of the patient as a whole,
sentient being and not just as the cholecystectomy in bed 4, means that it is unsuitable
for evaluation via this reductionist methodology; the Changing Childbirth initiative,
too, which was predicated on the assumption that having a named midwife throughout the ante-, peri- and post-natal periods leads to better outcomes, does not easily
lend itself to evaluation via the randomized controlled trial (although many attempts
have been made to do so). Such comments underline the point that in a relentless
quest for gold standard science and objectivity, clinical studies are often distorted to
fit a randomized controlled trial paradigm, a captive clinical problem on the Pro-
crustean bed of scientific method, a point made succinctly by Rogers (2002). Given
that the randomized controlled trial originated in agriculture, perhaps we should
not be surprised that the procedures used to assess optimal growing conditions for
cabbages do not readily apply to more complex human problems.

All these points notwithstanding, the randomized controlled trial has managed to
pervade just about every corner of medical and health care research, however potentially inappropriate. Indeed, a glance at the content subheadings of the journal
Evidence-based Health Care reveals that alongside 'evidence-based clinical practice',
there is also 'evidence-based public health', 'evidence-based health-care management'
and 'evidence-based health care promotion', all of which carry articles that review
randomized controlled trials conducted with highly complex interactive health
issues, such as de Fine Olivarius and co-workers' (2001) study on diabetes (see above).

The problem within these health interventions is what Plsek and Greenhalgh call
'a complex adaptive system', which they define as:

> A collection of individual agents with freedom to act in ways that are not always
> totally predictable and whose actions are interconnected so that one agent's
> actions change the context for other agents. Examples include . . . just about any
> collection of humans (for example, a family, a committee or a primary health care
> team).
>
> (Plsek and Greenhalgh 2001, p. 625)

In a highly useful discourse, Plsek and Greenhalgh suggest that these complex systems have fuzzy boundaries, with changing membership, role functions and social
contexts, and that every individual in the group interprets and responds to their
environment according to a set of personal rules, constructs, intuitions, hunches and
the like. The rules are not necessarily explicit or logical, which means that other
members of the group do not share the same understanding of any given situation and
consequently do not respond in the same way. And most importantly, each individual
has a degree of behavioural autonomy – a point that will be returned to later. Moreover, each complex adaptive system interacts with others, such that the primary care
team as a system will interact with the acute hospital, the community team, the work-
force confederation, the Department of Health and so on, each of which constitutes
another complex system. Therefore, the understanding and investigation of one system cannot take place without full consideration of the other systems that impact

upon it. In addition, the behaviour of a complex system is a result of the interaction between the individuals that comprise it, and is of necessity unpredictable. However, many circumstances in health care provision demand that the system's behaviour should respond in an adaptive way to externally imposed demands, such as the adoption of clinical guidelines in the treatment of stroke patients. These circumstances have been called 'the edge of chaos' (Langton 1989), or the zone of complexity, in that they are characterized by only moderate to low levels of agreement and certainty among the system's members about what should be done when confronted by a patient suffering from a defined medical condition. Where there is a high level of agreement and certainty among members about a course of action, the problem and its solution are relatively simple (for instance, management of chronic lymphocytic leukaemia); where there is no agreement or certainty, there is complete chaos (e.g. treatment programmes for people with eating disorders) (Kernick 2002). The purpose of conventional scientific reductionism and the randomized controlled trial is to tease out the component parts of the zone of complexity, and to test the suitability of each of these before recommending a course of action. While the impact and efficacy of the cytotoxic drugs and corticosteroids used for chronic lymphocytic leukaemia can be evaluated in this way, the psychotherapeutic input into the treatment of individuals with eating disorders cannot be so readily broken down for componential investigation. So called 'Complexity science' suggests that multifactorial explanations and approaches are more productive in these sorts of situation (e.g. Schon's reflective practitioner and Kolb's experiential learning cycle). Complicated, multi-layered interventions do not lend and bend themselves to evaluation and study by randomized controlled trials, which means that a considerable proportion of health care activity is removed from this type of research investigation. Because health care operates as a system of non-linear relationships across and between layers (e.g. from the individual patient and practitioner, through the multidisciplinary team, to the Trust and various NHS management strata) it must be classified as a chaotic system (Kernick 2002). The assumption of the randomized controlled trial that it is suitable for evaluating health care interventions because there is a simple linear cause and effect relationship between treatment input and clinical outcome must therefore be challenged.

What is also of particular interest in the context of evidence-based health care is the zone of simplicity, the area of high agreement and high certainty about what to do next. A classic example might be the decision taken by a multi-professional obstetric team to deliver a severely distressed foetus by Caesarian section. The situation is relatively unambiguous and the choice of action for each individual is clear. But where this situation prevails, the decision making and response also become mechanistic, with individuals abandoning their professional autonomy or right to 'clinical judgement'. Yet it is this clinical judgement that allows a patient or a situation to be treated as unique. The dilemma is obvious: very few health care situations can be reduced to such an unambiguous set of decisions and behaviours, yet the current thinking demands that there are treatment protocols based on randomized controlled trials for a great number of interventions. Not only is the concept highly dubious, but the methodology on which these protocols are founded may be highly inappropriate for complex adaptive systems. Indeed, the inherent complexity of health care provision would explain that where simple linear analyses have been used to inform care delivery, they have been unsuccessful (Kernick 2002). Health care delivery is essentially a social system that is non-linear and cannot therefore be forced into a linear analytical framework.

Many analysts have raised concerns about the domination of health care by the evidence-based health care culture (Walshe and Rundall 2001), some of which emerge from the foregoing discussion. It is clear that adhering to research-guided protocols stifles innovation, deskills the clinician, sidelines his or her judgement and overrides the individual patient's choice. Other critics focus on the preoccupation of the new culture with experimental research, almost to the exclusion of all others, an oversight that is especially concerning in the light of the poor quality of much of the published experimental research (Walshe and Rundall 2001). Moreover, much of the experimental work in health care is so obsessed with quantifiable outcomes that the global picture of the patient is overlooked. Yet despite the objections, the randomized controlled trial paradigm continues to gain momentum. The reasons why (both official and unofficial) have been articulated many times before, but without doubt one major driver continues to be the mounting cost of the health service, which can only begin to cope with a concomitant rise in demand for high-quality care if cost-effective treatments are used routinely rather than haphazardly and ineffective treatments are eliminated. Another driver, of course, is fear of litigation.

The foregoing argument suggests that the topics that can be usefully investigated using a randomized controlled trial are, of necessity, small and medium scale ones (Jadad 1998). Because of the degree of control that is required to eliminate extraneous variables that may impact on the results, looking at holistic problems via a randomized controlled trial is rendered meaningless. In other words, such trials are useful for looking at the component parts of complex wholes, but have little relevance for an investigation of the whole. Moreover, reductionist approaches typically concentrate on physical phenomena, since these are considered to be the only real data. This latter point alone makes the experimental study of any non-organic mental disorder impossible, yet this does not seem to have deterred the advocates of randomized controlled trials (Adams 2002). Many other examples come to mind, but one of the most interesting is that of restoration of sight for the congenitally blind – despite the clinical success of the procedure, many patients suffer serious post-operative mental health problems (Gregory 1977), highlighting clearly the point that quality of life and outcome cannot always be measured in simple clinical and numerical terms. The value of reductionist approaches has been subject to much debate, especially in the social sciences, whose foci of interest are the human psyche, groups of people, societies and the like, which tend to render the experiment in all its forms somewhat irrelevant. Since the main sources of health care research are also people, organizations and groups with similar medical problems, the same argument could similarly be levelled at the application of the randomized controlled trial in this domain. However, Rose (1976) uses semantics to reconcile the position to some extent, differentiating between the need to explain and the need to explain away. If reductionist approaches are used to understand the core components that together make the whole, but are used in a complementary way with holistic methods that address the more global picture, then together proper research progress is possible. If, on the other hand, reductionism is construed and used as the only valid method of obtaining research

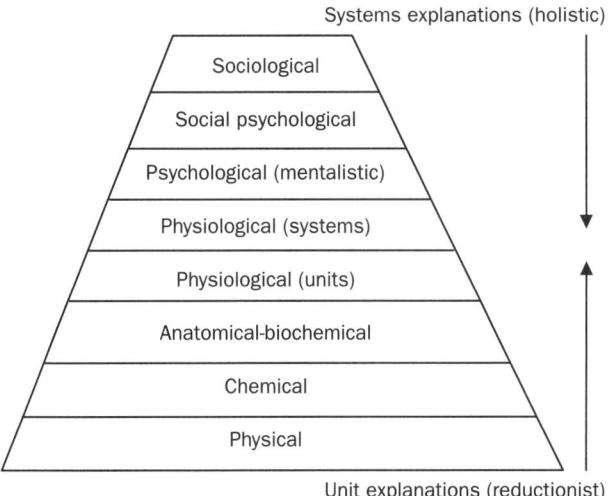

Figure 5.1 The hierarchy of levels of explanation (from Rose 1976).

evidence, then progress will be confined only to an understanding of the part and not the whole. Rose portrays his conceptualization as a hierarchy of levels of explanation (see Figure 5.1).

The different levels equate with different scientific disciplines, with the lower levels relating to the classical sciences of physics and chemistry, and the higher ones to the more modern social sciences. The knowledge gained from each level can inform any other, but cannot replace it, since their purpose and functions are different. Rose refers to this as the universe of discourse, a set of concepts, terminologies, methodologies and means of conceptualizing events. Each level has its own universe of discourse that is appropriate for its purpose. Such an explanation has immediate appeal for health research and permits co-operation and co-existence between different methodologies, which together increase the possibility that useful research-driven knowledge can be obtained at every level. What is also clear is that where the point of interest is the patient, the group of patients, the health care professional, the organization or whatever, the randomized controlled trial cannot be acclaimed as the 'gold-standard' approach. It is clearly appropriate for investigating some of the lower levels of the hierarchy, but cannot satisfy the sorts of questions that need to be addressed at the upper levels. It is perhaps time for a paradigm shift.

Conclusion

The randomized controlled trial has frequently been held up as the only valid route both to medical truth and to improved health provision. Yet far from being objective and impartial, the scientific method is as riddled with value-judgements as the less esteemed qualitative approaches. The question of what is researched, how and by whom all introduce bias, which together with additional decisions about what is published and how the research results are implemented, collectively add cumulative layers of potential distortion. This is not to say that the methodology isn't useful, or that other research techniques are superior. What this chapter and the previous one have aimed to achieve instead is an element of caution, whereby the reader can bring a healthy degree of scepticism and informed judgement when confronted with the claims of statistics and experimental research. And, of course, the evidence cited to support the arguments throughout this chapter and the last is unlikely to be objective and value-free either. The only conclusion that can realistically be drawn is that all knowledge and research are susceptible to bias and all are driven by a value-system that is often unacknowledged – and this claim applies to any discipline that is founded on a bedrock of research evidence. But within health care, the problem is compounded by the inherent complexities of the systems and multi-layered interactions that are involved. Clinical interventions cannot be reduced to simple linear cause/effect relationships and, as a result, the application of the randomized controlled trial may have limited relevance. In conjunction with other sources of evidence, the randomized controlled trial has its place in contributing to medical knowledge and in informing interventions, but of itself cannot be considered to be either a sufficient fount of wisdom or a wholly objective one. Complementarity and multi-disciplinarity are the current names of the health care game; the concepts should apply equally to the research on which it is founded.

References

Acheson, D. (1998) *Independent Inquiry into Inequalities in Health*. London: The Stationery Office.

Adams, C. (2002) What have we learned from 50 years of randomised controlled trials for people with schizophrenia?, in L. Duley and B. Farrell (eds) *Clinical Trials*. London: BMJ Books.

Altman, D.G. and Dore, C.J. (1990) Randomisation and baseline comparisons in clinical trials, *Lancet*, 335(8682): 149–53.

Archer, J. (1992) Gender stereotyping of school subjects, *The Psychologist*, 5: 66–9.

Bagenal, F.S., Easton, D.F., Harris, E., Chilvers, C.E. and McElwain, T.J. (1990) Survival of patients with breast cancer attending the Bristol Cancer Help Centre, *Lancet*, 336(8715): 606–10.

Barloon, T.J. and Noyes, R. Jr. (1997) Charles Darwin and panic disorder, *Journal of the American Medical Association*, 277(2): 138–41.

Bartholomew, R.E. and Wessely, S. (2002) Protean nature of mass psychogenic illness: from possessed nuns to chemical and biological terrorism fears, *British Journal of Psychiatry*, 180: 300–6.

Berge, E. and Sandercock, P. (2002) The nuts and bolts of doing a clinical trial, in L. Duley and B. Farrell (eds) *Clinical Trials*. London: BMJ Books.

Bernard, C. (1885) *An Introduction to the Study of Experimental Medicine*. Paris: Henry Schuman.

Blanks, R.G., Moss, S.M., McGahan, C.E., Quinn, M.J. and Babb, P.J. (2000) Effect of NHS breast cancer screening programme on mortality from breast cancer in England and Wales 1990–1998: comparison of observed with predicted mortality, *British Medical Journal*, 321: 665–9.

Bordieri, J.E., Scotolongo, M. and Wilson, M. (1983) Physical attractiveness and attributions for disability, *Rehabilitation Psychology*, 28: 207–15.

Brawley, O.W. (1999) The study of untreated syphilis in the Negro male, *International Journal of Radiation Oncology, Biology, Physics*, 40(1): 5–8.

Burns, V.E., Carroll, D., Ring, C., Harrison, L.K. and Drayson, M. (2002) Stress, coping and hepatitis B antibody status, *Psychosomatic Medicine*, 64(2): 287–93.

Campbell, A., Gillett, G. and Jones, G. (2001) *Medical Ethics*, 3rd edn. Oxford: Oxford University Press.

Cleverly, D. (1998) Nursing research – taking an active interest, *Nurse Education Today*, 18(4): 267–72.

Corter, C. (1978) Nurses: judgements of the attractiveness of premature infants, *Infant Behaviour and Development*, 1(4): 432–9.

Cowles, M. and Davis, C. (1987) The subject matter of psychology: volunteers, *British Journal of Social Psychology*, 26: 289–94.

Cox, D.C.T. (2002) Histories of controlled trials, in I. Chalmers, I. Milne and U. Troher (eds) *Controlled Trials from History* (www.rcpe.ac.uk/controlled_trials).

Darbyshire, P. (1986) When the face doesn't fit, *Nursing Times*, 24 September.

David, F.N. (1962) *Games, God and Gambling*. New York: Hafner.

Davies, C. (1998) *Gender and the Professional Predicament in Nursing*. Buckingham: Open University Press.

de Fine Olivarius, N., Beck-Nielsen, H., Andreasen, A.H., Horder, M. and Pedersen, P.A. (2001) Randomised controlled trial of structured personal care of type 2 diabetes mellitus, *British Medical Journal*, 323: 970–5.

Dixon, M. and Sweeney, K. (2000) *The Human Effect in Medicine: Theory, Research and Practice*. Abingdon: Radcliffe Medical Press.

Downie, R.S. and Macnaughton, J. (2000) *Clinical Judgement: Evidence in Practice*. Oxford: Oxford University Press.

Duley, L. and Villar, J. (2002) Big is still beautiful: why we still need large simple trials, in L. Duley and B. Farrell (eds) *Clinical Trials*. London: BMJ Books.

Durkheim, E. ([1897] 1953) *Suicide* (translated by J.A. Spaulding and G. Simpson). London: Routledge & Kegan Paul.

Edwards, D., Ashmore, M. and Potter, J. (1995) Death and furniture: the rhetoric, politics, and theology of bottom line arguments against relativism, *History of the Human Sciences*, 8(2): 25–49.

Evans, D. (2003) *Placebo: The Belief Effect*. London: HarperCollins.

Feyerabend, P. (1999) *Knowledge, Science and Relativism: Philosophical Papers*, Vol. 3 (edited by J. Preston). Cambridge: Cambridge University Press.

Fibiger, J. (1898) On treatment of diphtheria with serum, *Hospitalstidende*, 6: 309–25.

Fox, N.J. (1993) Discourse, organisation and the surgical ward round, *Sociology of Health and Illness*, 15(1): 16–42.

Frenkel-Brunswick, E. (1949) Intolerance of ambiguity as an emotional and perceptual personality variable, *Journal of Personality*, 18: 108–43.

Gamarnikov, E. (1978) Sexual division of labour: the case of nursing, in A. Kuhn and A.-M. Wolpe (eds) *Feminism and Materialism*. London: Routledge & Kegan Paul.

Gamble, V.N. (1997) The Tuskegee syphilis study and women's health, *Journal of the American Medical Women's Association*, 52(4): 195–6.

Gregory, R.L. (1977) *Eye and Brain*. London: Weidenfeld & Nicholson.

Guttenplan, D.D. (2001) *The Holocaust Trial, Justice and the David Irving Case*. London: Granta.

Hacohen, H. (1998) Karl Popper, the Vienna Circle, and Red Vienna, *Journal of the History of Ideas*, 59(4): 711–34.

Harwood, R. (1978) *Did Six Million Really Die?* Southam, Warwickshire: Historical Review Press.

Hayes, R.J., Smith, P.G. and Carpenter, L. (1990) Bristol Cancer Help Centre: Letter to the editor, *Lancet*, 336(8724): 1185.

Health Service Journal (2002) News in brief, *Health Service Journal*, 112(5823): 6.

Hicks, C. (1992) Of sex and status: a study of the effects of gender and occupation on nurses' evaluations of nursing research, *Journal of Advanced Nursing*, 17: 1343–9.

Hicks, C. (1996) Nurse researcher: a study of a contradiction in terms?, *Journal of Advanced Nursing*, 24: 357–63.

Hughes, J. and Sharrock, W. (1997) *The Philosophy of Social Research*, 3rd edn. London: Longman.

Irving, D. (1983) *The War Path: Hitler's Germany, 1933–1939*. London: Macmillan.

Jadad, A.R. (1998) *Randomised Controlled Trials: A User's Guide*. London: BMJ Books.

Kass, N.E. and Sugarman, J. (1996) Are research subjects adequately protected? A review and discussion of studies conducted by the Advisory Committee on Human Radiation Experiments, *Kennedy Institute of Ethics Journal*, 6(3): 271–82.

Kernick, D. (2002) Complexity in health care continued: on chaos, *British Journal of Health Care Management*, 8(10): 376–9.

Kiecolt-Glaser, J.K., McGuire, L., Robles, T.F. and Glaser, R. (2002) Psychoneuroimmunology and psychosomatic medicine: back to the future, *Psychosomatic Medicine*, 64(1): 15–28.

Kristensen, B.O. and Kornerup, H.J. (1982) Which arm to measure blood pressure?, *Acta Medica Scandinavica Supplementum*, 670: 69–73.

Kuhn, T.S. (1996) *The Structure of Scientific Revolutions*, 3rd edn. Chicago, IL: University of Chicago Press.

Langton, C.G. (ed.) (1989) *Artificial Life: The Proceedings of an Interdisciplinary Workshop on the Synthesis and Stimulation of Living Systems*. Redwood City, CA: Addison-Wesley.

Lyotard, J.-F. (1988) *The Differend: Phrases in Dispute* (translated by G. Van Den Abbeele). Minneapolis, MN: University of Minnesota Press.

Medawar, P. (1963) *The Art of the Soluble*. Harmondsworth: Penguin.

Meerabeau, L. (1997) Why are our grant applications continually rejected?, *Nurse Researcher*, 5(1): 5–13.

Moher, D., Fortin, P., Jadad, A.R. *et al.* (1996) Completeness of reporting trials in languages other than English: implications for the conduct and reporting of systematic reviews, *Lancet*, 347(8998): 363–6.

Monod, J. (1972) *Chance and Necessity: An Essay on the Natural Philosophy of Modern Biology*. New York: Random House.

Mulkay, M. (1979) *Science and the Sociology of Knowledge*. London: Allen & Unwin.

Olsen, O. and Goetzsche, P.C. (2000) There is something wrong in the studies of mammography! No support for the conclusions about the benefits of breast cancer screening. *Lakartidningen*, 97(4): 286–7.

Olsen, O. and Goetzsche, P.C. (2001a) Screening for breast cancer with mammography, *Cochrane database of Systematic Reviews*, 4 CD001877.

Olsen, O. and Goetzsche, P.C. (2001b) Cochrane review on screening for breast cancer with mammography, *Lancet*, 358(9290): 1340–2.

Pasnau, R.O. (1990) Darwin's illness: a biopsychosocial perspective, *Psychosomatics*, 31(2): 121–8.

Plsek, P. and Greenhalgh, T. (2001) The challenge of complexity in health care, *British Medical Journal*, 323: 625–8.

Polit-O'Hara, D. and Hungler, B. (1995) *Nursing Research: Principles and Methods*. (5th Edition) Philadelphia: Lippincott.

Popper, K.R. ([1935] 1959) *The Logic of Scientific Discovery*. London: Hutchinson.

Popper, K. (1968) *Conjecture and Refutations: The Growth of Scientific Knowledge*. New York: Harper & Row.

Popper, K. (1983) *Realism and the Aim of Science*. London: Hutchinson.

Prescott, R.J., Counsell, C.E., Gillespie, W.J. *et al.* (2002) Improving the quality, number and progress of randomised controlled trials, in L. Duley and B. Farrell (eds) *Clinical Trials*. London: BMJ Books.

Richards, T. (1990) Death from complementary medicine. *British Medical Journal*, 301: 510–11.

Robson-Scott, M. (1997) Be aware – but don't panic, *Independent on Sunday*, 28 September.

Roff, S.R. (2000) Human radiation experiments: what price informed consent?, *Medicine, Conflict and Survival*, 16(3): 291–301.

Rogers, W.A. (2002) Evidence-based medicine in practice: limiting or facilitating patient choice?, *Health Expectations*, 5: 95–103.

Rose, S. (1976) *The Conscious Brain*. Harmondsworth: Penguin.

Rosenthal, R. and Rosnow, R. (1975) *The Volunteer Subject*. New York: Riley.

Samei, E. and Kearfott, K.J. (1995) A limited bibliography of the federal Government funded human radiation experiments, *Health Physics*, 69(6): 885–91.

Schopenhauer, A. ([1851] 1974) *Parerga and Paralipomena: Short Philosophical Essays* (translated by E.F.J. Payne). Oxford: Clarendon Press.

Schultz, K.F., Chalmers, I., Hayes, R.J. and Altman, D.G. (1995) Empirical evidence of bias: dimensions of methodological quality associated with estimates of treatment effects in controlled trials, *Journal of the American Medical Association*, 273: 408–12.

Sepa, A., Frodi, A. and Ludvigsson, J. (2002) Could parenting stress and lack of support/confidence function as mediating mechanisms between certain environmental factors and the development of autoimmunity in children? A study within ABIS, *Annals of the New York Academy of Sciences*, 958: 431–5.

Sheard, T.A.B. (1990) Bristol Cancer Help Centre: Letter to the editor, *Lancet* 336(8716): 1185–6.

Shepherd, E., Rafferty, M. and James, V. (1996) Prescribing the boundaries of nursing practice: professional regulation and nurse prescribing, *Nursing Times Research*, 1(16): 465–78.

Silverman, W.A. and Chalmers, I. (2002) Casting and drawing lots, in I. Chalmers, I. Milne and U. Troher (eds) *Controlled Trials from History* (www.rcpe.ac.uk/controlled_trials).

Steen, M., Cooper, K., Marchant, P., Griffiths-Jones, M. and Walker, J. (2000) A randomised controlled trial to compare the effectiveness of ice-packs and Epifoam with cooling maternity gel pads at alleviating postnatal perineal trauma, *Midwifery*, 16: 48–55.

Stephan, C.W. and Langlois, J.H. (1984) Baby beautiful: adult attributions of infant competence as a function of infant attractiveness, *Child Development*, 55(2): 576–85.

Stewart, M. (2001) Whose evidence counts? An exploration of health professionals' perceptions of evidence-based practice, focusing on the maternity services, *Midwifery*, 17: 279–88.

Thomas, B.C., Pandey, M., Ramdas, K. and Nair, M.K. (2002) Psychological distress in cancer patients: hypothesis of a distress model, *European Journal of Cancer Prevention*, 11(2): 179–85.

Thomas, W.I. and Thomas, D.S. (1928) *The Child in America: Behaviour Problems and Programs*. New York: Knopf.

Townsend, P., Donaldson, N. and Whitehead, M. (1990) *Inequalities in Health: The Black Report and the Health Divide*. London: Penguin.

UK Breast Cancer Coalition (1997) Breast cancer: research without consent, *Journal of Medical Ethics*, 23(6): 372.

Walsh, M.P. (1998) What is evidence? A critical view for nursing, *Clinical Effectiveness in Nursing*, 2: 86–93.

Walsh, M. and Ford, P. (1994) *Nursing Rituals, Research and Rational Actions*. Oxford: Butterworth-Heinemann.

Walshe, K. and Rundall, T.G. (2001) Evidence-based management: from theory to practice in health care, *Milbank Quarterly*, 79(3): 429–57.

Webb, P.A. (1980) Effectiveness of patient education and psychological counseling in promoting compliance and control among hypertensive patients, *Journal of Family Practice*, 10: 1047–55.

West, C. (1854) *Lectures on the Diseases of Infancy and Childhood*. London: Longman, Brown, Green & Longman.

Williams, C.J. and Zwitter, M. (1994) Informed consent in European multicentre trials – are patients really informed?, *European Journal of Cancer*, 30A: 907–10.

Witz, A. (1992) *Professions and Patriarchy*. London: Routledge.

Wolpert, L. (1992) *The Unnatural Nature of Science*. Cambridge, MA: Harvard University Press.

Yoshioka, A. (1998) Use of randomisation in the Medical Research Council's clinical trial of streptomycin in pulmonary tuberculosis in the 1940s, *British Medical Journal*, 317: 1220–3.

6

Experiments in medicine and the health sciences

While experimental methods had been accelerating the productivity of chemists, physicists and biologists since the nineteenth century, medics, nurses and other health care workers were slow to catch on to the power of the experiment. In Chapter 5, we considered the role of the experiment in health care research and some of the issues relating to experimental methods, such as the difficulty in making observations with the required level of objectivity and the generalizability of results from the sometimes small and specialized samples involved. The peculiar case of experiments in health care requires some additional consideration, however, because the role of randomized controlled trials – the most high-profile manifestation of experimental design in medicine – represents a revolution in thinking about health and illness too. The experiment is not just a means to an end, in a naive, technical way, but is important in establishing and defining the very role of medicine itself. Experiments involve conceptualizing health and illness in particular ways, as a sequence of actions by pathogens and drugs, and also, by implication, help to carve out a particularly favourable niche for medicine within the human condition. Randomized controlled trials are fundamental in creating a role for health care professionals in contemporary life.

Thus in this chapter we shall investigate the special status of health care disciplines and discuss why their forms of enquiry, which once upon a time were so blatantly non-experimental, have come to be dominated by experimental designs. Perhaps the answer to this explosion of experimentation comes from having to justify the contribution medicine makes to human welfare. In the early twenty-first century, it is largely taken for granted that medicine is good for us as individuals and for populations. In the event of disaster, medical aid is sent just as urgently as food.

Yet there are many commentators who have called into question the role of medicine in the rapid rise in life expectancy seen in the industrialized world in the last 200 years. The most famous critiques of medicine's ability to improve the human condition were written by Ivan Illich (e.g. 1976), but others have questioned medicine's role, for example McKeown (1976) and Greenberg and Raymond (1999). Commentators such as these point out that, for example, tuberculosis rates were in decline well before the discovery of the bacillus responsible in 1880, and that the psychiatric hospital population was in decline before the use of neuroleptics became widespread. Instead, these authors point to the large contributions made to human welfare by public health improvements in diet and sanitation, modernization and industrialization rather than medicine *per se*. Aligned with these arguments, which minimize medicine's role, is a growing suspicion that many health care interventions are ineffective. For an industry that absorbs so much of the resources of the developed world (about one seventh of the gross national product of the USA in 1999, according to Greenberg and Raymond 1999), this could put the health care industry in a potentially embarrassing position.

There is therefore a pressing need to demonstrate medicine's effectiveness and that it gives value for money. The randomized controlled clinical trial is now a feature of the health care research landscape. It is so firmly entrenched that it appears to be inviolable. There is often a hierarchy of evidence established in a good deal of policy such that the evidence from randomized controlled trials is granted a special status, as if it had privileged access to the reality underlying heath care practice. In the UK and USA, the whole evidence-based practice movement is built around randomized controlled clinical trials. In a sense, they form a gravity well in the epistemological space time fabric. The predominant model seems to be that evidence is gathered in these experiments and is then applicable to clinical practice in the future. Experiments in health care are establishing that medical science is in dialogue with the very fabric of nature itself. The experiment borrows from the rhetoric of science as well as drawing upon a culturally entrenched rhetoric of reductionism (Dupre 1983). This involves the belief that phenomena can be specified and studied by making sense of them in terms of more basic elements or processes. In everyday life we might more or less be persuaded that, say, biology can be explained in terms of chemistry or that chemistry can be explained in terms of physics. This involves 'looking at reality in an analytical way, by decomposing the research object into aspects and particles' (Verschuren 2001, p. 389). In the case of experiments in health care, the leap is comparable between health and well-being and the processes that can be studied with experiments. They provide a sort of touchstone to our faith in science and if the practice of medicine can be based more completely on experiments as heuristic devices, then it can vouchsafe its credibility and social utility. Indeed, in recent years this rationale has become even more conspicuously formulated in the shape of 'evidence-based practice' initiatives in health and social care.

To understand the special role of experiments in health care, let us first go back a little way and describe some of the origins of this evidence-based spirit in health care and identify the role that these kinds of experiments can take in establishing the credibility and value of health care interventions. At present, this vogue for evidence-based practice has gripped clinical practitioners and policy makers, and researchers have been keen to lend their findings to this influential movement too.

The definition of evidence-based practice by Sackett *et al.* probably still commands considerable assent among practitioners and researchers:

> the conscientious, explicit and judicious use of current best evidence in making decisions about the care of individual patients, based on the skills which allow the doctor [*sic*] to evaluate both personal experience and external evidence in a systematic and objective manner.

(Sackett *et al.* 1996, p. 71)

The hierarchy of evidence that tends to be promoted in accounts of evidence-based practice on both sides of the Atlantic tends to place randomized controlled trials – experiments, in other words – at the top of the list. Here, for example, is the kind of typology of evidence presented by the UK's Department of Health (1996). In descending order of credibility it goes:

1   Strong evidence from at least one systematic review of multiple well-designed randomized controlled trials.

2   Strong evidence from at least one properly designed randomized controlled trial of appropriate size.

3   Evidence from well-designed trials such as non-randomized trials, cohort studies, time series or matched case-controlled studies.

4   Evidence from well-designed non-experimental studies from more than one centre or research group.

5   Opinions of respected authorities, based on clinical evidence, descriptive studies or reports of expert committees.

Thus the only thing better than a randomized controlled trial is a large number of these which are sufficiently similar that their data (or perhaps some measure of effect size) can be added together in a systematic review. This, then, is the evidence on which practitioners are encouraged to base their work.

The arguments in favour of evidence-based practice are made to sound persuasive on scientific, humane and economic grounds. The spectre of expensive and ineffective interventions falling to the astute gaze of empirical scrutiny is an attractive one. Given the support on the part of researchers, policy makers and managers for this approach to health care, it is perhaps surprising that it does not make even more rapid headway. In principle, it seems to be endorsed as a service philosophy among health care staff. Yet as we have shown elsewhere (Crawford et al. 2002), it is often not implemented because of difficulties in finding or interpreting the relevant research and lack of time to put the interventions suggested by the evidence into practice. The key part of the appeal of evidence-based practice is the way that it encourages us to think that health care is perfectible.

This enthusiasm for evidence-based practice gained in strength through the 1990s and into the twenty-first century despite some severe difficulties. First, there was a notorious difficulty in applying the formal models of evidence-based health care in some fields, such as mental health care and nursing in particular, because no matter how fully we try to specify the details of a psycho-social intervention, there will be aspects of the way it is delivered in practice that may vary in clinically significant ways and over which the researcher has no control (Parry 2000). By extension, this kind of problem may well affect other apparently more physically based therapies, too. So at the same time as randomized controlled clinical trials are being promoted as a way of making sense of the field of health care, their very identity as heuristic tools is subject to some scepticism.

This curious tension is perhaps one reason why randomized controlled clinical trials have a relatively recent history in the health care disciplines. Especially when we consider that the logic of randomized controlled clinical trials in their present form has existed for several centuries. However, there was a long and tortuous process before they emerged in their present early twenty-first-century form. There were a number of contributing factors to their evolution, derived from many different research techniques and epistemological tensions.

The earliest reference to a random process in assessing treatments in the European literature is cited by Richard Doll (1998), writing in a special issue of the *British Medical Journal* to mark the 50th anniversary of the randomized controlled trial in medicine. This kind of looking backwards to history is a potent means of establishing the authenticity of a practice, especially if it can be linked to some famous authority of days gone by. Doll, for example, argues that the idea for these kinds of experiments goes back three centuries rather than 50 years. The method was proposed originally, he says, by a chemist called van Helmont in 1662 when he challenged the academics of the day to test their treatments based on theory with his based on experience.

> Let us take out of the hospitals, out of the Camps, or from elsewhere, 200, or 500 poor People, that have Fevers, Pleurisies, etc. Let us divide them into half, let us cast lots, that one half of them may fall to my share, and the other to yours . . . We shall see how many funerals both of us shall have. But let the reward of the contention or wager, be 300 florens, deposited on both sides.
>
> (Doll 1998, p. 1218)

Sadly, the challenge was not accepted. This romantic evocation, a kind of modern-day consciousness in days gone by, is a literary device whose role has been noted in studies of romantic novels (Radway 1987). This rhetorical motif involves identifying the precursors of the present in the past, such that it looks like present-day attitudes, beliefs and ways of making sense of the world are adequate to make sense of everything. It is reassuring, says Radway, because no matter how far away people might be culturally or historically, it's still pretty much the same as the leafy suburbs of small town America. So, too, with science. If our forebears thought like us, then this consolidates and verifies the certainties of the present.

The primacy of the randomized controlled trial in health care research is a species of naturalism. As Danto puts it:

> Naturalism . . . is a species of philosophical monism according to which whatever exists or happens is natural in the sense of being susceptible to explanation through methods which, although paradigmatically exemplified in the natural sciences, are continuous from domain to domain . . . Hence, naturalism is polemically defined as repudiating the view that there exists or could exist any entities or events which lie, in principle, beyond the scope of scientific explanation.
>
> (Danto 1967, p. 448)

As we shall argue, the spirit of naturalism is alive and well in the health sciences. It exists in the implicit view that all the important elements of health care can be extracted from their ecological context and either controlled or manipulated in an experiment.

The early attempt by van Helmont to design a forerunner of the modern-day randomized controlled trial with an element of chance governing the assignment of patients to groups was not taken up in practice until some 250 years later. Health care, as we have seen, was often a discipline that relied on theory and practice rather than on science. Experiments were mostly done in laboratories rather than in hospitals until the latter part of the twentieth century.

There were, however, some notable exceptions. Experiments occasionally left the laboratory and were nurtured into life in clinics. A noteworthy example, again often used in histories of experiments in medicine, involved a trial of serum treatment in diphtheria conducted by a Danish doctor, Johannes Fibiger, in 1896–1897 (Hrobjartsson *et al.* 1998). Although not strictly random by today's standards, it allowed the researchers to systematically separate the decision about whether the patient was in the treatment or control group from anything that might influence the outcome. The method used depended on the day the patient attended. Patients arriving on alternate days were assigned to the different groups in the experiment. Thus, Monday's patients might be in the treatment group, whereas Tuesday's might be in the control group. They were tested to ensure that they did indeed have diphtheria. In Fibiger's experiment, 8 of 239 patients in the serum treated group and 30 of 245 in the control group died. No formal statistical analysis was performed but 'no objection can be raised against the statistical significance of the numbers', which were deemed correct by an inspector of the sick benefit association (Hrobjartsson *et al.* 1998, p. 1243). It was still four years before Karl Pearson would invent his famous Chi-square test, but had it been available at the time it would have yielded a P-value of 0.0003, well inside the usual 0.05 threshold familiar to researchers today. The results were decisive, however, even in the absence of formal statistical testing.

This study was performed early in Fibiger's career. He was only 28 years old at the time. Later he was to receive the Nobel Prize for a rather different piece of work, involving nematodes and cancer in rats, but even as a young man in his 20s his design of the diphtheria study set in motion a number of issues. Fibiger emphasized four methodological features of the trial that would be recognizable to researchers nowadays. 'Even with minimal knowledge of diphtheria epidemics, one will realise that it is necessary to have, firstly, large numbers and, secondly, a long study period.' Thirdly, he stated that 'To compensate for the large seasonal variation in mortality, the study should last at least one year.' His fourth contribution was an emphasis on random allocation and the avoidance of bias: 'Truly, the control cases in the earlier studies were selected to be as similar as possible to the ones treated with serum, but to eliminate completely the play of chance and the influence of subjective judgment, one had to use a different procedure. The only method which could be used rationally was to treat some patients with serum and every other patient in the usual way' (quotes from Hrobjartsson *et al.* 1998, p. 1244). Here we can see the liberal use of references to common knowledge in Fibiger's account, as if this new research method were merely the application of what any intellectual of the day would find commonsensical and universally agreeable. It is this readiness to exploit the folkways and lay theories of epistemology that has guaranteed the success of the randomized controlled trial in health care subsequently. Moreover, the epistemological persuasiveness of this manoeuvre has allowed a number of other subtle reconfigurations of the subject matter of medicine as if they were necessary casualties in the battle for truth.

In line with other aspects of modern clinical research, Fibiger tried to make sure the outcomes of his diphtheria research were defined as clearly and unambiguously as possible. Whether the patients lived or died, of course, was relatively easy to record, but other measures included croup, dislodgement of membranes, temperature, albuminuria and paralysis. He also tried to maximize the reliability of the observations by using 'concordant observations by the consultant and myself'.

The implications of this study were considerable. Even though the method was relatively novel, it clearly had enormous persuasive power. As a result of the visible success of serum treatment, the demand for the new treatment increased so rapidly that a whole new 'Serum Institute' was built. There was another important implication. The serum had unpleasant side-effects. 'Serum sickness' was feared so much that when doctors themselves contracted diphtheria from their patients, they would often refuse serum treatment (Hrobjartsson et al. 1998, p. 1243). The persuasive power of the study helped to override fears and objections such that the short-term difficulties of serum sickness were outweighed by the spectacularly lifesaving effects of the treatment itself.

This study by Fibiger formed part of an important shift in the design of experiments in both the laboratory and the field, commencing in the late nineteenth century. Other examples of probabilistic elements in research design from this period in history could be enumerated. In 1884, Charles Sanders Peirce used a deck of cards to determine the order in which stimuli were presented in an investigation of the threshold for perception for 'just noticeable differences' in weights (Peirce and Jastrow 1884). Peirce's innovation was not appreciated or widely adopted at the time and he is now best known for his contributions to philosophy and linguistics.

This technique of using a probabilistic assignment process was developing at around the same time as many of the statistical techniques in use in the human sciences. Karl Pearson and Charles Spearman were busy developing these techniques and Ronald Fisher made explicit use of the idea of randomization in his famous textbook of statistics, written when he was a researcher at the Rothamstead Laboratories in Harpenden in 1925. The spirits of probability, randomization and statistical inference grew side by side in the early twentieth century.

Whereas it would still be several years before randomization took hold in the medical and health sciences, researchers in other disciplines were demanding random numbers in the first half of the twentieth century. In her fascinating book *Randomness*, Deborah Bennett takes up the story:

> As Alfred Bork has pointed out, 'A rational nineteenth-century man would have thought it the height of folly to produce a book containing only random numbers.' Nevertheless, in 1927 Cambridge University Press did indeed publish a table of 41,600 digits that had been randomly arranged by Leonard Tippett . . . Rejecting the effectiveness of cards, tickets, balls, and dice, Pearson, Tippett's mentor, contended that statistical experimenters 'who have had to deal with the problems of random sampling' might benefit by 'a single system of numbers' . . . A mere ten years after its publication, Tippett's table of over 40,000 Random

Sampling Numbers was deemed inadequate for very large sampling experiments. In 1938 the mathematicians R.A. Fisher and F. Yates published 15,000 additional random digits . . . In 1939 M.G. Kendall and B. Babington-Smith published a table of 100,000 digits . . . In 1949 the Interstate Commerce Commission published a table of 105,000 random digits, . . . [and] in 1955 the RAND Corporation published a document entitled 'A Million Random Digits with 100,000 Normal Deviates'. RAND stated that the purpose of producing such large tables was to meet the growing need for random numbers in solving problems by experimental probability procedures.

(Bennett 1998, pp. 132–5)

Yet while so many investigations were subject to the new theories emerging from statistics, mathematics and the biological sciences, medicine remained curiously unmoved by these developments. This proliferation of random number series described by Bennett is an index of the importance of randomization in research design. Moreover, large samples required ever larger sets of random numbers. The twentieth-century proliferation of opinion polling is one such example. Longitudinal studies, where fresh samples had to be drawn from a sampling frame, repeatedly required fresh sets of random numbers each time, so that different participants might be chosen.

Only a few studies, however, made use of the technique of randomization in health care. For example, a study of the serum treatment of lobar pneumonia appeared in 1934 (Medical Research Council 1934) and another study by D'Arcy Hart concerned a trial of a compound called patulin for treatment of the common cold (Medical Research Council 1944). These developments in controlled, comparative clinical trials eventually involved importing a number of other methods from the researcher's armamentarium devised by Ronald Fisher. For example, the use of factorial designs in medicine was introduced by Wilson *et al.* (1946) to enable two comparisons to be made in the same group of patients. This involved four groups in a study of two treatments for hepatitis: a low fat diet and di-cysteine as a dietary supplement, two remedies that were currently in favour. A low fat diet had no measurable effect on hepatitis, but di-cysteine appeared to shorten an episode of acute hepatitis by a few days. Thus the experiment was able not only to establish the curative effect of treatments, in the face of possible scepticism, but was able to put a quantified value upon it.

In the middle years of the twentieth century, there was a good deal of opposition to these kinds of research methods in clinical research. Indeed, the spread of randomization in clinical trials was limited until it became an essential requirement in trials submitted to licensing authorities for the approval of new drugs. To give an example of the kinds of resistance to randomized controlled clinical trials that existed at the time, let us consider the opinion of the eminent physician Sir Thomas Lewis of what he called 'the statistical method of testing treatment' (Lewis 1934). Lewis was then responsible for the department of clinical research at University College Hospital, London, and a powerful figure in British medicine. Lewis did believe in comparative research to determine the effectiveness of treatments, but he was acutely aware of its limitations. In evaluating treatments, Lewis thought that two groups of patients that were as similar as possible should be treated at the same time in exactly the same way, with one group receiving the remedy and the other receiving a placebo. However, he added that

> it is to be recognised that the statistical method of testing treatment is never more than a temporary expedient, and that but little progress can come of it directly: for in investigating cases collectively, it does not discriminate between cases that benefit and those that do not, and so fails to determine criteria by which we may know beforehand in any given case that treatment will be successful.
>
> (Lewis 1934, p. 178)

This kind of scepticism of the experimental clinical trials perhaps stunted their growth in the mid-twentieth century. The point here is that the focus of Lewis and other clinicians and theorists of a similar kidney was on something different – individual differences in susceptibility to the medicinal effects of various treatments. This hints that a conceptual shift was necessary to make the issue of randomized clinical trials an interesting one. Many workers and researchers in health care had to reorient their thinking away from the individual to the class of patients of a broadly similar quality who could be probabilistically assigned to treatment or placebo conditions. Thus, while typically impregnable, the randomized controlled clinical trial subtly reconfigured the epistemological and personal terrain of medicine away from patients and towards kinds of patients that could meaningfully be randomized.

The cause of randomization was also boosted by concerns about bias. The development of experimental techniques and statistical methods has facilitated an intriguing conceptual split between data and theory, between objectivity and subjectivity. The fear was that clinicians working on trials might either consciously (or even worse, unconsciously) allocate patients preferentially to one condition or other depending on what they expected the results to be. Thus encouraged by the subtle communications from the researcher, the patients might flourish or languish, not because of the pharmacological properties of the drug, but because of the placebo effect. Moreover, if the clinician knew which condition the patient was in, expectations of the prognosis might somehow be communicated to the patient and influence the likelihood of recovery. The aim of the scientifically trained mind was to eliminate error, bias and subjective elements from the process of discovery, and yet to yield results with genuine humanitarian value. This spirit was to be found not only in health care but in a variety of projects and social movements in the 1930s and 1940s. For example, there are curious parallels between this movement and the 1939 World's Fair in New York. Both were born with a nineteenth-century plan and the latter's futuristic slogan – 'Building the World of Tomorrow with the Tools of Today' – could equally well be applied to the enthusiasm for clinical trials which developed in the mid-twentieth century. This movement had its first major breakthrough in a study by the Medical Research Council (1948) published in the *British Medical Journal* of a trial of streptomycin for pulmonary tuberculosis. As Yoshioka (1998) notes, the statistician involved, Professor (later Sir) Austin Bradford Hill, had been vigorously promoting the use of random allocation since before the Second World War (Hill 1937, 1990). Remarkably, however, the word 'random' appeared nowhere in the Medical Research Council's files on streptomycin for 1946. Yet with the benefit of hindsight, this study has become a landmark, meriting a 50th anniversary special issue of the *British Medical Journal* in 1998.

It is significant that the field where randomized controlled trials first developed was tuberculosis research. This disease has had a special role in the development of research methodology, partly because patients sometimes exhibit spontaneous recovery. Tuberculosis had also been subject to a variety of different treatments over the preceding decades and clinicians were concerned to try to develop a foolproof method of evaluating them. Thus, the randomized controlled trial rapidly came to have a debunking role. In this respect, it suited Popper's idea of hypothesis testing very neatly, and its appeal as a 'gold standard' for medical knowledge can readily be understood today. As an example of its debunking role, in the case of tuberculosis, a previously popular treatment involved sanocrysin, a gold compound that flourished as a treatment in the 1920s and 1930s. In 1931, a team in Detroit divided 24 patients into two groups, with groups of patients paired as closely as possible according to criteria such as age and severity of disease. A coin was tossed to decide which group would receive sanocrysin and which group injections of distilled water. The control group fared better (Amberson *et al.* 1931; Yoshioka 1998, p. 1222). Thus, at a stroke the claims about the effectiveness of sanocrysin were demolished, and this established the experiment as a means of debunking potentially spurious claims in medicine. The process of finding things out was made into a cybernetic, impersonal process, fully manualized with established procedures to make it into a ruthless sword of truth cutting through the nonsense.

Thus, with the publication of the trials of streptomycin, one of the last big killers of the nineteenth and early twentieth centuries was felled by the combination of new treatment and new research methodologies to demonstrate its superiority over any-thing that had been available before. This was fortunate for the cause of randomized controlled trials, in that rates of tuberculosis were in decline at the time, and the trials in question entered the sphere of debate of scientists and practitioners in such a way as to make it seem that the randomized controlled trial had helped to finish off the last big killer. This 'giant killer' reputation for randomized controlled trials was to finish off the residual objections to their use and establish them as the gold standard in health care research.

One possible reason why randomized controlled trials were adopted relatively late in medical research might be to do with the nature of the treatments that the health care professions used. That is, as the twentieth century wore on, the kinds of therapies under test were a good deal more subtle than those used in previous generations. It was possible for patient, clinician and evaluator to be blind as to whether the patient had received the treatment or not. Unlike the more heroic treatments of days gone by where 15-second limb amputations, bleeding and purging had been practised, medi-cine could now do its work invisibly. The spectacular events that had been astonishing audiences in dissection and operating theatres from the Renaissance to the Age of Reason had been superseded by this new molecular-level medicine. The foundations laid in microbiology by Pasteur and Koch in the nineteenth century were finally coming to fruition. Morbidity and mortality had yielded up their secret pathogenic agents, and experimental medicine had scientifically selected the best available treatments to conquer them.

From a philosophical point of view, there were even more issues brought to the surface by the development of randomized controlled trials. There were important ethical issues to be discussed and worked through. As Richard Doll (1998) reminds us, at the time that streptomycin was first used in a clinical trial of this kind, there was a strong suspicion that it would do the patients some good. Thus, what should we think about the unfortunate patients who believed they might be getting a treatment but were merely in the control group? In the streptomycin trial it was debated whether it was ethical to withhold from the control patients a drug that had already been effective in animal experiments and had yielded encouraging results in clinical studies on humans. In the event, as reported by the eminent medical statistician Austin Bradford Hill, the Medical Research Council's Streptomycin in Tuberculosis Trials Committee agreed that 'it would have been unethical not to have seized the opportunity to design a strictly controlled trial which could speedily and effectively reveal the value of the treatment' (Hill 1963, p. 1043). The committee thus agreed that it was ethically permissible to withhold the drug from the patients assigned to the control or placebo condition. At the same time, of course, the notorious Tuskgee Study was under way in the United States, where treatment was being withheld from syphilis sufferers so that US public health officials could study the 'natural course of the disease'. However, the nature of the randomized controlled trial as it was constructed in the UK was such that it went hand in hand with these ethical sensibilities, which appeared to be absent on the other side of the Atlantic. This relates to the sense of meticulous care with which the trials were created and is thus important in the credibility they rapidly gained.

The reconfiguration of the ethical issues represented an important moral transformation for health care research. It was difficult for the committee to reconcile the intentional withholding of treatment in the randomized controlled clinical trial with the principle that the doctor must always 'do for his patient whatever he really believes to be essential for that patient to return him to health' (Hill 1963, p. 1043). The solution they reached in this trial was that if the patients in the study were likely to benefit from the best existing treatment other than streptomycin, it should be given, even if it upset the balance of the treatments and control group. Thus, the principles of ethical medicine were subtly modified, but at the same time were allowed to remain more or less intact despite this innovation in research.

Another issue that these kinds of experiments raise which is germane to philosophy is the question of informed consent. The idea that patients should be fully informed of the likely risks as well as the benefits of their treatment or their involvement in the study was not yet evolved to its present state at the time that the streptomycin trials were being undertaken. Bradford Hill argued against obtaining formal consent if this involved giving a frightening account of the risks:

Does the doctor invariably seek the patient's consent before using a new drug alleged to be efficacious and safe? If the answer is No, then what process, one may ask, makes it needful for him to do so if he chooses to test the drug in such a way that he can compare its effects with those of the previous orthodox treatment?

(Hill 1963, p. 1043)

As Doll (1998) notes, the issue would be seen in rather different terms today. The idea that obtaining informed consent might scare patients and, more importantly, scare them off the study, would not persuade any ethics committees today. The ascendance of the randomized controlled trial has gone hand in hand with the rise of a meticulous ethics, to lend it a kind of moral authority.

Whereas the principle of informed consent is supposed to be central to experimental medicine, it is in practice rather difficult to be sure that it is followed. The principle that informed consent should always be obtained from competent patients was widely, though not universally, accepted (Benson *et al.* 1991; Williams and Zwitter 1994; Edwards *et al.* 1998). However, there is some doubt as to whether it is universally obtained. According to Taylor and Kellner (1987) and Williams and Zwitter (1994), as many as one in five doctors regularly entered competent patients in trials without even obtaining informed consent.

In the review by Edwards *et al.* (1998), several studies are mentioned in which the experimenters were asked whether they were confident that the participants had grasped the key issues. As many as 47 per cent of the responding doctors thought that few patients understood they were taking part in a controlled experiment. This was even though the patients typically provided written consent and even signed an agreement outlining the study and their role in it. Even more extreme results concerning the issue of patients not understanding their role in a study have been noted in the literature. In two studies, more than three-quarters of the doctors responding thought their patients rarely understood the information they were given (Spaight *et al.* 1984; Blum *et al.* 1987; Edwards *et al.* 1998).

Thus randomized controlled trials occupy a peculiar social space. They widely command the confidence on the part of the researchers and clinicians who conduct, publish, read and review them, yet, if these figures about the patients' comprehension are to be believed, they are being conducted in a way that is invisible to patients, at least in important respects. The idea of informed consent is often in practice compressed into a brief description of the study and a space to sign on a form for the patient or the patient's carer.

That was the position a few years ago. There are intimations that the situation is changing and there are some signs that 'consumers' (as the recipients of health care are increasingly called) are playing an increasingly important role in the planning and conduct of clinical trials. This sort of involvement is also increasingly encouraged by a number of bodies whose job it is to promote research. In the UK, for example, both the Medical Research Council and the United Kingdom Co-ordinating Committee on Cancer Research have established consumer liaison groups (Hanley *et al.* 2001). The Medical Research Council's trial management guides encourage the involvement of consumers, and were written with help from consumers.

This involvement of consumers in research fits in with a growing enthusiasm for soliciting the views of consumers and involving them in decision making about resources, treatments, service planning and so on. The rationale for involving consumers in research is a means of avoiding the problems outlined above, where they may apparently know very little about the research process. It is argued that if consumers are involved in randomized controlled trials, they will become 'knowledge-empowered' (Epstein 1996) and thus enabled to inform, challenge and transform the beliefs and practices of researchers. The idea of consumer and public involvement in trials has itself been actively pursued by consumers themselves. For example, Thornton (1997) is a passionate advocate of the importance of trials and argues that professionals and the public should share responsibility throughout the trial process and work together to solve the problems that arise. This point of view is echoed from within the medical establishment too. Jadad (1998) argues that 'the clinical relevance of randomised controlled trials could be increased, easily and substantially, if researchers and funding agencies were willing to involve consumers . . . as active members of research teams' (p. 17).

This idea of empowering consumers through clinical trials is one which is rapidly gaining ground. The 50-odd years since Bradford Hill argued against telling patients too much about the research they were involved in have seen some profound changes. Perhaps the consumers' role in them is a kind of therapy in itself. This might especially be the case in trials of treatments in mental health. Trivedi and Wykes (2002) discuss the state of user involvement in experiments in the mental health field and note that user involvement in the trials lead to a focus on keeping the interventions user-friendly and may involve the use of more user-relevant outcome measures. However, user involvement exacts a price from the trials themselves, such that they typically become longer and more costly.

More interestingly, the idea of this active participation of consumers in research seems to be redolent of a rather different ethos on the part of both practitioners and patients than there has been in the past. This notion of the practitioners and patients or consumers being active agents in the process of establishing the best treatments and in implementing them has a curious resonance with the current policy initiatives in the UK that emphasize clinical governance, a way of organizing the delivery of health care services that is closely aligned with evidence-based practice and, with it, the randomized controlled trial. Clinical governance has been promoted as a way of managing the organization, resourcing and delivery of health care in the UK for several years now and it is a process that has grown in strength and popularity during that time.

The standard definition of clinical governance that is promoted in the literature is one which takes its cue from the seminal 'First class service' (Department of Health 1998): 'A framework through which NHS organisations are accountable for continuously improving the quality of their services, and safeguarding high standards of care, by creating an environment in which excellence in clinical care will flourish.' In addition to this, the precise pathways under which this was to be achieved were elaborated in an earlier document 'The new NHS: modern, dependable' (Department of Health 1997), which outlined three major planks in the strategy. First, there was to be a set of clear national standards, delivered through national service frameworks (e.g. Department of Health 1999) and the National Institute for Clinical Excellence. Second, the local delivery of quality services was to be undertaken via the mechanism of clinical governance and a statutory duty of quality, and this was to be supported by lifelong learning programmes and professional self-regulation. Third, the services themselves were to be monitored via the Commission for Health Improvement and the NHS Performance Framework (Lilley 1999, p. 6).

In line with this plethora of regulation and monitoring, the aim of the whole process, like that of evidence-based practice itself, was to ensure that the treatments were based on the best evidence available, and implemented through this multi-layered framework of self-regulation and statutory oversight called clinical governance.

The point, from our perspective, is that the past few years of burgeoning enthusiasm for randomized controlled trials, under initiatives like evidence-based practice and clinical governance, is that the randomized controlled trial is not merely about testing a hypothesis in an open-minded way. It is embedded in a socially organized framework of rationality and the results of these kinds of trials have a kind of coercive force. It is as if the practitioner and patient have to be governed by the results of such research endeavours. Moreover, this new spirit of trialling in medicine has involved some interesting rewriting of the consumer of research. Consumers – no longer merely patients – are, according to the views we have reviewed above, supposed to be hard at work participating with the researchers in designing studies. They are enlisted into the self-same ubiquitous logic of the randomized controlled trial. The experiment in medicine is now more than just a technique, it is a whole ideological system to which researchers, practitioners and patients alike are subject.

This brief sketch should be sufficient to establish that this process of clinical governance, backed up by experimentally derived findings, emphasizes classical processes of rationality. Human ills and their amelioration are, in this view, subject to the same laws of nature as may be detected by the rational scientist working in the Enlightenment paradigm of sceptical enquiry. Moreover, it contains an implicit message that this rational, accountable process can and should be extended to all areas of nursing care. There are rational processes of governance at work with directives and policies as well as frameworks and mechanisms for ensuring that the process is implemented and inspected with some degree of efficiency.

There is thus an uncompromising modernity to clinical governance. It emphasizes – like Karl Popper's theories of scientific enquiry – the value of testing clinical interventions against evidence as to their effectiveness. It urges the responsibility on staff for making sure their practice is based on knowledge of what works and what does not. Like many systems of management that have taken root in the commercial sector, from Taylor's scientific management of the late nineteenth century (Taylor [1911] 1967) to total quality management in the 1980s (Boje and Windsor 1993; Ross 1993), it emphasizes how the pursuit of excellence and efficiency are goals which can be accomplished by means of these rational processes and by enlisting the members of the organization as agents of change.

Thus as well as the scientific rationale for randomized controlled trials, our attention is drawn also to the social processes involved in maintaining the roles of doctor, researcher, nurse and patient or 'consumer', in an evidence-based health care culture. In connection with this, we are also concerned with how the knowledge used in health care might reflect and contribute to the inequalities of power in the clinical situation. More broadly, we can also begin to understand how the presence of particular knowledge at work in the clinic or the community is not merely a scientific accident – the result of self-evident facts which speak for themselves. Instead, it is part of a regime of truth, where what counts as knowledge is seen as being related to the history, cultural context and power relations in the organization and in society as a whole (Foucault 1980).

In this way, the idea of evidence-based practice is not simply the straightforward application of knowledge from experimental clinical trials which pre-exists in the research literature, but is a political process of deciding what is relevant, how it applies in the case of the patients in question, and how this regime of truth might be implemented around them so as to achieve a therapeutic benefit. Indeed, there are power processes at work in deciding that the people concerned are indeed patients, that they have a condition which can be colonized by medico-nursing knowledge and that the effects of this upon them are therapeutic. No matter how self-evident and common-sensical this seems, it still behoves us as researchers to examine how this is achieved in the social practice of health care. For example, an increasing proportion of the consumers of mental health care are being diagnosed as having 'personality disorder' or 'borderline personality disorder' (Coid 2003). Once such a diagnosis has been made, there are concerns that patients with this diagnosis are neglected because of the lingering belief that it is 'untreatable', and perhaps to save money. To reiterate, we are not concerned with the literal truth of what the patient's problem 'really is'. This is what the researchers and clinicians do, using their own formal and folk techniques. Neither are we concerned with the literal effectiveness of scientific experiments or clinical governance initiatives in delivering better or more cost-effective patient care. Again, that is decided largely by other people using their own criteria. What we are concerned with is the way that a different kind of practitioner is brought into being by this experimentally informed, evidence-based culture in health care, and that both practitioners and patients themselves are enlisted in this new process of being.

Thus there have been transformations of language and culture in health care to accommodate this new spirit. As Wellsby (1999) remarks, we have guidelines rather than advice, protocols rather than instructions and meta-analyses rather than reviews. Evidence-based medicine used to be called 'clinical scepticism'. The changes in language have ushered in a new era where the reliance on clinical trials and medical experiments means that practitioners are faced with having to exercise a constant self-scrutiny and vigilance about their work. Practitioners are not simply constructed through an educational process at the start of their careers. Rather, there is an ongoing process of being constantly remodelled and reinscribed with differing professional practices and ideologies throughout their working lives, based on the yield of this continual process of updating the research, feeding it through into the literature and incorporating it into practice.

Clinical governance is thus very close to the notion of 'governmentality', a term employed by scholars who study processes of regulation and social control (Dean 1999). The term is especially likely to be used where the conduct of individuals is being regulated in line with policies, statutes, imperatives from 'science' and governmental initiatives, which may emanate from a variety of sources. In addition, the relationship between power and the processes that shape and govern the psyche or 'soul' of the individual in late twentieth-century society have been discussed by Nikolas Rose (1990), who contends that the development of new ways of talking about the self, and about the relationship between the state and the individual, have helped to construct a different kind of selfhood. In particular, the idea of an autonomous, self-aware, self-disciplined, self-governing individual has become the dominant way of making sense of the person, especially as a result of the promotion of ideologies of self-reliance through the 1980s. In this view, individual empowerment itself is seen as a micro-technique of surveillance and control – a form of governance – rather than a genuinely emancipatory experience (Thorogood 2000). In addition, this mode of being involves a good deal of introspection, self-disclosure and reformulations of one's inner psychic space. The insight from this literature is that policy changes initiated by the government or through a complex of knowledge-bearing, organizing processes of regulation may well have effects on the mindset of the practitioners and patients. It may alter how they see themselves, their jobs and their role within the larger polity. Thus the reliance on clinical trials and experimental research in health care could be seen as having revolutionized not only the discipline but also the mindset of the practitioners and researchers who work in it.

Perhaps we could make a further provocative suggestion: the change in mindset is the most significant legacy of this revolution in medicine. The use of randomized controlled trials, one might expect, should be to settle questions about which treatment is better or more cost-effective. Moreover, the use of systematic reviews, meta-analyses and convenient digests of findings by the UK's National Institute of Clinical Excellence and the Cochrane Collaboration should surely mean that the weight of evidence will readily determine optimal clinical treatments. Health care will come to embody that which is effective, efficient and excellent, in rehearsal of the conventional up-the-mountain story of science itself.

A quick glance at the pattern of research and treatment in health care will disclose that this is certainly not the case. Of course, in some cases, like the story of tuberculosis treatment above, the general pattern is portrayed as favourable. However, it is possible to see many cases of areas which are rich in randomized controlled trials where the pattern of treatment, prognosis and outcome remains resolutely unclear and controversial.

Let us examine a couple of these areas in a little more detail. The first example relates to an area of cancer care, that of prostate cancer. Cancer treatments in general have been subject to rigorous investigation along the lines recommended by randomized controlled trial enthusiasts. Yet, at the same time, there are a number of controversial issues left unresolved. Neither patients nor practitioners can easily make decisions about the best course of action. The incidence of prostate cancer is increasing in Western nations where increases in longevity and advances in detection technology have made its presence more likely and its detection easier (Gray et al. 2002). Indeed, in many Western nations it is the most common cancer among men (National Cancer Institute of Canada 1999). According to Gray et al. (2002), it is the second leading cause of cancer death among men in developed nations. At the same time, it is clear that many of those with the disease live relatively unaffected lives and the majority of those in whom it is diagnosed die of other causes.

Despite the research efforts around the disease, patients diagnosed with prostate cancer are faced with a variety of options. A few of the more widely known ones within the conventional clinician's armoury include prostatectomy, radiation therapy or 'watchful waiting' (Phillips et al. 2000). The choice is not clear-cut for either patient or physician, as controversy surrounds the probabilities of long-term survival, recurrence, complications and impact on quality of life (Phillips et al. 2000). In particular, some treatments, especially surgery, carry substantial risks of incontinence and erectile dysfunction (Fowler *et al.* 1995; Gray *et al.* 1997). These side-effects can be both debilitating and humiliating. Moreover, clients who have the operations are often particularly distressed at the incontinence afterwards (Moore and Estey 1999).

The point here is that even where an established disease entity such as prostate cancer is concerned, which has been subject to a great many carefully researched therapeutic initiatives, the best course of action is by no means clear-cut. Thus in an area where trials have been an established method of adjudicating between different treatment options for some time, this has not narrowed down the choice but rather opened it up. Moreover, it is increasingly the case that the clients themselves are involved in the decision to proceed with treatment or undertake 'watchful waiting'. That is, the proliferation of randomized controlled trials has developed in tandem with increased responsibility on the part of the client to make choices. Experiments have thus opened up uncertainty rather than reduced it and opened up new kinds of responsibility for the client who has to act as a kind of entrepreneur amidst the treatment possibilities.

This is an odd state of affairs given the ambitions of experimentalists, hypothesis testers and many practical researchers. The situation is sometimes no clearer at the end of a series of randomized controlled trials than at the beginning. Moreover, as well as survival rates, there are complex social, moral and ethical questions that inform treatment choice. Thus, how do we measure the quality of life issues that clients identify as significant and weigh them against the mortality and morbidity statistics? For example, measures of disease progression do not take into account the human costs of living with urinary incontinence (Fossa *et al.* 1994; Moore and Estey 1999). Reductions in physical activity may lead to a poorer reported quality of life and marital adjustment. Over half of post-surgery patients reported distress at loss of erectile function when followed up 18 months after surgery (Pedersen *et al.* 1993). To complicate matters even further, when following up people who have had prostatectomy, it appears that the rate of satisfaction with the choice declines over time. Herr (1994) notes that up to three years after surgery, 83 per cent of those who have had their prostate gland removed would choose a radical prostatectomy again, whereas of those more than three years post-surgery, only 47 per cent would do so. As two of Moore and Estey's participants said:

> Even though the urologist spent a long time with me and answered all my questions before surgery, the only thing I ever heard was cancer. The biggest shock is to find I am incontinent. It just hadn't penetrated and is devastating.

> I think he told me about incontinence but I didn't know he meant this.
>
> (Moore and Estey 1999, p. 1125)

The situation is thus one which is difficult to resolve using randomized controlled trials. The situation at the start is only a little less ambiguous than what we now know after several decades of research. To illustrate this, let us return to look at the rationale for randomized controlled trials. As Edwards *et al.* put it:

> The scientific rationale for conducting a trial rests in collective equipoise, which means that the medical community as a whole is genuinely uncertain over

which treatment is best. The key point, however, is that future patients benefit at no cost to participants, provided that participants are in personal equipoise and give informed consent on this basis. In these circumstances, the trial arms are an equally good bet prospectively.

(Edwards *et al.* 1998, p. 1209)

This is all well and good. The researchers, clinicians and patients are unsure which course of action is best, so the study or studies set out to compare treatment over no treatment or different treatment modalities. Yet in some areas, as we have outlined, the situation is pretty much one of equipoise afterwards. Controversy, in other words, does not abate.

In some of our own work looking at how health care practitioners made sense of their working lives (Crawford *et al.* 2002; Brown and Crawford 2003), evidence from the research literature has a rather ambiguous status for practitioners. In looking at the nature of evidence that might be brought to bear on the process of health care, it is clear that within the respondents' work context this is not a uniform commodity. Evidence is structured into a hierarchy of prestige depending on what kind it is and where it comes from. The more prestigious, credible and important evidence is often the least accessible. Either it is available only via computer links, which are not accessible from the ward, or it is sufficiently esoteric to be opaque to the practitioner. The more remote it is, the more highly valued it will be. Indeed, the evidence that is most readily accessible – that which emerges from experience with patients – is not valued highly. Practitioners are apt to distrust their own perceptions of what patients might want, and feel that these are not taken seriously as 'evidence' – at least when compared with the material available in the literature. In fieldwork conducted by two of the authors (B.B. and P.C.) one participant said:

Yes I am not sure I have been told by, again the organisation I was talking about before, they asked how they could improve the service and I canvassed a couple of clients on the ward that day, and they had given me a couple of things they wanted to do or things they thought which would be useful and I was told there was not evidence to support that, and I said well here is the evidence. So and so and so said, this is what they would like to do. But because it hadn't come from a text book or a published paper or recognised document it didn't seem to class as evidence.

Again we can see how this tendency under regimes of evidence-based practice and clinical governance to locate evidence in the research literature creates hierarchies of knowledge where experimental evidence trumps experience. Because in these studies our respondents were nurses, and they had limited access to the largely computer-based research evidence, the effect of this hierarchy of evidence quality was to push them out of the mainstream of clinical knowledge. At the same time as nurses are being invited to become responsible participants in the drive for evidence-based practice, they are reminded of their marginality to the knowledge/power axis of the medical enterprise.

The second major point to emerge on this issue appears to operate in contradiction to the first aspect outlined above. This second strand locates the sources of knowledge, evidence and expertise in the patients themselves. The sources of recovery for patients are issues which the patients themselves should be knowledgeable of. In the case of prostate cancer outlined above, it is somehow the patients' responsibility to decide on the best course of action. In the case of nurses in our studies, they are involved in a quest for this knowledge of cure which can apparently be retrieved from the patients themselves: 'It's evolving in such ways that we've got the team now looking at patients who are able to identify areas that made them better or made it worse in the NHS.' Thus the 'patient' is no longer the recipient of care in any simple sense but has been re-engineered too, into a new, entrepreneurial subjectivity. Indeed, it is almost as if patients are obligated to be experts on their own treatment: 'What we really want is asking the patients what made them better. What is it? (. . .) a lot of them can't tell you what it is. And sometimes that does let the nurses down.'

There is a sense, then, that patients who find the question of what might help them to be difficult or unanswerable are 'letting the nurses down'. The patient under this new regime is someone morally obliged to be a technologist of the self – or, in Rose's (1990) terms, to be an expert in the 'orthopaedics of the soul'. Installing the mechanisms of self-regulation has a long history in the disciplines which have sought to understand and reform deviance, from Bentham's prisoners developing consciences in the Panopticon through to the contemporary patient monitoring themselves for signs of their 'relapse profile' recurring. Clinical governance and evidence-based practice, then, as they are implemented, attempt to enlist the patient as a member of the therapeutic team, and patients' inability to play the role assigned to them is a sign of moral failing.

Whereas clinical governance might purport to enhance the influence users have over their treatment and involve them in care planning, it may have the opposite effect, as the following quote demonstrates:

> It gives lip service to the idea that the clients are involved in their care because they have signed that bit of paper that says this is what you are going to do for me, and I understand that I can make changes or additions if I want to, but I have never known anyone to make any changes or additions. We sit with people to try to design care plans but it tends to be nurse led by and large, with prompting and things like that.

Here, the process of involving sometimes indifferent or reluctant clients provides another way in which the clients are subject to the regime of the hospital and rendered docile within it. We can see also how the process of clinical governance predisposes a new consciousness and subjectivity for the clients too – one which is avowedly entrepreneurial in the same way as the nurse's – inasmuch as they are responsible for planning their care. In a sense, they are responsible for knowing. The knowledge has been individuated and placed back within the patient. The epistemological drift of much of this reliance on randomized controlled trials is to return responsibility to the individualized, privatized clients of the health care system to make choices about their own health.

This, then, is what we mean by the transformation that has been wrought by the dominance of randomized controlled trials. It has meant that practitioners and clients must be rather different people than they were 50 years ago. They have new responsibilities and new frames of consciousness. The grip of the randomized controlled trial in health care could be likened to the notion of epistemic enslavement, rather than offering liberation.

David E. Cooper identifies the different versions of the liberation versus enslavement argument in *Philosophy and Technology* (edited by Fellows 1995). To Cooper there are three main camps on each side of the debate. On the liberation side there are those that argue technology grants us 'freedom from' things, there are those who see the technology as a force of political freedom, and there is the Faustian man, moving forward with technology towards liberty. On the enslavement side there is the 'Frankenstein thesis', the argument that technology endangers political freedom, and the argument of epistemic enslavement (Fellows 1995, pp. 10–13). Epistemic enslavement occurs when the technologies, forms of knowledge and techniques for problem solving form a kind of conceptual cage from which the individual or the scientific community cannot break out. That is, once medical science is understood as a matter of randomized controlled trials, then it becomes difficult for researchers and clinicians to see the generation of more medical knowledge in anything other than these terms.

The epistemic enslavement in health care is not solely formulated in and through controlled clinical trials. We have seen how, in the case of prostate cancer, the scientific evidence from controlled clinical trials is the starting point of a process of decision and debate. In some areas of health care, however, the epistemic enslavement comes from established practice and technique as much as from evidence *per se*.

A good example of this kind of issue is the practice of episiotomy, where a cut is made in the perineum, allegedly to facilitate the delivery of the baby. As we shall see, if one takes the results of large-scale controlled studies at face value, then the indications are that episiotomies do not necessarily aid the delivery or improve foetal or maternal health, and may be associated with a variety of difficulties afterwards. However, despite research questioning the operation's utility being available since the late 1980s (Sleep *et al.* 1989), this procedure has remained very popular with clinicians.

To make sense of this retention of a practice that is not supported by research evidence from large-scale clinical trials, we must look at the history of the practice and understand how it has embedded itself in the modern medical consciousness as a desirable procedure. This kind of intervention to aid childbirth and preserve foetal health was popularized in the early twentieth century by a number of authorities who relied for their rationale on an understanding of the mechanical forces on the foetus during delivery. The eminent American obstetrician Dr Pomeroy delivered the following peroration in the *American Journal of Obstetrics* in 1918:

A long second stage has destroyed innumerable children by prolonged pressure effects and varying degrees of asphyxia. Why should we consider it other than reckless to allow the child's head to be used as a battering ram?

(Pomeroy 1918, p. 211)

This advice was diligently repeated for most of the next 70 years, appearing up until the 1989 edition of the widely used textbook *Williams' Obstetrics* (Eason and Feldman

2000). The health of the mother was cited as a reason for surgical intervention too. Another famous American obstetrician, Dr De Lee, gravely advised his colleagues as follows: '[Perineotomy] undoubtedly preserves the integrity of the pelvic floor and introitus vulvae and forestalls uterine prolapse, rupture of the vesicovaginal septum and the long train of sequelae' (De Lee 1920, p. 34).

The conviction of authorities such as these appears to have contributed to the popularity of the practice throughout the twentieth century (Low et al. 2000). However, evidence began to emerge in the late twentieth century that all was not well with this assumption on the part of practitioners. Episiotomy had been evaluated by means of randomized controlled clinical trials rather late in the day because it had simply been assumed that it was good for mothers and children. But in the early 1990s, evidence had begun to mount up that poor perineal outcomes were not the result of factors relating to the mother, the child or the labour, but were the result of episiotomies themselves (Klein et al. 1995, 1997). Indeed, the better designed trials revealed higher rates of severe perineal lacerations and perineal pain in those who had undergone episiotomy (Klein et al. 1992; Labreque et al. 1997). Thus as Low et al. (2000, p. 87) summarize: 'the scientific evidence that routine use of episiotomy can endanger rather than protect a woman's health suggests that the routine use of this procedure should be abandoned'. Yet in the closing years of the twentieth century, it was still the most common surgical procedure performed on women (Low et al. 2000). There is evidence to suggest that a sober evaluation of the risks of the delivery is not the deciding factor in whether a woman has an episiotomy. The belief of the doctor attending her about the value of episiotomy makes the most difference, according to a study of 6522 women in childbirth and their doctors by Labreque et al. (1997). Thus, even when there is good evidence from the epistemologically privileged randomized controlled trials, this does not always inform practice or practitioners.

So far, then, the role of experiments in medicine and the health sciences has been to effect only a partial intervention in the process of health care. Despite the claims to superior rationality and soundness of knowledge, they are still only one piece in the mosaic, despite their being valued under evidence-based regimes.

To delve further into the question of what role experiments play in medicine and the health sciences, let us consider the role of 'lifestyle' in health care. In the early twenty-first century, there has been a good deal of interest in the role of lifestyle and health. Previously, researchers and practitioners might have been concerned with single variables like smoking, diet, stress or exercise as contributors to mortality and morbidity. More recently, however, a variable of crucial interest is 'lifestyle'. Certainly, it contains many of these earlier variables whose effect on health has been subject to research and intervention, but it consolidates them into a single issue.

Lifestyle studies and lifestyle management programmes are appearing at universities in the UK. These are often directed at people who would wish to be personal trainers, coaches or mentors, and short lifestyle management courses are also available so that companies can send their stressed and distressed employees to have their lifestyles remodelled. This kind of intervention is part of a broader process of creating lifestyle as if it were a variable. Once upon a time when people discussed lifestyles, these involved qualitative concerns about such matters as work, leisure, preferred means of spending spare time and so on. In its original form, it does not readily turn itself into something that is measurable or identifiable as an experimental variable.

However, recently, clinicians and researchers have begun to consolidate the notion of lifestyle into something more like a variable in an experimental paradigm. For example, a recent paper by Lear *et al.* (2002) describes an 'extensive lifestyle management intervention' as part of a cardiac rehabilitation programme. These kinds of interventions attempt to minimize future cardiac risk by encouraging participants to exercise, control their weight, give up smoking and so on. The lifestyle management intervention in this case involved assigning participants to a programme where these kinds of lifestyle changes were intensively encouraged over a long period of time. These kinds of interventions to promote cardiovascular health are, of course, not new. What is most interesting from our point of view is that in this case the lifestyle interventions are part of a randomized controlled trial. This represents a conceptual shift. The power of lifestyles is such as to make a difference to the mortality and morbidity of people and has become corralled into the experimentalist armoury as something that can be manipulated or so that people can be assigned to a particular kind.

This, then, is one of the effects of the experimentalist outlook: psychosocial and cultural issues can be made to look like the kinds of variables that are beloved of experimentalists. Doses of lifestyle are like doses of a drug. Moreover, like any other experimentally validated treatment, once the procedure has been established as having a therapeutic value, then the next question relates to whether people can be persuaded to follow it (Feldman *et al.* 2002). Thus, compliance with lifestyle becomes like compliance with a drug regime – something that can be enforced and encouraged. It turns lives into variables in a treatment protocol.

The nature of experimental methods then tends to affect the kind of lens through which health and well-being are seen. The epistemology and methodology in this case are not socially neutral but are spreading out over a variety of health care surfaces to transform the way we think about health and disease.

Perhaps even more interesting is the way that the experimental approach to medicine has paralleled a number of social changes in the past 50 years. The influential social theorists Bataille (1985) and Baudrillard (1988) characterize this as a shift from a production-oriented industrial capitalism to that of a consumption-based economy. That is, a change has taken place whereby the Protestant work ethic with its emphasis on hard labour and endless toil combined with ascetic self-denial has been reversed in the past half century, with the development of Western societies so as to stress non-utilitarian expenditure, consumption, and the gross, expulsive or excretory features of the human condition.

As we have seen in earlier chapters of this volume, it was during the Renaissance that anatomy was turned into an observational discipline, where careful dissection and drawing progressively replaced the previous incarnations of medicine. As this was happening, the feudal order of the Middle Ages was being replaced by the carnivalesque disorder and multiple transgressions of Renaissance cities. Rabelais, who characterized the transgressive spirit of these kinds of events and incorporated the low, bodily humour of the carnival into his works of fiction, was also a doctor – which may be more than coincidence. The development of towns and cities throughout

Renaissance Europe, with abundant marketplaces and social spaces that were not governable through the traditional feudal hierarchies, facilitated this revolution in consciousness (Bakhtin 1968). Perhaps also it facilitated the Renaissance revolution in the way the body was seen, the way its functions were mapped and its expulsions of urine and faeces rendered humorous (Larsen 2001).

We could argue that a similar economic, political and cultural shift accompanied the growth of experimentation in medicine in the late twentieth century. The orderliness which was progressively imposed on disease in the nineteenth century when the pathogens responsible for many of the world's major killers were identified was followed by the mid-twentieth century when the agents responsible for bringing them under control were put to the test. Leprosy, for example, was the first major disease whose bacterial causes were firmly established by G.A. Hansen in 1873 with his discovery of *Mycobacterium leprae*. This was eventually found to respond to the drug dapsone, one of the revolutionary new 'sulfa drugs' that transformed medicine in the middle years of the twentieth century. As we have seen, it was the 1940s which saw the development of randomized controlled clinical trials to test the effectiveness of anti-tuberculosis drugs. These were drugs whose action was so subtle that the patients would not be able to tell whether they had taken them or not, unlike the more invasive treatments of days gone by. The subtlety of the modern medicines facilitated the possibility of a control group who would also be unaware of whether they had taken the active drug.

It might also be worth noting that nursing has striven for many years to throw away the handmaiden mantle and get itself recognized as a profession, independent of doctors. Yet expertise based on a specific body of scientifically derived knowledge is a central determinant of any claim to professionalism. Unless and until nursing generates its own body of scientific knowledge, in the eyes of many critics it will remain a quasi-profession. In this sense, because science and research are male-gendered, so professionalism too is masculinized (Davies 1998). A paradigm shift within health care research methodologies would go some way towards facilitating their bid, but the organizational and cultural odds are stacked against it. The territoriality inherent in the doctor/nurse arena means that medics will attempt to keep their stranglehold over health care provision through the limitation of nursing activities. This has been amply evidenced by their opposition towards the introduction of the Advanced Nurse Practitioner and nurse prescribing (e.g. Saul 1996). Indeed, McCartney *et al.* (1999) suggest that the official reasons provided for the deregulation of medical prescribing are peripheral to the true motivations, namely to save money, to transfer basic medical activities to nurses and to 'challenge the professional monolith of medicine' (p. 348).

Medical supremacy can be further buttressed by retaining control over research activities and the distribution of research monies, especially if the scientific method and the randomized controlled trial maintain their position as the methods of choice.

The medicalization of health care research is clearly apparent in the topics selected for study and the methods used to study them. A review of all papers submitted to *Nurse Education Today* by Long and Johnson (2002) found that the majority of data collection techniques used derived from the qualitative methodologies – interviews, focus groups, reflective diaries and the like – while there was a marked absence of experimental work and inferential analysis. Nor is the problem a local one, since

Schlomer (1999) found that Medline and CINAHL searches over an 11-year period produced just 15 nursing randomized controlled trials written in German. Bonell (1999) also notes the reluctance of nurses to use experimental and quantitative research approaches.

If the subject matter of health care could be mined satisfactorily by means of randomized controlled trials and this was all there was to medicine, the picture of health would perhaps have changed more rapidly over the past half century and there would be more evidence of progress. There would have perhaps been much more evidence of diseases being conquered. However, the late twentieth century saw an explosion of new illnesses and conditions that are not so readily resolvable. A scan of press reports at the time of writing reveals the enigma of new diseases emerging that are not susceptible to resolution through the careful study of experiments already accomplished. For example, in March 2003 reports emerged in the press of a new illness with pneumonia-like symptoms, severe acute respiratory syndrome (SARS). 'Worldwide alert as air travellers spread killer bug' reports the usually understated UK *Daily Telegraph* (17 March 2003, p. 13). The nature of disease, then, appears to be protean and escapes the confines we place on it:

> The best evidence is that its causative agent is a coronavirus, which is normally the second-commonest cause of the common cold . . . That may be a premature conclusion, because scientists are not yet certain that the coronavirus is the cause. Some laboratories have also found traces of paramyxovirus, which is known to cause respiratory disease. There is speculation that the two viruses might even be conspiring to cause the disease together.
>
> (*Times T2*, 1 April 2003, p. 4)

Once upon a time, experimental medicine allowed us to conquer tuberculosis, yet the present day throws up new forms and variants of disease that attack the same body systems. In addition, the measures to control disease itself are themselves often highly controversial. Reports in the UK press about possible hazards of the combined immunization for measles, mumps and rubella (MMR) continue unabated. The *Daily Mail* carried a feature article by journalist Melanie Phillips (12 March 2003, p. 36) in which she rehearsed some of the controversy around this immunization.

This latter example is worth pausing over because it invites a number of issues about the social spaces of scientific controversy in health care and the role of experimental designs in the resolution of controversy. Here the concern is that the combined MMR vaccine is associated with pathologies of the intestines and in addition neurological and psychological problems such as autism and learning difficulties. One of the leading academic opponents of this vaccine is Andrew Wakefield, who at the time of writing was at the Royal Free Hospital, London. In a series of articles, he has challenged claims as to the safety of this vaccine (e.g. Wakefield *et al.* 1998; Wakefield and Montgomery 2000). Moreover, Phillips (2003) reports that there have been claims of associations between bowel disease, measles and autism from researchers in a number of locations, from the USA and Ireland too. A good deal of the argument hinges on the evidential claims of Wakefield and his colleagues. This relates to the clinical trials of the MMR vaccine and the causal inferences possible from findings of measles virus and measles antibodies in the intestines of autistic children.

There are even controversies about the kind and nature of research that has been done on the subject. After Wakefield's claim, a savage critique of his work was published by three authors from the UK's Medicines Control Agency, claiming that Wakefield had misrepresented some studies, made elementary mistakes in interpreting evidence and got other studies completely wrong (Arlett *et al.* 2001).

Thus even where there are a multitude of studies, the controversy still exists, because of differing opinions as to which studies are relevant or what the original research actually might have said. Wakefield's position hinges on the possibility that pathogens and vaccines act in hitherto undisclosed and unimagined ways to cause diseases. In the face of the relentless sociality of twenty-first century life, there appears to have been an increase in autism. The Medical Research Council recently reported that the incidence of autism in the UK now appeared to be six in every 1000 children, whereas once it was believed to be merely one or two (Young 2001). Arguably this is because studies designed to identify the condition epidemiologically are more thorough, but there are some who believe that there has been an explosion in the condition. Speculations about the causes for this have included MMR vaccination itself, as well as the presence of mercury compounds in a range of common vaccines. With the present state of knowledge, we cannot point the reader in the direction of any correct interpretation of the debate. However, the purpose of mentioning this is that the complexity of issues and the debates that arise from them rapidly outstrip the scientific evidence that can be brought to bear on them. The questions about MMR, gastrointestinal disorders and autism are shot through also with concerns about the immune system, whose imagined complexity, as we have seen, has expanded by leaps and bounds in the latter years of the twentieth century. The historical asceticism of the tireless experimental workers is effaced by the omnipotence of doubt and the prevalence of panic concerning the effectiveness and safety of medicines which had previously been researched and approved.

New forms of illness and bodily disorder continuously erupt onto the social scene. The stable disease topographies of the nineteenth century, with their orderly microbial illnesses whose pathogens were identified, have been replaced. In the opinion of more post-modern theorists, these have been replaced by expulsive self-digesting human topographies of the late twentieth and early twenty-first centuries (Kroker and Kroker 1987; Larsen 2001). The human bodies called into being by the new panics about viruses and vaccines are not the rationally organized factories of the nineteenth century but lack comforting boundaries. The bounded systems of the rational nineteenth century body, the conceptual models of bodies where the immune system was differentiated from the gut and that both were different from the brain, are thwarted and transcended by the vision of the body conjured up in the MMR scare, where all these systems are interlocked and interdependent. The apparently unchanging flesh and blood body continues to thwart the technologies set up to investigate it and subjugate its malfunctions. The attempts to impose health and orderliness are subverted by the protean, illness-rich body.

In the face, then, of their short history and their many controversies and problems, it is perhaps odd that randomized controlled trials have achieved their current predominance in medicine, especially as there is some doubt as to exactly what the body involves and how it works. Experimental, randomized controlled trial approaches are often used as debunking mechanisms where scientifically oriented researchers seek to undermine the claims of other practitioners whose treatments they see to be outmoded, harmful or lacking in evidential support. Experiments, then, are often done in an atmosphere of controversy, so it is usual to find them being subject to criticism, re-evaluation and attempts at replication. Rather than putting a stop to controversy in the health sciences, experiments are often the very things that spark it off in the first place.

These kinds of problems of medicine, where experiments attempt to discern how the body works and how it responds to medication, show how the body itself slithers out of the experimentalist's grasp to malfunction in new and sometimes iatrogenic ways. One of the most interesting effects of the experimentalist movement in medicine with its emphasis on randomized controlled clinical trials is the kind of assumptions it has encouraged about the nature of the body and its pathologies and how we may think about them.

The historian and philosopher of science Ian Hacking (1981) argues that scientists need not be realists concerning at least some elements of theory – but experimentalists become realists once they learn to manipulate and use entities (such as drugs, operations and other interventions), especially if these are used to learn something about other entities (such as the response of the body to diseases and vaccines). The technology of finding out, then, predisposes the kinds of assumptions we make about reality.

At a more fundamental level, we need to make some important assumptions for the experiments that are conducted to be meaningful. We must, for example, assume a certain distinction or separation between theory and observations, such that the two may be independent of one another. We must assume the effectiveness of our own agency on the experimental situation. The causal inferences about phenomena possible from experiments presuppose that an underlying matrix of causal relationships is already in place in some bodily reality which is independent of and pre-existent of the experimenter. And, more to the point, outlasts the experiment itself. A body must not merely produce measles antibodies on one occasion and brain damage on another, for example. For experimental medicine to work, the body must be real and be stable. Hacking (1981) distinguishes between realism at the level of theory – the debate about which, he suggests, in the face of now familiar feminist and social constructivist critiques, is inconclusive – and realism at the level of experiment, which is our concern here. From his argument, we may surmise that realism concerning entities such as microbes and molecules is plausible in so far as we can manipulate these entities in experiments designed to help us learn more about other entities (in our case, the body's responses to disease). This places Hacking in the unusual position of somehow being a realist with regard to entities manipulated in experiments and also an instrumentalist.

An anomaly is generated when an observation or experimental result does not agree (to some specified degree of accuracy) with a prediction of a theory. One might be able to resolve the anomaly by showing that there is a problem with the data. In the case of Andrew Wakefield's work, his critics point to the highly self-selected nature of his samples of children, and the difficulty in linking measles, gut disorders and autism in a coherent manner, given the causal inferences that our observations allow us to make and the theoretical models of human disease metabolism that are currently in vogue. As we have already discussed, another kind of reaction to the situation of finding that events outstrip our theory is to decide that the anomaly is sufficiently serious as to require complete abandonment of the theory, and as Kuhn describes it, a change in the paradigm (Kuhn 1970).

The life sciences themselves have a tradition of being relatively flexible about theories and models, and there are a number of examples of theories being discarded almost casually, without plunging the field into a revolution or paradigm shift in the way that physics was revolutionized about 100 years ago. The tradition in the basic life sciences seems to be one of quiet revolution. An example of this is given by the retrospective accounts of the discovery of DNA. James Watson and Francis Crick received the Nobel Prize in 1962 for their double helix model of DNA, constructed in Cambridge nearly ten years previously, in 1953. After the discovery of the structure of the molecules, Crick went on to develop what he called a 'pretty, almost elegant' version of the genetic code, called 'the comma free code' (Crick 1988, p. 99). This theory, eventually discarded, was described as 'an idea of Crick's that was the most elegant biological theory ever to be proposed and proved wrong' (Judson 1996, p. 314). Crick attempted to test his own hypothesis with genetic experiments, with little success (Judson 1996). Later, Marshall Nirenberg, using biochemical methods, cracked the genetic code (Nirenberg [1968] 1972). Crick then magnanimously acknowledged the success of the alternative experimental method and accepted the code that the biochemists deciphered. His own genetic experiments later produced independent evidence for some of the details (Crick 1988). Crick's own reflection on the events was as follows:

> Theorists in biology should realize that it is . . . unlikely that they will produce a good theory at their first attempt. It is amateurs who have one big bright beautiful idea that they can never abandon. Professionals know that they have to produce theory after theory before they are likely to hit the jackpot. The very process of abandoning one theory for another gives them a degree of critical detachment that is almost essential if they are to succeed.
>
> (Crick 1988, p. 142)

This, then, is a model of enquiry that is curiously reminiscent of some sort of sporting activity like cricket. Certainly there is competition, and the participants and spectators have an interest in the outcome of the various plays in the game but we can see that people build on one another's ideas, share each other's successes and the spirit of competition does not break apart the sense of fraternal common enterprise among the different workers in the field. This is rather a different picture than one might find if one looked at the debate over the safety of the MMR vaccine. Some participants such as John O'Leary at Coombe Women's Hospital in Dublin have argued that there is now 'compelling evidence' of a link between MMR and autism, whereas the UK's Department of Health says that O'Leary's research did not prove anything and there is no evidence to suggest there is any link between the MMR jab and autism (Mayor 2001). Indeed, the head of the UK's immunization programme David Salisbury was quoted as saying that Wakefield's views 'have no support from experts in vaccines' and that 'Dr Wakefield is on a crusade' (Mayor 2001). So, despite research having been conducted there are people with a stake in the field who are not acting like gentlemanly participants.

To make sense of what is going on here we need to draw on some other traditions in the history and philosophy of science. Rather than the revolutions seen by Kuhn, some writers such as Lakatos (1974) and Laudan (1977) have suggested alternative world-view models. Perhaps making sense of these issues might be helped by outlining Laudan's concept of a 'research tradition', which attempts to investigate the position of rationality in theory development and selection by expanding the concept of rationality itself.

Like Kuhn and Lakatos, Laudan sees science operating within a conceptual framework that he calls a research tradition (Anderson 1982). The research tradition consists of a number of specific theories, along with a set of metaphysical and conceptual assumptions that are shared by those scientists who adhere to the tradition. Within this approach the philosopher or historian of science makes the assumption that scientific decision making is performed rationally by scholars in a particular tradition. An important function of the research tradition is to provide a set of methodological and philosophical guidelines for the further development of the tradition (Anderson 1982).

Following both Kuhn and Popper, Laudan argues that the objective of science is to solve problems – that is, to provide 'acceptable answers to interesting questions' (Laudan 1977, p. 13). On this view, the 'truth' or 'falsity' of a theory is irrelevant as an appraisal criterion. The key question is whether the theory offers an explanation for problems that arise when we encounter something in the natural or social environment which clashes with our preconceived notions or which is otherwise in need of explanation (Anderson 1982). It is assumed that scientific questions are resolved at the time by people acting rationally and that rationality leads just as readily to conclusions that are subsequently believed to be false as it does to conclusions that are believed to be true (Collins 2002). This, then, resembles the symmetry thesis in the 'strong programme', which we have already seen, in the work of Bloor and his colleagues.

For example, the interactionist interpretation of the mind/body divide is predicated on the notion that there is a reciprocal impact of both entities and while it has its advocates, it also has its opponents. For example, there is a school of thought that contends that the only distinction between the mind and body is the semantics used to describe them. For example, Ryle (1949) claimed that nouns and pronouns were used to describe tangible, physical, body-related issues, while verbs, adverbs and adjectives were used to describe the intangible properties of the mind – the concrete versus the abstract.

One of the difficulties in resolving the problems that occur when experimental results do not resolve debates is that research traditions often contain their own rationalities. For example, within the mainstream Western tradition in the life sciences, it is widely supposed that thought precedes and anticipates action, that conjectures and hypotheses precede experiments designed to test them and that science is a means of developing a rational understanding of nature, which technologies merely embody. Thus in science, tools and technologies are seen to be consequences of creative, intentional, purposive thought but have no role in enabling or shaping thought. The pre-eminence of mind is also expressed by the priority assigned to representations and reasoning processes in cognitive psychology and, similarly, to ideas and arguments in the history of science, with its corollary that technologies emerge from the application of scientifically discerned principles (Gooding 2001). This kind of implicit model of human enquiry is often to be found haunting the warp and weft of the fabric of science. It is this, perhaps, that leads to some of the fervour that exists within scientific debates on, for example, MMR safety. If the experimentally derived evidence is part of a particular tradition, then this is what gives it meaning. If, for example, we rely on epidemiological data, we may conclude that the risks of vaccination are far less than the risks of the diseases. On the other hand, other traditions with proponents such as Wakefield, privilege instead the accounts from parents and patients. These two traditions are both present in contemporary medicine and it is partly as a result of these co-existing traditions that conflicts emerge and different bodies of evidence are produced in support of the different positions.

The fact is that conflicts and controversies have proliferated despite there being a comparable proliferation in evidence derived from experiments and other scientific techniques. Perhaps some salvation for this problem comes from the position of scientific realism. This is not the same kind of realism as was understood in classical positivistic approaches, but instead we shall turn to a newer variety of realism which appeared in the 1970s (Suppe 1977). This variant of realism involved the reasoned pursuit of truth, but refrained from making strong statements about the exact nature of reality. A fundamental tenet of modern-day scientific realism is the classical realist view that the world exists independently of its being perceived (Hunt 1990). This is in contrast to a relativist position (Olson 1981): realism proposes that there really is something 'out there' for science to theorize about (Hunt 1990). However, the newer variants of scientific realism do not necessarily involve 'direct' realism that holds that our perceptual processes result in a direct awareness of, or straightforward confrontation with, objects in the external world. Advocates of scientific realism, though agreeing that our perceptual processes can yield genuine knowledge about an external world, emphatically reject direct realism. They argue for a fallibilistic and critical realism. Hence scientific realism is a middle-ground position between direct realism and relativism. Scientific realism is also a critical realism, contending that the job of science is to use its method to improve our perceptual or measurement processes, separate illusion from reality, and thereby generate the most accurate possible description and understanding of the world (Hunt 1990). The practice of developing multiple measures of constructs and testing them in multiple contexts in social science stems from this critical orientation (Cook and Campbell 1986). In short, scientific realism proposes that: (1) the world exists independently of its being perceived (classical realism); (2) the job of science is to develop genuine knowledge about the world, even though such knowledge will never be known with certainty (fallible realism); and (3) all knowledge claims must be critically evaluated and tested to determine the extent to which they do, or do not, truly represent or correspond to that world (critical realism). In conclusion, with respect to truth and scientific realism, the perspective of Siegel (1983) seems a fair summary statement: 'To claim that a scientific proposition is true is not to claim that it is certain; rather, it is to claim that the world is as the proposition says it is' (p. 82).

This, then, is perhaps the best characterization of the position of experimental research within health care. The emphasis here is on researchers permanently striving towards an ever elusive truth whose existence, while credible, can never be grasped with certainty.

References

Amberson, J.B., McMahon, B.T. and Pinner, M. (1931) A clinical trial of sanocrysin in pulmonary tuberculosis, *American Review of Tuberculosis*, 24: 401–35.

Anderson, P.F. (1982) Marketing, strategic planning and the theory of the firm, *Journal of Marketing*, 46: 15–26.

Arlett, P., Bryan, P. and Evans, S. (2001) A response to 'Measles mumps, rubella vaccine: Through a glass darkly' by Drs A.J. Wakefield and S.M. Montgomery and published reviewers' comments, *Adverse Drug Reactions and Toxicology Reviews*, 20(1): 37–45.

Bakhtin, M.M. (1968) *Rabelais and His World*. Cambridge, MA: MIT Press.

Bataille, G. (1985) *Visions of Excess: Selected Writings 1927–1939*. Manchester: Manchester University Press.

Bauldrillard, J. (1988) *Jean Baudrillard: Selected Writings*. Oxford: Polity Press.

Bennett, D.J. (1998) *Randomness*. Cambridge, MA: Harvard University Press.

Benson, A.B., Pregler, J.P., Bean, J.A. *et al.* (1991) Oncologists' reluctance to accrue patients onto clinical trials: an Illinois Center study, *Journal of Clinical Oncology*, 9: 2067–75.

Blum, A.L., Chalmers, T.C., Deutch, E. *et al.* (1987) The Lugano statement on controlled clinical trials, *Journal of International Medical Research*, 15: 2–22.

Boje, D.M. and Windsor, R.D. (1993) The resurrection of Taylorism: total quality management's hidden agenda, *Journal of Organisational Change Management*, 6(4): 58–71.

Bonell, C. (1999) Evidence-based nursing: a stereotyped view of quantitative and experimental research could work against professional autonomy and authority, *Journal of Advanced Nursing*, 30(1): 18–23.

Brown, B. and Crawford, P. (2003) The clinical governance of the soul: 'deep management' and the self-regulating subject in integrated community mental health teams, *Social Science and Medicine*, 56: 67–81.

Coid, J. (2003) Epidemiology, public health and the problem of personality disorder, *British Journal of Psychiatry*, 182 (suppl. 44): 3–10.

Collins, H.M. (2002) The experimenter's regress as philosophical sociology, *Studies in History and Philosophy of Science*, 33: 153–60.

Cook, T.D. and Campbell, D.T. (1986) The causal assumptions of quasi-experimental practice, *Synthese*, 68: 141–80.

Crawford, P., Brown, B., Anthony, P. and Hicks, C. (2002) Reluctant empiricists: community mental health nurses and the art of evidence based praxis, *Health and Social Care in the Community*, 10(4): 287–98.

Crick, F. (1988) *What Mad Pursuit: A Personal View of Scientific Discovery*. New York: Basic Books.

Danto, A.C. (1967) Naturalism, in P. Edwards (ed.) *The Encyclopaedia of Philosophy*, Vol. 5. New York: Macmillan.

Davies, C. (1998) *Gender and the Professional Predicament in Nursing*. Buckingham: Open University Press.

Dean, M. (1999) *Governmentality: Power and Rule in Modern Society*. London: Sage.

De Lee, J.B. (1920) The prophylactic forceps operation, *American Journal of Obstetrics and Gynecology*, 1: 34–44.

Department of Health (1996) *Promoting Clinical Effectiveness: A Framework for Action In and Through the NHS*. London: Department of Health.

Department of Health (1997) *The New NHS: Modern, Dependable*. London: Department of Health.

Department of Health (1998) *A First Class Service: Quality in the New NHS*. London: Department of Health.

Department of Health (1999) *The National Service Framework for Mental Health*. London: Department of Health.

Doll, R. (1998) Controlled trials: the 1948 watershed, *British Medical Journal*, 317: 1217–19.

Dupre, J. (1983) The disunity of science, *Mind*, 92: 321–46.

Eason, E. and Feldman, P. (2000) Much ado about a little cut: is episiotomy worthwhile?, *Obstetrics and Gynaecology*, 95: 616–18.

Edwards, S.J.L., Lilford, R.J. and Hewison, J. (1998) The ethics of randomised controlled trials from the perspective of patients, the public and health care professionals, *British Medical Journal*, 317: 1209–12.

Epstein, S. (1996) *Impure Science*. Berkeley, CA: University of California Press.

Feldman, S.R., Chen, G.J., Hu, J.Y. and Fleischer, A.B. (2002) Effects of systematic asymmetric discounting on physician patient interactions: a theoretical framework to explain poor compliance with lifestyle counselling, *Medical Informatics and Decision Making*, 2(1): 8–16.

Fellows, R. (ed.) (1995) *Philosophy and Technology*. New York: The Press Syndicate of the University of Cambridge.

Fossa, S.D., Aass, N. and Opjordsmoen, S. (1994) Assessment of quality of life in patients with prostate cancer, *Seminars in Oncology*, 21: 657–61.

Foucault, M. (1980) *Michel Foucault: Power/Knowledge: Selected Interviews and Other Writings, 1972/1977*. Brighton: Harvester Wheatsheaf.

Fowler, F.J., Barry, M.J., Lu-Yao, G. *et al.* (1995) Effect of radical prostatectomy for prostate cancer on patient quality of life: results from a Medicare survey, *Urology*, 45: 1007–15.

Gooding, D.C. (2001) Experiment as an instrument of innovation: experience and embodied thought, Keynote lecture to the *Annual Conference of the Cognitive Technologies Society*, University of Warwick, August.

Gray, R.E., Klotz, L.H. and Iscoe, N.I. (1997) Results of a survey of Canadian men with prostate cancer, *Canadian Journal of Urology*, 4: 359–65.

Gray, R.E., Fitch, M.J., Fergus, K.D., Mykalovskiy, E. and Church, K. (2002) Hegemonic masculinity and the experience of prostate cancer: a narrative approach, *Journal of Aging and Identity*, 7(1): 43–62.

Greenberg, H.M. and Raymond, S.U. (1999) *Medical Education Meets the Marketplace*. New York: New York Academy of Sciences.

Hacking, I. (1981) *Scientific Revolutions*. Oxford Readings in Philosophy Series. Oxford: Oxford University Press.

Hanley, B., Truesdale, A., King, A., Elbourne, D. and Chalmers, E. (2001) Involving consumers in designing, conducting and interpreting randomised controlled trials: questionnaire survey, *British Medical Journal*, 322: 519–23.

Herr, H.W. (1994) Quality of life of incontinent men after radical prostatectomy, *Journal of Urology*, 151: 652–4.

Hill, A.B. (1937) Principles of medical statistics: the aim of the statistical method, *Lancet*, i: 41–3.

Hill A.B. (1963) Medical ethics and controlled trials, *British Medical Journal*, i: 1043.

Hill, A.B. (1990) Memories of the British streptomycin trial in tuberculosis, *Controlled Clinical Trials*, 11: 77–9.

Hrobjartsson, A., Gotzschem, P.C. and Glund, C. (1998) The controlled clinical trial turns 100 years: Fibiger's trial of serum treatment of diphtheria, *British Medical Journal*, 317: 1243–5.

Hunt, S.D. (1990) Truth in marketing theory and research, *Journal of Marketing*, 54: 1–15.

Illich, I. (1976) *Limits to Medicine: Medical Nemesis: The Expropriation of Health*. Harmondsworth: Pelican Books.

Jadad, A. (1998) *Randomised Controlled Trials*. London: BMJ Books.

Judson, H.F. (1996) *The Eighth Day of Creation: The Makers of the Revolution in Biology*. Cold Spring Harbor, NY: Cold Spring Harbor Laboratory Press.

Klein, M., Gauthier, R. and Jorgensen, S. (1992) Does episiotomy prevent perineal trauma and pelvic floor relaxation?, *Online Journal of Current Clinical Trials*, 1992: Doc. 10.

Klein, M., Kaczorowski, J., Robbins, J. *et al.* (1995) Physicians' beliefs and behaviour during a randomised controlled trial of episiotomy: consequences for women in their care, *Journal of the Canadian Medical Association*, 153: 769–79.

Klein, M., Janssen, P., MacWilliam, L., Kaczorowski, J. and Johnson, B. (1997) Determinants of vaginal perineal integrity and pelvic floor functioning in childbirth, *Journal of Obstetrics and Gynaecology*, 176: 403–10.

Kroker, A. and Kroker, M. (1987) *Body Invaders: Panic Sex in America*. New York: St. Martin's Press.

Kuhn, T.S. (1970) *The Structure of Scientific Revolutions*, 2nd edn. Chicago, IL: University of Chicago Press.

Labrecque, M., Baillargeon, L., Dallaire, M. *et al.* (1997) Association between episiotomy and severe perineal lacerations in primiparous women, *Canadian Medical Association Journal*, 156: 97–102.

Lakatos, I. (1974) Falsification and the methodology of scientific research programs, in I. Lakatos and A. Musgrave (eds) *Criticism and the Growth of Knowledge*. Cambridge: Cambridge University Press.

Larsen, D. (2001) South Park's Solar Anus, or Rabelais returns: cultures of consumption and the contemporary aesthetic of obscenity, *Theory, Culture and Society*, 18(4): 65–82.

Laudan, L. (1977) *Progress and Its Problems*. Berkeley, CA: University of California Press.

Lear, S.A., Ignaszewski, A., Linden, W. *et al.* (2002) A randomized controlled trial of an extensive lifestyle management intervention (ELMI) following cardiac rehabilitation: study design and baseline data, *Current Controlled Trials in Cardiovascular Medicine*, 3(1): 9–23.

Lewis, T. (1934) *Clinical Science Illustrated by Personal Experiences*. London: Shaw & Sons.

Lilley, R. (1999) *Making Sense of Clinical Governance: A Workbook for NHS Doctors, Nurses and Managers*. Oxford: Radcliffe Medical Press.

Long, T. and Johnson, M. (2002) Research in *Nurse Education Today*: do we meet our aims and scope?, *Nurse Education Today*, 22(1): 85–93.

Low, L.K., Seng, J.S., Murtland, T.L. and Oakland, D. (2000) Clinician specific episiotomy rates: impact on perineal outcomes, *Journal of Midwifery and Women's Health*, 45(2): 87–93.

Mayor, S. (2001) The MMR saga: blinding or fooling the public with science?, *The Scientist: Daily News*, 24 January, p. 13.

McCartney, W., Tyrer, S., Brazier, M. and Prayle, D. (1999) Nurse prescribing: radicalism or tokenism?, *Journal of Advanced Nursing*, 29(2): 348–54.

McKeown, T. (1976) *The Modern Rise of Population*. New York: Academic Press.

Medical Research Council Therapeutic Trials Committee (1934) The serum treatment of lobar pneumonia, *British Medical Journal*, i: 241–5.

Medical Research Council Patulin Trials Committee (1944) Clinical trial of patulin in the common cold, *Lancet*, ii: 373–4.

Medical Research Council (1948) Streptomycin treatment of pulmonary tuberculosis. *British Medical Journal*, ii: 769–82.

Moore, K.N. and Estey, S.A. (1999) The early post operative concerns of men after radical prostatectomy, *Journal of Advanced Nursing*, 29(5): 1121–9.

National Cancer Institute of Canada (1999) *Canadian Cancer Statistics 1999*. Toronto: National Cancer Institute of Canada.

Nirenberg, M. ([1968] 1972) 'The Genetic Code', *Nobel Lectures: Physiology or Medicine, 1963–1970*. New York: Elsevier.

Olson, J.C. (1981) Towards a science of consumer behaviour, in A.A. Mitchell (ed.) *Advances in Consumer Research*, Vol. 9. Ann Arbor, MI: Association for Consumer Research,

Parry, G. (2000) Evidence based psychotherapy: special case or special pleading?, *Evidence Based Mental Health*, 3: 35–7.

Pedersen, K.V., Carlsson, P., Rahmquist, M. and Varenhorst, E. (1993) Quality of life after radical retro pubic prostatectomy for carcinoma of the prostate, *European Urology*, 24: 7–11.

Peirce, C.S. and Jastrow, J. (1884) On small differences of sensation, *Memoirs of the National Academy of Science*, 3: 73–83.

Phillips, C., Gray, R.E., Fitch, M.E. *et al.* (2000) Early postsurgery experience of prostate cancer patients and spouses, *Cancer Practice*, 8(4): 165–71.

Phillips, M. (2003) This baby suffered brain damage and epilepsy after the MMR jab. So why did doctors ignore warnings that it might be unsafe?, *Daily Mail*, 12 March, p. 36.

Pomeroy, R.H. (1918) Shall we cut and reconstruct the perineum for every primipara?, *American Journal of Obstetrics*, 78: 211–19.

Radway, J. (1987) *Reading the Romance*. Chapel Hill, NC: University of North Carolina Press.

Rose, N. (1990) *Governing the Soul: The Shaping of the Private Self*. London: Routledge.

Ross, J.E. (1993) *Total Quality Management: Texts, Cases and Readings*. Delray Beach, CA: St Lucie Press.

Ryle, G. (1949) *The Concept of Mind*. London: Hutchinson.

Sackett, D.L., Rosenberg, W.M., Gray, J.A., Haynes, R.B. and Richardson, W.S. (1996) Evidence-based medicine: what it is and what it isn't, *British Medical Journal*, 312: 71–2.

Saul, P. (1996) News: prescribing the reality, *Community Nurse*, 2(3): 10.

Schlomer, G. (1999) Randomised clinical trials and systematic reviews in nursing literature, *Pflege*, 12(4): 250–8.

Siegel, S. (1983) Brown on epistemology and the new philosophy of science, *Synthese*, 14: 61–89.

Sleep, J., Roberts, J. and Chalmers, I. (1989) Care during the second stage of labour, in I. Chalmers, M. Enkin and M.J.N.C. Keirse (eds) *Effective Care in Pregnancy and Childbirth*. Oxford: Oxford University Press.

Spaight, S.J., Nash, S., Finison. L.J. and Patterson, W.B. (1984) Medical oncologists' participation in cancer clinical trials, *Progress in Clinical and Biological Research*, 15: 49–61.

Suppe, F. (1977) *The Structure of Scientific Theories*, 2nd edn. Chicago, IL: University of Illinois Press.

Taylor, F.W. ([1911] 1967) *Principles of Scientific Management*. New York: Norton Library Harper & Row.

Taylor, K.M. and Kellner, M. (1987) Interpreting physician participation in randomized clinical trials: the physician orientation profile, *Journal of Health and Social Behaviour*, 28: 389–400.

Thornton, H. (1997) Randomised clinical trials: the patient's point of view, in M.J. Silverstein (ed.) *Ductal Carcinoma In Situ of the Breast*. Baltimore, MD: Williams & Wilkins.

Thorogood, N. (2000) Sex education as disciplinary technique: policy and practice in England and Wales, *Sexualities*, 3(4): 425–38.

Trivedi, P. and Wykes, T. (2002) From passive subjects to equal partners: qualitative review of user involvement in research, *British Journal of Psychiatry*, 181: 468–72.

Verschuren, P.I.M. (2001) Holism versus reductionism in modern social science research, *Quality and Quantity*, 35: 389–405.

Wakefield, A.J. and Montgomery, S.M. (2000) Measles, mumps and rubella vaccine: through a glass, darkly, *Adverse Drug Reactions and Toxicology Reviews*, 19(4): 265–92.

Wakefield, A.J., Murch, S.H., Anthony, A. and Linnell, J. (1998) Ileal-lymphoid-nodular hypoplasia, non-specific colitis and pervasive developmental disorder in children, *Lancet*, 351(9103): 637–41.

Wellsby, P.D. (1999) Reductionism in medicine: some thoughts on medical education from the front line, *Journal of Evaluation in Clinical Practice*, 5(2): 125–31.

Williams, C.J. and Zwitter, M. (1994) Informed consent in European multicentre randomized clinical trials – are patients really informed?, *European Journal of Cancer*, 30: 907–10.

Wilson, C., Pollock, M.R. and Harris, A.D. (1946) Diet in the treatment of infectious hepatitis, *Lancet*, i: 881–3.

Yoshioka, A. (1998) Use of randomisation in the Medical Research Council's clinical trial of streptomycin in pulmonary tuberculosis in the 1940s, *British Medical Journal*, 317: 1220–3.

Young, E. (2001) Autism 'no longer a rare condition', *New Scientist*, 13 December.

7

Epistemology II: interpretation and hermeneutics

So far, we have examined the rise of science as applied to health care. In the previous two chapters we have attempted to give the reader a sense of how the present guise of scientific medicine has come about. In this chapter, we describe the rise of a different way of looking at the world which scholars have adopted and which has been influential in research on illness and health. For the past century and a half, interpretive or hermeneutic approaches have been making headway in the social sciences, and latterly they have become popular in the health care disciplines too. To a number of nineteenth-century social thinkers, notably Max Weber, the social sciences could not proceed in the same way as the natural sciences. Because of the centrality of meaning to human life, it was necessary, in his view, for the social scientist to engage in a kind of interpretive understanding or *Verstehen*, where the goal of the researcher is to reconstruct the subjective social experience of people. Whereas we can discern patterns in health behaviour by looking at life in the way that a positivist would – by examining the antecedents of morbidity or looking at what factors predispose people, for example, to use GP services or attend breast screening clinics – we cannot penetrate the activity unless we consider the meanings people attach to their behaviour, what they think is wrong with them and why they think that the health care system can offer them some hope. In this chapter, we also consider the special problems facing the researcher attempting to discern regularities in social life. How can we infer rules in social behaviour? What part does language or discourse play in interpreting and making sense of the world?

In practical terms, there has been a recent growth of interest in qualitative methodology, especially in nursing, where researchers have sought to clarify the nature of the nursing process through a fine-grained attention to language, interaction and subjectivity in health care encounters. This spirit of qualitative enquiry has been theoretically eclectic, drawing on methods and theories from phenomenology, grounded theory, feminist research and many more. The practical activity of health care, especially as it is practised and studied in nursing, is a rich mosaic of different styles of knowing and action and is formulated into practices of human enquiry through a complex and often confusing potpourri of theory which is sometimes grafted on in a haphazard or *ad hoc* fashion. Thus, one of the tasks of this chapter is to examine the role of health care practitioners as practical philosophers and methodologists as they go about the everyday tasks of health care, and discuss some of the recent scholarly attempts to provide interpretive descriptions of the health care process.

We shall, rather roughly, call all this emphasis on description 'phenomenology' and interpretation 'interpretivism' and, equally roughly, we can view interpretivism as an alternative to positivism and natural science approaches to health care. In this chapter, we begin to unpick the philosophy underpinning descriptive approaches to research. We identify key arguments in support of the interpretivist's view of the social world. In particular, we hope to illustrate just how central language theory is within this approach. If we take an interpretivist view of the world, we buy into the belief that the social world is constructed by humans and that we are forever involved in making sense of or interpreting our social environments or settings. Thus, interpretivism is at heart a catch-all for a collection of approaches broadly called 'qualitative' – it says 'go forth and qualify' as opposed to positivism's 'go forth and quantify'.

Interpretivism brings with it a dose of scepticism concerning the possibility of attaining objective certainties. It foregrounds human creativity in terms of human history and society; it interrogates simplified or reductive views of reality – it focuses on the fluid, more open and creative engagement of human beings and the world and seeks knowledge and understanding that is ultimately less concrete or objectified yet deserving of rigorous enquiry. Ultimately, it involves an investigation and interpretation of human behaviour. Edmund Husserl viewed knowledge of the world as an act of consciousness (phenomenology). The world is experienced and given meaning by acts of consciousness. The task of phenomenology is to describe this experience of what can be called the 'life world': the world as given in immediate experience and independent of and prior to scientific or other interpretation. Of course, such processes are always going to have their limitations.

Interpretivism had rather unusual beginnings. One of the important strands in contemporary interpretive social science is hermeneutics. In the late nineteenth century and then again in the late 1960s, hermeneutics flourished, prompted originally by the problems faced by theologians in interpreting the Bible. Hermeneutics was concerned with difficulty over literal meaning of the Bible, due to multiple translations, multiple gospels, loss of the actual words of Christ (*ipsissima verba*), which would originally have been in Aramaic, not Greek, Latin or the later vernacular languages of English, French and so on. As a result, scholars debated which translation was the most authentic. This early hermeneutics, which involved exegesis or critical explanation of written texts, developed into a much wider application of interpreting human society and history. In essence, the notion of 'text' widened to include spoken language and the diverse ways that peoples or societies represent themselves, not least in a symbolic way. In effect, humans and what they did could be 'read' and interpreted like you would read and interpret a piece of writing or set of symbols or images.

The central concerns of hermeneutics – the study of interpretive practices – are important to any account of interpretation and description. If we are to delineate the meaning of what people say about their state of health, the treatments that health professionals administer and patients receive or any other health-related matter, we must deal with the processes of interpretation. In a sense, the issue of health care is hermeneutic on a number of levels. People as they suffer and heal are hard at work making interpretations about what is happening and what they are doing. Similarly, health professionals engage in interpreting their own actions. Moreover, the researcher or philosopher who attempts to make sense of all these diverse processes is engaged in a hermeneutic practice too.

Giddens (1984) reminds us that the social sciences are in a subject–subject relationship with their object of study. This could equally be said of many health care disciplines. Social scientists and health care researchers usually have to interact with their objects of study to implement their research, and the subject–subject relationship also implies that the social world can be transformed by research and theory in the social and health care sciences. Change can take place as the seepage from academic life to the broader community occurs. The patient in the GP's surgery nowadays may come armed with a sheaf of notes downloaded from the internet, for example. This relationship between knowledge and society is what Giddens identifies as the 'double hermeneutic', defined as: 'a mutual interpretative interplay between social science and those whose activities compose its subject matter' (Giddens 1984: pp. xxxii and 348). In agreement with this, Sayer (1992) explains: 'social phenomena can be changed intrinsically by learning and adjusting to the subject's understanding' (pp. 28–9). Thus, the health care disciplines, like the social sciences, are embedded in their subject matter and are therefore almost bound to have some sort of interaction with it. Describing the world may well tend to change it, once people get wind of, support and respond to that description. The rise in dissociative identity disorder or 'multiple personality', for example, has puzzled and perplexed many clinicians and researchers. In the USA and Canada, as many as 2 per cent of the population are believed to meet the diagnostic criteria (Casey 2001). This is a huge leap, for up until about 1980 or so, less than 300 cases had been identified. Casey herself points to cultural differences, inasmuch as clinicians on the European side of the Atlantic treat the whole idea with much greater scepticism and there are much lower rates of diagnosis. Authors such as Casey (2001) and Spanos (1994) put this down to a greater awareness on the part of patients and clinicians and the increasing attention given to such problems in the media over the past 40 years. This seems to have created a new framework within which people can interpret their difficulties. Now this is not to say that the people turning up in therapists' consulting rooms are deliberately 'faking' in any obvious sense. Rather, the contemporary interest in such problems has allowed the formulation of problems in a particular way. There is a link, then, between the scientific aspects of mental health, the popular representations of these, and the kinds of symptoms which are displayed by individuals in distress.

The cynic might conclude that all these individual, idiosyncratic hermeneutic moments as people delivering or receiving health care interpret their experiences are so fragmented that they cannot add up to a rigorous, systematic or scientific activity. However, the impact of hermeneutic practices on literary studies, social science and even health care practices requires some coverage if we are to make sense of the interpretive activity that goes to make up health care.

As already noted, hermeneutics originated in European philosophers' accounts of the interpretive problems faced in theology, history and the 'human sciences'. Hermeneutics is motivated by a desire to make the most defensible reading of a relatively obscure text – however widely we define the latter. It involves sifting competing readings of that text, weighing their respective merits in the light of what is given in that text. Hudson (1984) admits that hermeneutics is 'little more than a slogan' (p. 66) but is characterized by its concentration on what is 'tangibly, incontrovertibly *there*' in a text (p. 66). Hudson takes some specific artistic images and unpacks the meaning with which they are freighted, as in his book *Bodies of Knowledge* (1982), where he concentrates on representations of the body in art and literature, attempting to render them in their full complexity.

But, as Hudson admits, we need to know more to make interpretations. For example, the public outrage when Edouard Manet's painting 'Olympia' was first exhibited in 1865 is difficult to deduce from the picture alone. This famous painting of a naked reclining woman gazing at the viewer, attended by a maid offering her a bunch of flowers, might have been shocking for a variety of reasons. The suspicion that this was a picture not of a classical theme, as was implied by the title, but of a prostitute had something to do with the horror of polite Parisian society. The high prevalence of prostitution in Paris at that time meant that Manet was offering a kind of social commentary too. The turn away from a classical style of painting with fine brushwork towards a style with bold, large brushstrokes was also controversial at a time when many artists were still trying to achieve realism in competition with the camera. Even knowing something of the historical situation, it would still be difficult to proceed with any definiteness to a conclusion as to why the painting was 'shocking'. Hudson exhibits a curious tension, one which is perhaps inherent in hermeneutics, between the desire to work on what is uncontrovertibly there in the 'text' or artefact and the need for some interpretive licence, for 'nuance and innuendo' (Hudson 1982, p. 69). Moreover, in hermeneutics we cannot refer to comfortable bodies of rules and received procedure. Yet it is possible to salvage a description of the method:

> In interpretive or hermeneutic work, whether applied to dreams or to more public texts and signs, one advances not by reference to more public texts and signs but by fastidious respect for what the text says. If the hermeneut is impatient of its fine grain, the progress he [*sic*] makes will be illusory.
>
> (Hudson 1982, p. 48)

This, then, was the kind of route that hermeneutics took into the human sciences, via projects on art history, imagery and culture. More recently, the fine-grained texts to which scholars are turning their attention are medical as well as artistic or literary. There is a growing interest in seeing 'patients as texts' too (Svenaeus 2000).

Ambiguity need not be fatal to the hermeneutic project provided it is acknowledged and built upon as an analytic topic in its own right, rather than glossed over. Ambiguity might give us access to recesses of experience which other means of research would fail to reach, yet it must remain centred on what the 'text' actually says.

While we might accept that hermeneutics is concerned to develop the best and most defensible interpretation of a text, the possibility of a unitary hermeneutic method is elusive, as Ricouer [1968] (1976) confesses: 'there is no general hermeneutics, no universal canon for exegesis, but only disparate and opposed theories concerning the rules of interpretation. The hermeneutic field . . . is internally at variance with itself' (p. 194). Some of the internal variance might be compressed into a distinction between two different kinds of hermeneutics: 'According to the one pole, hermeneutics is understood as the manifestation and restoration of a meaning addressed to me in the manner of a message . . . according to the other pole it is understood as a demystification, a reduction of illusion' (p. 194). Or, as Ricouer later calls them, 'interpretation as a recollection of meaning' and 'interpretation as an exercise of suspicion'. That is, in the first type we attempt to define the meaning of the object, whereas in the second we are suspicious, rather as Marx, Nietzsche and Freud were suspicious of the contents of consciousness. A general theory of interpretation would have to accommodate these two different approaches – a difficult mode of analysis to achieve. It is not situated easily within a Popperian 'science of health'. A great deal of what the hermeneut might seek to present in his or her analysis might be dismissed on the pretexts that it contains too much of their personality. This objection was of concern to Bultmann (1986):

> The question of whether exegesis without presuppositions is possible must be answered affirmatively if 'without presuppositions' means 'without presupposing the results of the exegesis'. In this sense exegesis without presuppositions is not only possible but demanded. In another sense however, there is no exegesis [that] is without presuppositions, inasmuch as the exegete is not a *tabula rasa* [or blank slate].
>
> (Bultmann 1986, p. 242)

We may suggest further that some of the problems for hermeneutic theory reside in its very specificity. It is not a unified body of expertise and method which can itself be set down in the form of a textbook. Even when the presuppositions are limited, however, there are concerns that interpretation represents some kind of loss over the original. As Susan Sontag (2001) argues, interpretation is a 'vicious and cowardly' form of translation. It involves the work of art – or anything else – being stripped of its 'sensuous life' and being reduced to a series of statements. Subsequently, these weakened, eviscerated statements are processed through the categories of various schools of criticism (for instance, Marxism, Freudian analysis, Judeo-Christian thought) into a message that is all too familiar, thereby denaturing the radical potential of the original.

A further complication arises in that there will be some distance between the originator of discourse or action and the prospective interpreter, such that the intended subjective meaning of the author or actor will remain opaque (Ricouer 1971, p. 203). Hirsch describes the procedure which will then become necessary:

> The act of understanding is at first a genial (or mistaken) guess and there are no methods for making guesses, no formal rules for generating insights, the methodological activity of interpretation commences when we begin to test and criticise our guesses.
>
> (Hirsch 1976, p. 25)

Ricouer argues that the means by which guesses are tested follows a logic of probability rather than a logic of empirical verification. In the hermeneutic cycle of moving from guess to validation and back to refined guess, we must always retain the possibility of disconfirmation of our hypotheses, of being surprised. Our favoured interpretation must be more likely than any other.

> The logic of validation allows us to move between the two limits of dogmatism and scepticism. It is always possible to argue for or against an interpretation, to confront interpretations, to arbitrate between them and to seek for an agreement, even if this agreement remains beyond our reach.
>
> (Ricouer 1971, p. 207)

Thus Ricouer defies the possibility that for any manifestation there are a multiplicity of possible causal models or possible interpretations. But at least he allows the possibility of differing interpretations without imposing a closure unwarranted by the data. We must ensure that an adequate number and variety of possible competing interpretations are generated, particularly when the character of the material is alien. We would need to study the contexts of production and reception, before being able to suggest its meaning.

The process of validation may well have a polemical character, since the 'context of argumentation' for our conclusions will be more conspicuous than the context of proof. So perhaps the judicial metaphor for the validation of interpretations is appropriate (Hart 1948). Yet a single analyst cannot be at the same time opposing counsel, judge, jury and executioner. While no human heuristic process can be exhaustively specified by systems of rules, this does not eliminate the trust between the hermeneut and his or her audience.

Even so, Markovic (1984) argues that an interpretive science does more justice to the subject matter of social research than the hypothetico-deductive method. Interpretation is an open-ended search for consensus in a dialogue between conflicting interpretations. Unlike legal practice, though, hermeneutics does not have verdict and execution: 'Neither in literary criticism nor in social science is there such a last word. Or, if there is any, we call that violence' (Ricouer 1971, p. 84). But then any conclusion, by that token, is violence. When do we know when we've done enough? This is particularly perplexing as he describes the hermeneutic method as one of validation. The problems of hermeneutics are compounded by ill-informed criticisms. In defiance of the above quote, Shklar (1986) says that 'We are simply told that, first of all, a text, any text is fixed, unalterable and just obdurately there' (p. 459). Whereas Ricouer identifies text not in this latter positivistic sense, but as a thing brought into being by our understanding process.

Thus, the problem of hermeneutic procedures does not inhere solely in the vagueness with which they are specified, nor entirely in the trust which they depend on between the hermeneutic author and his or her audience. Some of the critical points about hermeneutics having no theory of the production and use of meaning ring true. But even so, Hudson (1984) claimed to be doing hermeneutics, even though his discussion of the human body in nineteenth-century art describes the preoccupations of French society. These cannot be deduced from 'reading' the paintings; they have to come from other documentary sources. Perhaps, then, Hudson is able to circumvent the criticism of hermeneutics by Habermas (1980) and Outhwaite

(1987) that its focus on the text leads it away from the possibility that the text may misrepresent some grander reality. That is, what Ricouer calls the truth of symbols might be a naive assumption. For example, enthusiasts for evolutionary theory in the nineteenth century were interested in the way that human foetuses appeared to have features which suggested earlier periods in the development of life on earth. This idea was originally formulated by Darwin's ally Ernst Haeckel (1834–1919), who noted that foetuses appeared to have gill slits and a tail. Indeed, it has been suggested that he carefully doctored photographs, illustrations and specimens to make his interpretation appear the most likely. More contemporary opinion has it that the apparent gill slits are in fact vessels carrying blood to and from the head and that the fact that the lower limb buds are initially seen some distance from the base of the spine is more to do with their needing a good blood supply rather than being a vestige of a former tail. Indeed, the tailbone or coccyx in modern humans is not necessarily a 'vestigial organ', as it forms an anchorage point for ligaments and muscles controlling the anus. The idea that 'ontogeny recapitulates phylogeny' was a powerful component of Haeckel's thought, yet has now almost entirely fallen into disuse as different theories of human development come to predominate and functions are discovered for what were previously thought of as vestigial organs, such as the thymus gland. The point here, then, is that we cannot make sense of Haeckel's illustrations solely by looking at them as pictures. We have to know something about what he was trying to do with the pictures. However, the limitation of hermeneutic theory and practice is that we don't necessarily have the benefit of additional information about the content of the text with which to judge this.

It is therefore difficult to present a manifesto for hermeneutics, or an explicit definition of it. Still less can we appropriate it verbatim as a method having the conventionally respectable means of adjudicating between competing claims in the way that self-identified empiricists suppose occurs in the conventional Popperian model. We are not in a realm of received procedure. When Ricouer speaks of 'rules', they may very likely not materialize as such in his subsequent discussion (e.g. Ricouer 1971, p. 185). Yet there must presumably be a hermeneutic moment in all research; where we identify the salient aspects of the field or are interpreting the results, be there ever so much rigorous quantification in between. And in doing so there is little in the way of precise practical guidance for the researcher.

That said, many philosophically astute scholars, such as Wilhelm Dilthey, have argued that an understanding or knowledge of human phenomena was unobtainable through 'positivism'. In other words, in the work of accruing knowledge about human activity and its meanings, we have little choice but to get messy in the world of interpretivism. 'Positivism' simply could not put a handle on the diverse activity of humans in creating their own societies and indeed histories. In other words, the positivist focus on objects – study of natural and material bodies – could not do justice in explanatory terms for the subjective, mindful aspects of human society and history – the play of the human mind as a creative force in the world and at the heart of 'real' phenomena such as morality, values, social institutions, law, literature and so on. The emphasis of 'interpretivism' was on how the human mind determined or constituted the lived experience of social reality. Dilthey was of the view that any objectivity in terms of mind, culture and society has to come through the 'intersubjective' agreement about the status of 'out there' social reality.

Back in the nineteenth century, Max Weber tried to strengthen the bond between interpretative understanding and the more positivistic rigours of science, through *Verstehen* – that is, 'the attempt to reconstruct the subjective experience of social actors' (Hughes and Sharrock 1997). This rested on two principles: value neutrality, which involved trying not to pass off value judgements as scientific truths; and ideal types, which were abstractions used as thinking tools – artificial, abstract patterns for subjectively held meanings. You can never see a 'Protestant work ethic', for example, yet it remains a useful tool for making sense of the religious asceticism, self-denial and hard work that characterized many predominantly Protestant countries through the industrial revolution.

Traditional, positivistic social science derives stable elements such as social 'institutions' from patterns of social action that may themselves be derived from feelings, beliefs and attitudes of individuals and social rules external to those individuals. From an interpretive perspective, on the other hand, the researcher or theorist begins with a different set of premises:

- Our descriptions of social actions will always be limited and incomplete.
- The study of human action will not yield the kind of rigid framework that positivists desire.
- The description and explanation of human action will always come from interpretation of various 'texts', and interpretation is governed by a whole variety of influences or constraints – not least language and schemas that people hold and through which they view reality in one of many possible ways.

Moreover, from an interpretivist viewpoint:

- Human social life is seen as something constituted through the activity and social interaction of language.
- Language is seen as action – shaping and constructing human realities.
- We talk the world into existence in a particular way.

While we may share with others a particular language, and meanings about phenomena, there will inevitably be a great deal of fluidity in terms of how we interpret what other people say or write about the world, how the world is constituted in language by other people, differences in the way we receive and interpret the words, signs, symbols or actions of others. In short, there is no neutral language to describe reality – there is no neutral position from which to perceive social reality in an objective fashion. We cannot escape the selectivity of our knowledge, our explanations.

Hans-Georg Gadamer (1981) thought that it is our nature as human beings that we are defined and limited by language and time – we cannot step out of the 'hermeneutic circle' to see the whole of reality and have a complete view of it. We only interpret reality in part, not as a whole. The most we can do is be open to other people's ways of interpreting things and aim for a 'fusion' of our own horizon and that of others – a coming together, if you like – between our interpretation of 'reality', of 'texts', presentations and representations and those of others. Thus we are involved in an endless conversation with others and the past – an unending dialogue. Since there is no experience of the world, independent of language, there is a straitjacket upon our knowledge of the world.

There are other legacies from Gadamer's project which are important to hermeneutic approaches in the health sciences. The usual practice in conventional hermeneutics is to see the thing that one is interpreting as a text on which to exercise one's interpretive powers. In this sense, then, a medical encounter, a patient or an X-ray are all 'texts' of one sort or another. From the point of view of Gadamer, and a number of recent writers on the subject, this is not adequate as a conceptualization of what goes on.

The clinicians and clients are involved together in creating a joint understanding of what happens in clinical encounters, what the problem is and what matters. Svenaeus (2000), for example, draws on Gadamer's philosophy to get away from thinking about medicine as text and think instead of a dialogical social activity. Whereas existentialists have stressed 'being in the world', Svenaeus would add to this and stress that human life is about 'being in the world together'. Gadamer further stresses the importance of reflecting on the relationship between the interpreter and the things being interpreted, because, it is argued, this relationship or dialogue is crucial in helping to create the meanings and interpretations (Harrington 2000).

Yet such interpretative or hermeneutic dialogue, which can be positive and equitable, and even incorporate Gadamer's 'fusion of horizons', can still be unsatisfactory. Take, for example, the whole field of biography or life writing. This area is fraught with interpretive difficulty about what information captures the real, fleshy, embodied selves. Do we not suspect that many of the biographies or life interpretations of celebrities of all kinds are far from truth-bearing? Or when we read biographies that seem candid and unadorned, do we not suspect that even these might be less than truthful in representing 'real' lives? But before we get the sense that biography is far from our concerns as health practitioners, we might want to reflect on how much life-writing occurs in health practice settings in the form of case notes, reports, care plans and so on. Whether we like it or not, health professionals are in the thick of negotiating the realities of other people, of making sense of them for good and ill. We need to be vigilant about our interpretative dialogue with patients, since the greater portion of our encounters will be asymmetrical – in other words, the professionals will often assume superior interpretive power over and above the views, interpretations or perspectives of patients.

Interpretive social science was taken up with a vengeance in the middle of the twentieth century. The sociologist C. Wright Mills (1959) saw the overly positivistic approaches that were sometimes taken in sociology as being rather like a 'cookbook', whereas social science is better practised with imagination and flexibility; and Erving Goffman (1961) likened positivism to a child's chemistry set – follow the instructions and you too can be like a real scientist. Interpretivists do not necessarily deny the role of evidence in scientific activity, but they also highlight how much of our knowledge of the world is confined to interpretation and the restrictions of language – that the social world is actively constructed by human beings and we are continuously involved in making sense of or interpreting our social environment. Broadly speaking it opposes the 'positivist' study of humans as objects.

A further contrast can be seen in relation to the attitude of interpretivism and positivism to the foundations of scientific knowledge. Positivism, traditionally at least, was associated with some degree of foundationalism. That is, the belief that knowledge rests on a set of unquestionable truths or a solid reality that is somehow 'out there'. Anti-foundationalists subscribe to the belief that unquestionable truths and knowledge do not exist, that perhaps the phenomenal world of our experience is a human construction.

A good deal of interpretive social science draws on the method of analytic induction where laws and regularities are induced – that is, drawing conclusions or theorizing based on a large number of observations of any particular phenomenon, which may include almost any object or occurrence perceived by the senses. Analytic induction aims to provide a causal explanation by specifying the individually necessary and jointly sufficient conditions necessary for the emergence of some part of social life. Like hypothetico-deductive science as described by Karl Popper, the analytic inductive method seeks to challenge the initial findings by looking for more problem cases that might not fit the emerging hypotheses. It was originally proposed by Znaniecki (1934), who was famous for his studies of the immigration experience from Poland to the United States. It was 'analytic' because of this search for problem cases of the phenomenon that might refute the hypotheses. The idea is to undertake a progressive redefinition of the explanandum (the thing to be explained) and of the explanans (the explanatory factors) so that a perfect or 'universal' relationship is maintained. For example, one feature that a number of researchers have identified is the presence of turning points in people's lives. This may be told to the researcher with considerable detail and poignancy, perhaps especially when it is a turning point in the participant's commitment to activity that is socially defined as delinquent, deviant or discreditable. This might appear in accounts of opiate addiction (Lindesmith 1968), embezzling (Cressey 1953), marijuana use (Becker 1953), conversion to a religious cult (Lofland and Stark 1965) and seeking an abortion (Manning 1971). All these turning points and processes of commitment were described by those who had done them. What happens, though, when people turn away from a socially deviant or discreditable path? Let us try looking at this different kind of event to see how universal our inducted feature is. Sure enough – fortunately for the idea of turning points – similar experiences are reported by those who desist from crime (West 1978) and those who realize they have 'a problem' with alcohol, give up drinking and start attending Alcoholics Anonymous (Denzin 1989). Denzin even gives these experiences a new name – 'epiphanies'. That, then, is how analytic induction works. Induction goes from the specific to the general, pulling observations together to create a new theory.

As we have indicated, the interpretive approach to health phenomena looks to the meanings that people attach to their behaviour, what they think is wrong with them and why they think that the health care system might be of benefit to them. Let us examine a few cases of where such an approach has been applied.

1. 'Soundscapes of everyday life' and the 'killing machines'

Komatra Chuengsatiansup's (1999) ethnographic study of women in the Kui communities of Northern Thailand provides a strong model of the interpretive approach to knowledge acquisition, not least because it avoids the more obvious world of visual appearances and examines instead how the 'soundscape of everyday life' affects the women's 'lived experience' of symptoms such as sleeplessness, shortness of breath, feeling frightened, loss of appetite and chronic fatigue. By examining their life stories and experiences, Chuengsatiansup was able to identify how various harsh sounds, such as motorcycles, quarrelling neighbours, machinery or the noises made by drunkards, promoted somatic symptoms. These 'meaning-endowed sonic icons' acted as triggers for intense feelings of 'marginality, vulnerability, and defencelessness' that presented as uncomfortable bodily illness (Chuengsatiansup 1999, pp. 283, 275). For example, the sound of motorcycles provoked anxiety and worry among the women because of high fatalities and accidents among their teenager population who sought the high prestige of owning or riding them. The threat this posed was such that villagers spoke of the 'Suzuki Disease' or 'Yamaha Disease'. By investigating this and other aspects of the women's soundscape, Chuengsatiansup was able to show powerfully the impact of disharmonious sounds on health and well-being. Also, this work alerts us to the cultural privileging of vision and the possibility that various soundscapes may be endowed with all kinds of political and cultural meanings. Various sounds, Chuengsatiansup maintains, can be seen as 'embodied symbols of human relations' (p. 297).

The focus of Chuengsatiansup's anthropological study may seem a long way from the concerns of Westernized health care. So what if certain sounds spark certain symptoms in a variety of women in Northern Thailand? What has that to do with us? Well, this study alerts us to how the interpretive approach – examining here life histories and stories – affords new insights into how people experience illness. We might wish to replicate this approach in contemporary Western health care sites, for example a cardiology unit or an acute mental health unit. What soundscapes occur here? How might these impact on patients? At some time or other, most of us have had cause to complain about 'noise pollution' often from neighbours or mobile phones, but how seriously do we take soundscapes in relation to health and illness? Here, we can consider extending this interpretive approach that 'works to point to possibilities in order to enrich human existence through increasing understanding of the everydayness of being human' (Darbyshire *et al.* 1999, p. 23).

2. Interpreting pain – 'isn't pain supposed to be what the client says it is?'

In David Morley's (2002) collection of prose and poetry, *The Gift: New Writing for the NHS*, Susan Crawford, a nurse and sickle cell sufferer, writes an acrostic about pain:

Acrostic

Shards of pain coursing through your body –
Inconvenient I'm sorry pain can't tell the time.

Counting the seconds, minutes, hours for pain relief,
Knuckles aching, your fists are clenched so tight.
Lord I pray please guide me through this;
Eyes wild, tears streaming; to have my mother's arms around me.

Compassion – I know they wouldn't treat an animal this way;
Empathy, I've yet to see it, isn't pain supposed to be what the client says it is.
Lethargy, I haven't got the strength to cry.
Listen to me please: if I didn't need to be here, I'd be at home.

In her poem, Crawford reveals not simply the subjective nature of pain, but how disturbingly the scientific approach of medicine often fails to treat it with the seriousness it deserves. This undertreatment of pain has been noted by scholars, not least Resnik *et al.* (2001), who point out that medicine is often slow to respond to pain 'because: (1) pain is subjective, not objective; (2) the causal basis of pain is often poorly understood; (3) pain is regarded as a "mere" symptom, not as a disease; (4) there often are no "magic bullets" for pain; (5) pain does not fit the expert knowledge model' (p. 277). In many ways, the phenomena of pain, so central to the experience of illness, does not sit well with the positivist philosophy driving the scientific enterprises of modern medicine. In the grip of positivist science, medicine frequently relegates pain to the bottom of clinical priorities.

The experience of pain, as with other experiences of illness, falls more into a wide-ranging and inclusive interpretivist approach to phenomena. As Resnik *et al.* note:

Pain is subjective, private and highly variable. Only the person sensing the pain can determine whether they are having that sensation. In a clinical setting, pain is what the patient says it is and exists whenever the patient says it does (McCaffery and Beebe, 1989). The response to pain may vary a great deal from one person to another.

(Resnik *et al.* 2001, p. 278)

Importantly, there are diverse psychosocial and cultural aspects to the experience of pain and how we attend to it or interpret it:

A person who is enjoying the pleasant taste of hot pepper may be paying less attention to the pain it inflicts. A person who is receiving a massage for lower back pain may pay less attention to the pain and more attention to the massage . . . A person may believe that pain is an indicator of disease, of impending doom, or of a loss of control or dignity. Another person may believe that their pain is a sign of a desirable event, such as childbirth or muscle fatigue due to weightlifting . . . Cultural beliefs, social groups, and religious traditions can play an important role in the response to pain by affecting how we interpret and attend to pain.

(Resnik *et al.* 2001, pp. 280–1)

Whichever form the subjective experience of pain takes, the measurement and understanding of pain looks unlikely to emerge from positivistic enquiry. As conveyed in

Crawford's poem, we must rely on first-person reports. Understanding and interpreting these reports is by no means easy, as Resnik *et al.* (2001) note: 'We can no more experience another person's pain than we can experience their joy, their love of Mozart, their aversion to anchovies, or their suffering' (p. 283). However, interpretive research can help bring subjective, psycho-social and cultural perspectives to the fore in developing better pain management. Through a rich and detailed understanding of the diverse manifestations of pain experience, practitioners might be less likely to adopt limited and unsatisfactory responses.

3. *Textual practices: clinical hermeneutics*

Medicine's apparent devaluation of subjective accounts of pain seems strangely at odds with the overall hermeneutics of medicine and, indeed, nursing – where so much clinical practice is steeped in interpreting 'texts', be they medical charts, case reports or patients. In other words, while medicine and nursing present themselves as scientific and driven by the latest technologies for curing people of diseases, they are largely engaged in dialogue and interpretation. This irony is not lost on Svenaeus (2000), who, while disliking the concept of hermeneutics that focuses on 'textual readings', supports the view of medical practice as inescapably hermeneutic as it is scientific:

> characteristic of the hermeneutics of medicine is rather a distinct and unique form of dialogic interpretation enveloping the explanational methods of the *natural* sciences. The specific methods that are applied in the clinical encounter indeed seem to belong to the natural sciences rather than the humanities. But, and this is the important point, the meeting between doctor and patient from which this applicational machinery – X-rays, lab tests, ECG etc. – evolves can indeed be said to be hermeneutical – interpretative – *in itself.*
>
> (Svenaeus 2000, p. 173)

For Svenaeus, 'the dialogic aspect of clinical practice is downplayed by the metaphor of reading [texts]. Patients are indeed partners in the medical meeting and not objects, not even textual objects' (p. 175). But whether we are viewing medicine as concerned with 'reading texts' or being in dialogue – both amount broadly to the same – science-driven medicine is immersed in clinical hermeneutics or interpretation. Yet, by and large, this interpretivist activity is frequently discounted as little more than a transmission issue of 'white-coat' scientific objectivity and facts. The materiality of dialogue and 'text', however widely we define it, is often dismissed as a commonplace tool in the service of facts rather than facts in and of themselves that deserve serious scrutiny. At every turn, it appears, positivistic science prefers to overwrite the interpretivist dimension. Yet as Svenaeus suggests *à la* Gadamer, a 'merging of the horizons' of the two different life worlds of the doctor and patient should feature in clinical encounters: 'Through the explication of clinical practice as a dialogue based hermeneutics it is possible to point out the significance of this type of "life world knowledge" in medicine, as opposed to what would be the case if one restricts oneself to a model of clinical practice as applied biology' (Svenaeus 2000, p. 184).

This focus on clinical hermeneutics and interpretation in terms of dialogue betrays an increasing interest or focus on communication and language in the processes of health care delivery. Yet if the latter half of the twentieth century saw an increased focus upon language, there was also great uncertainty and scepticism about the meaning in language – the limitations of language – and the relationship of language to reality. There has been an ongoing debate between those who hold the view that reality is constructed by language and those who wish to hold on to the notion of an external, material world. The idea that language constructs reality, or is constitutive of the social world, has led to the idea of 'multiple realities'. People have their own conceptions of what they are doing, and the world they are in. This may be radically different from the conceptions of other people. A culture different to our own can be seen as a distinctive realm of discourse with its own logic and standards of rationality – discourse being a structure governed by a set of rules which identifies what things people can speak about and who has the right to speak about those things. Just think here of the discourse of medicine or law. Because of differences in discourse, someone else's cultural reality, in other words, may not be our own. The way that a doctor talks or writes will be different from that of a lawyer, or the discourse, say, of miners, and so on.

Edward Sapir and Benjamin Lee Whorf noted how language difference reflects different world views. For example, in an insurance case that Whorf was investigating, some people said that fuel drums without fuel in them were empty, while for others, including Whorf as an insurance loss adjuster, these drums without fuel in them were 'full' of fuel vapour and very much combustible. The different conceptions had implications for safety. A further twist to the tale was added by Potter (1996), who noted that the people in question were making an insurance claim, and thus were likely to be keen to show that they had acted responsibly. Their garage had burned down and it was likely that their claim would be disallowed had they been storing gasoline in it. Describing the drums as empty was probably a strategically advantageous move on their part. The Sapir-Whorf hypothesis, then, was that vocabularies are organized by their grammars, and thus help to organize the forms of thought of the speakers of the language.

Wittgenstein (1889–1951) alerted us to the strong sense that many people have that the meaning of a word was the thing the word stood for – that is, something external to language (Wittgenstein 1981). He advanced the notion that language is not as clear as this, but that the meaning of any word is given by its position in a city-like complex of relationships with other words and the things that we do. In other words, language is far trickier than being simply a system for naming objects in the external world.

Ludwig Wittgenstein, Peter Winch and Thomas Kuhn all argue that the study of social life must be as much the study of language use – language is the pre-eminent medium of the conduct of social life – and advance the rather relativistic and disturbing view for some, that reality is what a particular scientific community hold it to be or, indeed, describe it in language as being.

The problem of translation was taken up by the post-empiricist W.V.O. Quine (1990) and others, who attacked the simplistic, physicalist view of the world – that it is only worth examining physical things. For Quine, to give the meaning of any sentence is merely to substitute it with another one – that there is no intrinsic meaning to any sentence and, indeed, language as a whole – just a kind of pass the parcel with words and sentences. When someone speaks or writes, a translation of it can be given by the speaker themselves but that translation has no authority – it provides only one translation among many possible translations.

In the 1950s and 1960s, there was a great deal of interest in the structure of language and social life. Chomsky's emphasis on grammars and deep structures in language not only revolutionized linguistics, but also is believed to be responsible for toppling behaviourism from its dominant position in psychology (Chomsky 1957). In anthropology, structuralists like Claude Lévi-Strauss (1969) looked at the system of language as one of contrasts, rules and ideologies. In this view, there was a fairly clear correspondence between the structure of social life and the nature of language. People who were related or lived together tended to have the same sorts of names. Language, then, described the kinds of goods that were exchanged, the deities that were important and how the children were raised. There is a long tradition of exploring the common features of language, myths and folktales. Chomsky famously contended that all human beings speak pretty much the same language, such that all utterances are capable of being parsed into a structure consisting of subject–object–verb or subject–verb–object. Vladimir Propp ([1928] 1976), perhaps rather less famously, contended that all stories consist of seven roles and thirty-three functions. Lévi-Strauss (1969) focused on common features and structures in South American myths. The aim of these kinds of analyses was to identify common features, especially at the level of sentence or story structure – hence the term 'structuralism'.

In contrast to these ambitions to discern an intelligible structure, a far more sceptical and doubt-filled approach to language emerged in the last three decades of the twentieth century. This had a number of names, such as 'deconstruction', 'postmodernism' or 'poststructuralism'. What many of these more sceptical scholars such as Paul de Man (1986) and Jacques Derrida (1977) did was to bring a kind of vertigo to the notion of texts, discourse or language meaning anything at all, and foregrounded the contradictory nature of texts. Even the kind of neutral description of rules that the structuralists aimed at was itself tendentious and ideological, fired up with 'science'; and as such left out a variety of marginal, repressed discourses. A text, theory or item of knowledge may itself be riddled with contradictions. Resistance may itself be assimilated into the master discourse. Dominant discourses mask the more marginal and less powerful ways of viewing the world. Scepticism about meaning and language joined a whirl of scepticism surrounding the ambitions of reason, the progressive rational dream of the Enlightenment. Science and rationality were challenged by those who argued that they were instruments of domination rather than liberation. These 'big stories' – or grand narratives as Jean-François Lyotard (1991, 1993) called them – such as the progress of humanity through rationality and science, were undermined. Emphasis was placed upon the fragmentary, flawed, difficult nature of reality or realities – and on the vast number of competing forces and discourses that are part of our world; in other words, there was an intense focus on the various disunities of 'reality' rather than unifying and certain features of reality.

This movement involved 'reading' the world and its texts – that is, its writing, its images, its whole presentation of itself – in a massively sceptical way. By reading the world in a sceptical way, like reading a piece of writing or an advertisement, we begin to locate all sorts of contradictions, and missing viewpoints or angles, on any chosen subject. In all, the scepticism that emerged powerfully towards the end of the last century can be seen as a loss of faith in our ability to represent the truth about reality and provided a sobering note to all interpretive practices. History itself is problematical. Who writes it? Who decides what it is? Whose interpretation of 'history' is valid? Furthermore, Thomas Kuhn, Michel Foucault (1970), Richard Rorty (1991) and Quentin Skinner (1985) have attacked the notion of trans-historical, eternal truths – that is, they appreciate the limitations that historical context places on knowledge. In this view, there is no beautiful truth, progressing and rolling out across history and into the future. It is far messier than that. Just so with interpretation. All we can hope for is the accumulated probability that our best interpretations approximate the truth of any given phenomenon – that we produce credible results that command respect.

Writers like Foucault have brought to our attention the power issues in terms of our culture, our writings, our institutions. He foregrounded the power issue of institutions controlling people, and the project of setting apart abnormal or deviant members of society through the discourse of normality. Foucault (1965) subverted the authoritative status of Reason and brought into question the operation and ethics of knowledge and power in society, not least in terms of discourse – that is, the system of what is sayable, and who has the right to speak and who must keep silent. For example, what about the power of psychiatry, its discourse – who speaks and who cannot speak? Psychiatry and its discourse have no absolute right to exist based on a traditional scientific understanding of the issues. They have emerged as a response to particular social forces and conditions. Language and institutions arising out of these discourses have helped to construct the idea of the 'mental patient' as pathological, as abnormal and deserving social control. Mental health care, in this view, is 'successful' inasmuch as it pins pathological identities on vulnerable people. Psychiatry is not natural and logical. It is an ideological position or viewpoint that has gained authority. But it might not keep this. It could be undermined. As Foucault has claimed, 'where there is power there is resistance'. Whether resistance could uproot psychiatry's entrenched power is doubtful, but it remains open to critique and change.

Jacques Derrida (1977), like Wittgenstein, saw language as an open system and not a closed system with definite meanings. He argued, rather alarmingly for some, that there is no ultimate meaning to language, only the perpetual regression of the meanings of words. To say what one word means is to use other words, which, in turn, need to be defined by other words that need to be defined by other words and so on, endlessly. In other words (pun intended), Derrida finds it problematic to establish the definitive meaning of a text.

Derrida argues that whatever web of spoken or written words is made by humans, they will necessarily promote certain viewpoints while excluding others – and that any discourse, written or otherwise, will be an operation of inclusion and exclusion. What is present will also be a story about what is absent. We might think of exclusion in terms of the 'Other', the marginal or the outcast.

Derrida wrote about 'deconstruction', which involves revealing the shaky, indefinite, divided or contradictory nature or character of texts (speech, writing, images, etc.) – in fact, any signifying system. Deconstruction pluralizes the voices that are present and absent from any text. Imagine a construction – a building of a particular kind – and then imagine pointing what is left out of it, its weaknesses, its poor foundations, the people it might be excluding, the people it is for or includes, and its contradictory nature (e.g. a building for the disabled that does not have ramps). The same can be done with what people say or write, or the images they use.

For example, examine the following descriptions of psychiatry in the 1970s which offer radically different 'readings' or constructions of reality. The second description can be seen as a deconstruction of the first, pointing out what is absent or excluded in its account of psychiatric 'reality':

> . . . discouraging sick behaviour and encouraging healthy behaviour through the selective granting of rewards; the availability of seclusion, restraints, and closed wards to grant a patient a respite from interaction with others and from making decisions, and prevent harm to himself or others; enabling him to think about his behaviour, to cope with his temptations to elope and succumb to depression, and to develop a sense of security; immobilising the patient to calm him, satisfy his dependency needs, give him the extra nursing attention he values, and enable him to benefit from peer confrontation; placing limits on his acting out; and teaching him that the staff cares.
>
> (Edelman 1974, p. 302)

> . . . deprivation of food, bed, walks in the open air, visitors, mail, or telephone calls; solitary confinement; deprivation of reading or entertainment materials; immobilising people by tying them into wet sheets and then exhibiting them to staff and other patients; other physical restraints on body movement; drugging the mind against the client's will; incarceration in locked wards; a range of public humiliations such as the prominent posting of alleged intentions to escape or commit suicide, the requirement of public confessions of misconduct or guilt, and public announcement of individual misdeeds and abnormalities.
>
> (Edelman 1974, p. 300)

The interpretation of texts in terms of what is included or excluded also has ramifications for history itself, not least in light of late twentieth-century postmodernity, which Eagleton neatly summarizes as:

> . . . a style of thought which is suspicious of classical notions of truth, reason, identity and objectivity, of the idea of universal progress or emancipation, of single frameworks, grand narratives or ultimate grounds of explanation. Against these Enlightenment norms, it sees the world as contingent, ungrounded, diverse, unstable, indeterminate, a set of disunified cultures or interpretations which breed a degree of scepticism about the objectivity of truth, history and norms, the givenness of natures and the coherence of identities.
>
> (Eagleton 1996, p. 37)

Some theorists, like Bell (1974), Lyotard (1984) and Jameson (1991), have highlighted how post-war Western democracies appeared to be suffering from a changing, fragmented world economic order, increasingly driven by multinational companies, and fused with new consumerism and mass media, rather than old-style capitalist production. This post-industrial society appeared to offer as yet newly unfolding, and therefore unsettling, social and economic structures. Eagleton (1996) defines post-modernism as 'a style of culture which reflects something of this epochal change, in a depthless, decentred, ungrounded, self-reflective, playful, derivative, eclectic, plural-istic art which blurs the boundaries between "high" and "popular" culture, as well as between art and everyday experience' (p. vii). Thus we are in a dizzy-making zone of multiple interpretations about nearly everything.

We might investigate, for example, the recalcitrant history of the Jewish Holo-caust as a case in point. Any act of retrieval in the historical study of this awful event is fraught with difficulty, largely because the status of history has been problem-atized by sceptical approaches to historiography. Here, opposing voices can be heard. On the one hand, there are pessimists who see epistemological crisis and cultural diversity as exploding the value of history. On the other hand, we have optimists, such as Theodore K. Rabb, who draws an upbeat parallel between the upheaval in histori-ography in the 1990s and scientific revolution in the seventeenth century: 'disputes should be heartening: signs of vitality and engagement, not disintegration' (Rabb 1993, p. 75).

Perhaps we need to remember that historical interpretation will always be limited by its modes of knowledge. After all, objective truth is simply a tantalus to interpreting historical events. It is, as Rushdie (1992) writes, the 'unattainable goal for which one must struggle in spite of the impossibility of success' (p. 101). This struggle is all about delivering the most plausible explanations and interpretations.

The term 'historicism' has been widely used in the study of social phenomena. The study of history has often involved speculation as to how specific histories have to be. Are there general laws and regularities, or is each historical episode unique? Thus, historians of health care face much the same dilemma as we have just out-lined in the study of language and social phenomena. Historicism originally referred to a position in the study of history that emphasized the need to recognize the individuality of historical phenomena, which needed an empathetic grasp of the conditions that gave them life and meaning in a social context. For our purposes, it is also important to consider the wider interpretation of the term, which has relativ-ist implications, which highlights the possibility that the nature of any phenomenon can only be adequately comprehended by considering its place within a process of historical development. If we accept historicism in a strong form we cannot attain objective truth, but this does have the advantage of competing against discourses that prefer to lose sight of history, especially history as disturbing and uncomfort-able as the Holocaust. Such historical events, as Hamilton (1996, pp. 5–6) notes, can 'make a difference' in the realm of discursive practice. The political power or powerlessness of any discourse in relation to others is another question. Yet all that any historicist reading can do, as Porter (1988, p. 770) puts it, is 'inhabit a dis-cursive field'. This is a more humble position and one which 'does not', Scott (1988, p. 10) argues, 'acknowledge defeat in the search for universal explanation; rather it suggests that universal explanation is not, never has been possible'. As Benjamin writes:

> The true picture of the past flits by. The past can be seized only as an image which flashes up at the instant when it can be recognized and is never seen again . . . For every image of the past that is not recognized by the present as one of its own concerns threatens to disappear irretrievably.
>
> (Benjamin 1992, p. 247)

This 'living body' competes with those who would rather it did not make itself obvious in a kind of 'discursive friction'.

To return to the question of tragedies and outrages such as the Holocaust, making sense of the history around this is difficult. On the one hand, all that most people have to go on are other people's accounts – in the form of recounted personal experiences, television documentaries, photographs, historical literature and the like. On the other hand, it is still felt by many that to draw attention to the constructed, narrativized, quality of the stories is to discount or deny the full measure of the tragic events. There is a fine dividing line between saying that something is a story and saying it is 'just' a story or 'only' a story, as if that means it is somehow a piece of fiction. As Lipstadt (1994) argues, while historical interpretation 'cannot be purely objective', it is 'built on a certain body of irrefutable evidence: slavery happened; so did the Black Plague and the Holocaust' (p. 21).

In a sense, historicism has turned upon itself and eliminated the anchorage in reality that one finds in positivist or realist accounts of knowledge. With the conviction that events and the accounts people give of them have to be seen in their historical context, it is tempting to be anthropomorphic about the past and assume that people and the world they lived in were pretty much like us. Hence the way that the purported sayings of ancient Greek thinkers are regularly trotted out in academic writing today, as if they were our peers. Historicism calls this into question. However, followed to its conclusion, the historicist position says that virtually everything is merely some sort of historically local and culturally bounded story, including our own, and that of health care in the present day. 'Truth' is locally produced by the interactants in the present, and does not necessarily, in this view, tell us anything about nature or history. Historicist scholars are motivated ideologically from the present towards past events to evince correspondence between text and context, but with some kinds of events there is constraint operating. Yet at the same time there is a sense that the Jewish Holocaust and mass-extermination stand beyond the narrativization of history. The events are of such magnitude that perhaps no matter how hard we focus on the nature of the stories, there is still a sense that we must hang onto some sense that there is a truth lurking behind the stories. If we say otherwise, we are putting ourselves in the position of revisionist 'historians' like David Irving and Richard Harwood, who deny the scale of the Holocaust or even that it happened. Thus, even the arch relativists might want to place moral or epistemological limits on the fictional distance that can open up between past events and narration of those events. Faced with the likes of Irving and Harwood, most scholars would want to use historical evidence to counter the gross gestures of those who too readily blur fiction with history, and step back from the position which states that all stories are potentially true and must be treated with equal respect as truths in their own right. The strong form of the historicist or interpretivist position is stopped in its tracks by these recalcitrant events. Interestingly and ironically, while David Irving adopts a radically postmodern denial of the stories of Holocaustic massacre as having no foundation in historical reality, his historiography is invariably very foundational or realist when it comes down to the biographies of prominent Nazis or details of weapons used during the war. This reiterates how scholars and others can adopt both positivist and interpretivist stances when and as it suits them.

This issue of the relationship between tragedy and truth in health care has some interesting implications. Whereas there is a good deal of interest in the interpretations that patients and professionals make, does this mean that some events are so tragic and shocking that they cannot legitimately be studied in interpretive terms? That is, does it mean that a case of depression might be discussed in terms of the construction of meaning by therapist, client and researcher, but Dr Harold Shipman and his unfortunate patients must be dealt with in realist terms? Shipman, the reader may remember, was a Manchester doctor convicted in January 2000 of the murder of 15 patients. The inquiry into the events leading up to his arrest, chaired by Dame Janet Smith, concluded that the real death toll from Shipman was 215 cases, stretching back to 1975 and that she had a strong suspicion that he had killed a further 45 of his patients (Smith 2002). Now, from the point of view of the concerns we have outlined above about interpretation and history concerning the Holocaust, what can we do with tragic events on a grand scale? Whereas the Shipman case has not at the time of writing been subject to hermeneutic or interpretive enquiry, it is clear that it involves elements which scholars have ordinarily been keen to investigate. Terminal illness, assisted deaths and murders are certainly familiar territories for scholarship of this kind, and courtroom 'reality construction' is grist to the mill of interpretive enquiry. Interpretive scholarship often has a fascination with tragedy. Yet at the same time it is vulnerable to the accusation that it is trivializing, relativizing or even denying the tragic events themselves.

While it seems perfectly reasonable to discard monological accounts of history, and applaud all that is dialogical, there are brute, evidentiary resources of the past which may help to shape our future understanding. Terry Eagleton has attacked the 'hedonist withdrawal from history' which amounts to a 'liquidation of history' (quoted in Attridge *et al.* 1987, p. 4). Thus, there is a growing number of scholars who are impatient with the persistent focus on stories or narratives and the difficulty of knowing anything happened. This postmodern focus on the stories of history and the retreat from saying anything definite about nature or past events has been a source of disquiet for many scholars who, for epistemological or ethical reasons, wish to retain a sense of truth. Thus, for Eagleton and others, we cannot wish away historical events on the grounds that the interpretive process is necessarily flawed or limited. In his novel *A History of the World in 10½ Chapters*, Barnes (1989) describes the 'God-eyed version' of truth as 'a charming, impossible fake', but urges the reader to 'believe that 43 per cent objective truth is better than 41 per cent' and avoid the alternative of a 'beguiling relativity' in which 'we value one liar's version as much as another liar's' (Gasiorek 1995, pp. 192–3). The interpretivist approach will inevitably be a gesture towards this 43 per cent of truth.

Let us try to summarize and clarify the different orientations to the world and the different philosophies of research we have described so far. Let us imagine these different styles of research falling on a spectrum. Given what we have reviewed above, let us also imagine that the two ends of this spectrum can be referred to as positivism and interpretivism. Broadly speaking, 'positivism' seeks to establish universal laws, believing that all knowledge can be reduced to observable facts and the relations between them, and the overall methodological approach is that it 'goes forth and quantifies'. 'Interpretivism' highlights how much of our knowledge of the world is confined to interpretation and the restrictions of language – that the social world is actively constructed by human beings and we are continuously involved in making sense of or interpreting our social environment. Broadly speaking, it opposes the 'positivist' study of humans as objects. It may well be more interested in qualitative methodology as it 'goes forth and qualifies'. And it is the debate, battle even, between 'positivism' and 'interpretivism' that we are dealing with in this book as a whole. Characterizing the field of research rather crudely, then, we shall take 'positivism' and 'interpretivism' as the main research paradigms or philosophies in health and social research, and for ease of presentation try to indicate whereabouts on this spectrum the different research strategies fall.

Even as positivism was at its most powerful, there were a number of alternative points of view especially in the social sciences. Even when we seek to establish relationships between reasonably well-established facts and historical sequences, there is inevitably some use of interpretation. This was expressed most fully by Max Weber, who, among other things, was trying to explain how the development of Protestantism in Europe and the New World led to the Industrial Revolution. The spirit of hard work and self-denial encouraged by theologians such as John Calvin, he reasoned, must have had something to do with the rise of manufacturing industry (Weber 1904/1905). However, to grasp this link requires a kind of explanatory understanding, or *Verstehen*, which involves an intervening motivational link between the observed activity and its meaning for the actor. This motivation, and the explanation associated with it, may take a rational form such that we understand an action where the individual uses a means for a purpose. Alternatively, the irrational or emotional kind of motivational inference occurs if, for example, we observe someone burst into tears and know that he [*sic*] has suffered a bitter disappointment.

In explanatory understanding, the action is placed in an understandable sequence of motivation, the understanding of which can be placed within a 'complex of meaning'. The understanding of motivation involves embedding the conduct in question in a broader normative framework with reference to which the individual acts. The explanation of behaviour can be:

1   *Subjectively adequate*: the action concerned makes sense in terms of accepted norms. This, however, is incomplete because the same action may be promoted by different motivations and complexes of meaning.

2   *Causally adequate*: where it is possible to calculate a probability that a given observable event will result in another event. Here a special place is granted to 'consistent conjunction'. Explanatory significance involves relating the subjective meaning of the act to a specifiable range of determinable consequences.

To be part of interpretive sociology, an explanation must fulfil both of these criteria. The sociologist is not necessarily interested in interpreting events in psychological terms – Weber rejected the notion that social institutions can be explained in psychological terms. Certainly, an individual may 'have' the Protestant work ethic. Weber did himself, and spent his time almost exclusively in scholarly activity, pausing only to eat meals of 'raw chopped beef and four fried eggs' (Marianne Weber 1975, p. 105). However, to him, the Protestant work ethic was far more than an individual attitude. Weber, then, set the stage for an interpretive, non-reductive kind of explanation of human activity.

This kind of legacy, from Weber's sociology and from hermeneutics in biblical and literary studies, has left its mark on present-day intellectual endeavours in the social and health sciences. Elements of hermeneutics are seen to be important in grounded theory approaches to studying the social world (Rennie 2000). Here, the concern in grounded theory approaches to derive theory directly from data mirrors the concern in hermeneutics with the interpretation of social phenomena.

The legacy of hermeneutics has left its mark on health care research as well. For example, the role of nurses in forming therapeutic relationships with clients is susceptible to study in this way (O'Brien 2000). The approach of hermeneutic phenomenology enables researchers to uncover the experience of being in a particular health care situation. O'Brien's results suggest that nurses are also hard at work performing hermeneutic interpretations of their own in making sense of what they do. In describing her work with a client, one of O'Brien's informants disclosed the following: 'we both agreed that the best way to go was to use it as a learning experience firstly . . . about the stresses and her vulnerability, and secondly as a learning experience involving the kids – and to tailor it to their various levels of understanding' (O'Brien 2000, p. 190). Thus, hermeneutics can function at a number of different levels. The approach may inform research itself, and it may well be that such research uncovers a level at which practitioners are doing hermeneutics in their everyday work, making sense of health care situations (Svenaeus 2000). Hermeneutic activities on the part of health care staff also play a part in how they may work to transform the systems within which they find themselves. As one of Pejlert and co-workers' informants put it:

> Personally, I think that being aware of my own power and influence . . . as a staff member . . . and the possibility to delegate it . . . that there is nothing dangerous about giving it up. If I do I will only meet people . . . if I dare to do it . . . this feels like the heart of the matter.
>
> (Pejlert *et al.* 2000, p. 693)

This relationship between the nurses and the client was seen by Pejlert and co-workers' respondents as a 'we' relationship, such that the unity with clients was stressed and a sense of profundity was constructed that involved the participants feeling that the relationship went beyond words and that the client had hidden resources. Participants foregrounded notions of compassion and 'being with' others, especially those with whom the usual relationship with the consensual world of other people had been broken as a result of their illness or distress.

In connection with this, a related question arises of how the health care professional's phenomenological field or subjective organization is accomplished so as to facilitate this process. Moreover, how can the researcher discern patterns in this rich mosaic of thinking and practice? As McAlpine (1999) notes, there are some major difficulties in this field as the developing expertise of health professionals means they are doing a great many things that are not readily susceptible to being described and itemized. Hermeneutics, then, demands an interpretive field that is open to observation and inspection by the analyst. In the next chapter, we examine just how readily the analyst can achieve a descriptive account of the subject matter of health care research. In the meantime, let us sum up what we have discussed so far.

In terms of the contribution to the project of hermeneutics to health care research, we should perhaps note the following key features of the hermeneutic position. First, the hermeneutic position is predicated on the assumption that knowledge of the diverse forms of social life, though fallible, offers a rich source of information beyond the limited viewpoint of positivism. Second, intersubjective processes, language and making sense of the world are at the heart of complexities of social involvement and historical change. Finally, interpretive and hermeneutic approaches conceive of the world as socially constructed through language. This language may fall on a spectrum from liberatory to oppressive. And it is part of the hermeneutic project to shift the awareness of the analysts and readers away from the oppressive pole towards the liberatory one. Hermeneutics, then, is a fundamentally reformist discipline.

References

Attridge, D., Bennington, G. and Young, R. (eds) (1987) *Post-Structuralism and the Question of History*. Cambridge: Cambridge University Press.

Barnes, J. (1989) *A History of the World in 10½ Chapters*. London: Cape.

Becker, H.S. (1953) Becoming a marijuana user, *American Journal of Sociology*, 59: 235–42.

Bell, D. (1974) *The Coming of Post-Industrial Society*. London: Heinemann.

Benjamin, W. (1992) *Illuminations* (edited by H. Arendt and translated by H. Zohn). London: Fontana.

Bultmann, R. (1986) Is exegesis without presuppositions possible?, in K. Mueller-Vollmer (ed.) *The Hermeneutics Reader*. Oxford: Basil Blackwell.

Casey, P. (2001) Multiple personality disorder, *Primary Care Psychiatry*, 7(1): 7–11.

Chomsky, N. (1957) *Syntactic Structures*. The Hague: Mouton.

Chuengsatiansup, K. (1999) Sense, symbol, and soma: illness experience in the soundscape of everyday life, *Culture, Medicine and Psychiatry*, 23: 273–301.

Cressey, D.R. (1953) *Other People's Money*. Glencoe, IL: Free Press.

Darbyshire, P., Diekelmann, J. and Diekelmann, N. (1999) Reading Heidegger and interpretive phenomenology: a response to the work of Michael Crotty, *Nursing Inquiry*, 6: 17–25.

De Man, P. (1986) *Resistance to Theory*. Manchester: Manchester University Press.

Denzin, N. (1989) *Interpretive Biography*. London: Sage.

Derrida, J. (1977) *Of Grammatology* (translated by G.C. Spivak). Baltimore, MD: Johns Hopkins University Press.

Eagleton, T. (1996) *The Illusions of Postmodernism*. Oxford: Blackwell.

Edelman, M. (1974) The political language of the helping professions, *Politics and Society*, 4: 295–310.

Foucault, M. (1965) *Madness and Civilisation: A History of Madness in the Age of Reason* (translated by R. Howard). New York: Vintage.

Foucault, M. (1970) *The Order of Things*. London: Tavistock.

Gadamer, H.G. (1981) *Reason in the Age of Science* (translated by F.G. Lawrence). Cambridge, MA: MIT Press.

Gasiorek, A. (1995) *Post-War British Fiction: Realism and After*. London: Arnold.

Giddens, A. (1984). *The Constitution of Society: Outline of the Theory of Structuration*. Cambridge: Polity Press.

Goffman, E. (1961) *Encounters: Two Studies in the Sociology of Interaction*. Indianapolis, IN: Bobbs-Merrill.

Habermas, J. (1980) The hermeneutic claim to universality, in J. Bleicher (ed.) *Contemporary Hermeneutics*. London: Routledge & Kegan Paul.

Hamilton, P. (1996) *Historicism*. London: Routledge.

Harrington, A. (2000) Objectivism in hermeneutics? Gadamer, Habermas, Dilthey, *Philosophy of the Social Sciences*, 30(4): 491–507.

Hart, H.L.A. (1948) The ascription of responsibility and rights, *Proceedings of the Aristotelian Society*, 49: 171–94.

Hirsch, E. (1976) *The Aims of Interpretation*. Chicago, IL: University of Chicago Press.

Hudson, L. (1982) *Bodies of Knowledge*. London: Weidenfeld & Nicholson.

Hudson, L. (1984) Texts, signs and artefacts, in W.R. Crozier and A.R. Chapman (eds) *Cognitive Processes in the Perception of Art*. Oxford: North-Holland.

Hughes, J. and Sharrock, W. (1997) *The Philosophy of Social Research*, 3rd edn. London: Longman.

Jameson, F. (1991) *Postmodernism or, The Cultural Logic of Late Capitalism*. London: Verso.

Lévi Strauss, C. (1969) *The Raw and the Cooked*. London: Harper & Row.

Lindesmith, A. (1968) *Addiction and Opiates*. Chicago, IL: Aldine.

Lipstadt, L. (1994) *Denying the Holocaust: The Growing Assault on Truth and Memory*. New York: Plume.

Lofland, J. and Stark, R. (1965) Becoming a world saver: a theory of conversion to a deviant perspective, *American Sociological Review*, 30: 862–75.

Lyotard, J.-F. (1984) *The Postmodern Condition: A Report on Knowledge* (translated by G. Bennington and B. Massumi). Manchester: Manchester University Press.

Lyotard, J.-F. (1991) *Phenomenology*, Albany, NY: State University of New York Press.

Lyotard, J.-F. (1993) *Towards the Postmodern* (translated and edited by R. Harvey and M.S. Roberts). Atlantic Highlands, NJ: Humanities Press International.

Manning, P.K. (1971) Fixing what you feared: notes on the campus abortion search, in J. Hemslin (ed.) *The Sociology of Sex*. New York: Appleton-Century-Crofts.

Markovic, M. (1984) *Dialectical Theory of Meaning*. Dordrect, Holland: D. Reidel.

McAlpine, C.P. (1999) Expert thinking in nursing practice: implications for supporting expertise, *Nursing and Health Sciences*, 1: 131–7.

Mills, C.W. (1959) *The Sociological Imagination*. New York: Oxford University Press.

Morley, D. (ed.) (2002) *The Gift: New Writing for the NHS*. Birmingham: Stride Books in association with Birmingham Health Authority.

O'Brien, L. (2000) Nurse–client relationships: the experience of community psychiatric nurses, *Australian and New Zealand Journal of Mental Health Nursing*, 9: 184–94.

Outhwaite, W. (1987) *New Philosophies of Social Science: Realism, Hermeneutics and Critical Theory*. London: Macmillan.

Pejlert, A., Norberg, A. and Asplund, K. (2000) From psychiatric ward to home like setting: the meaning of caring as narrated by nurses, *Journal of Clinical Nursing*, 9: 689–70.

Porter, C. (1988) Are we being historical yet?, *The South Atlantic Quarterly*, 87(4): 743–86.

Potter, J. (1996) *Representing Reality*. London: Sage.

Propp, V.I. ([1928] 1968) *Morphology of the Folktale* (translated by L. Scott, 2nd edn). Austin, TX: University of Texas Press.

Quine, W.V.O. (1990) *Pursuit of Truth*. Cambridge, MA: Harvard University Press.

Rabb, T.K. (1993) Whither history? Reflections on the comparison between historians and scientists, in H. Kozicki (ed.) *Developments in Modern Historiography*. Basingstoke: Macmillan.

Rennie, D.L. (2000) Grounded theory methodology as methodical hermeneutics, *Theory and Psychology*, 10(4): 481–502.

Resnik, D.B., Rehm, M. and Minard, R.B. (2001) The undertreatment of pain: scientific, clinical, cultural, and philosophical factors, *Medicine, Health Care and Philosophy*, 4: 277–88.

Ricouer, P. (1971) The model of the text: meaningful action considered as text, *Social Research*, 39(3): 185–217.

Ricouer, P. ([1968] 1976) Hermeneutics: restoration of meaning or reduction of illusion?, in P. Connerton (ed.) *Critical Sociology*. Harmondsworth: Penguin.

Rorty, R. (1991) *Objectivity, Relativism and Truth*. Cambridge: Cambridge University Press.

Rushdie, S. (1992) *Imaginary Homelands: Essays and Criticism, 1981–1991*. London: Granta.

Sayer, A. (1992) *Method in Social Science: A Realist Approach*. London: Routledge.

Scott, J.W. (1988) *Gender and the Politics of History*. New York: Columbia University Press.

Shklar, J. (1986) Squaring the hermeneutic circle, *Social Research*, 53: 459–73.

Skinner, Q. (1985) *The Return of Grand Theory in the Human Sciences*. Cambridge: Cambridge University Press.

Smith, J. (2002) *The Shipman Inquiry*. London: HMSO.

Sontag, S. (1991) *Against Interpretation and Other Essays*. London: Picador.

Sontag, S. (2001) *Where the Stress Falls: Essays*. New York: Farrar, Straus & Giroux.

Spanos, N. (1994) Multiple identity enactments and multiple personality disorder: a socio-cognitive perspective, *Psychological Bulletin*, 116(1): 143–65.

Svenaeus, F. (2000) Hermeneutics of clinical practice: the question of textuality, *Theoretical Medicine and Bioethics*, 21: 171–89.

Weber, M. (1904/1905) *The Protestant Ethic and the Spirit of Capitalism*. New York: Scribner's.

Weber, M. (1975) *Max Weber: A Biography* (translated and edited by H. Zoltan). New York: Wiley.

West, W.G. (1978) The short term careers of serious thieves, *Canadian Journal of Criminology*, 20: 169–90.

Wittgenstein, L. (1981) *Remarks on the Philosophy of Psychology* (translated by G.E.M. Anscombe and G.E. Wright). Oxford: Blackwell.

Znaniecki, F.W. (1934) *The Method of Sociology*. New York: Farrar & Rinehart.

8

Philosophies of description

Researchers attempting to study health care are faced with a range of thorny philosophical issues when they attempt to characterize what it is they are studying. Straightforward clinical encounters may, upon closer inspection, disclose unforeseen complexities that may thwart the research programme. Accordingly, in this chapter we consider what it means to describe an object in the health care disciplines.

The social study of health care processes has often involved a good deal of reflection on the role of the observer and the way that observers may change or affect the thing they are observing. This chapter, therefore, includes several accounts of the ways in which the investigator's values and research commitments may impinge on the kinds of description achieved.

We shall focus on various accounts of descriptive methodology in health care contexts and consider some studies in medical sociology and psychology that have offered descriptions of different kinds. As well as descriptive research as an end in itself, we shall demonstrate how these descriptions are recruited to perform a number of important social scientific tasks, such as persuading the reader, supporting a theoretical model of health care encounters or justifying a course of action. Moreover, descriptions composed by health care practitioners, clients or their loved ones are important in creating a particular kind of disorder as a social object, and in deciding on a course of action. The kind of description the interactants formulate helps to decide, for example, whether a child has learning difficulties, whether a respiratory complaint merits a prescription or a person's genitalia need surgical intervention to make them more male or female. In many health care settings, the process of becoming professionalized is to a large extent the process of learning a particular way of describing nature. Howard Becker's (1957, 1993) classic study *Boys in White* about the training of doctors contained the example of medical students doing a ward round with a senior doctor when they encountered a patient with multiple yet non-specific complaints. The students commented disparagingly, 'that patient was a real crock'. On further enquiry by Becker to unpack the meaning of the term, the students were at first unsure of what it meant. Under questioning, they considered that it might be a term for a patient with psychosomatic complaints. Yet this was discounted, because in a nearby bed there was a patient with an ulcer and the senior doctor had used this as an occasion for some discussion of psychosomatic complaints. This was long before *Helicobacter pylori* had been identified as the likely culprit. Eventually it was decided that a crock was a patient with complaints but no identifiable physical pathology. This illustrates how the world-view, means of representing and using knowledge and attitudes to patients, shift as people move from being novice to expert practitioners. This may be reflected in their descriptions. It also shows how the descriptions themselves may operate on a number of barely conscious levels. There are terms that already contain a good deal of reasoning. Some terms, like 'crock' or 'heartsink patient', may be informal and whose use might be considered unprofessional, and others like schizotypal personality disorder, whose use may be professionally endorsed. Descriptions, then, are shot through with the norms, rules and social action of everyday life.

Description also enters into the lives of health care clients. There is an increasing interest in retrospective accounts, oral history, reminiscence therapy and the philosophical implications of having an autobiography. In theory at least, the concept of the person in health care has developed by leaps and bounds in the past few decades with the flourishing of literatures on illness experience, interpretive biographies and narratives of sufferers. All of these involve some sort of description by both the sufferer and by the researcher.

In psychology, philosophy and sociology, there has been a good deal of interest in whether it is possible to describe the contents of consciousness. Is looking at the world within as easy as looking at the world outside? Why is it important to look at the subjective realm? This kind of work sometimes draws on the approach taken by phenomenologists or cognitive scientists as they try to discern the contents of consciousness. In seventeenth-century European thought, Locke had much to say about the way that our gaze could be directed inwards to our inner world. Yet this itself relied on a good deal of prior work through the previous few centuries of Christianity to give shape and form to the inner world which it became fashionable to describe.

In terms of the various ways we can describe contemporary social life in health care, there seems to be a bewildering variety of brand names for approaches to description. Hermeneutic enquiry vies with hardy perennials like grounded theory and newcomers such as interpretive phenomenological analysis, as well as a variety of approaches that draw on literary theory in this chaotic cottage garden of research styles. There are, within the diverse buffet of approaches, a variety of different epistemologies and approaches to knowledge. In classical grounded theory, perhaps one of the more venerable approaches in the social sciences, there is an emphasis on the way investigators should try to take in their data in a raw, untheorized manner and attempt to build hypotheses that are 'grounded' in the data. On the other hand, there are those who have come more lately to the qualitative feast who emphasize the researcher's role and demand that it should be discussed through a process of reflexivity (Northway 2000). This emphasis on reflexivity partly answers the question of how we are to make sense of the investigator's values and prior theories as she or he investigates the social world and what effect these might have on the kind of theory that is generated. Reflexivity requires that a researcher's biases and prejudices are laid bare (Waterman 1998) and that the values and position of the researcher are made explicit (Hall and Stevens 1991). But how far can researchers make themselves aware of their own presuppositions? Researchers themselves and the processes of enquiry they deploy are often potent elements in the research setting and may affect what they observe in a variety of unexpected ways. Reflexivity thus requires that the research process itself is examined critically (Maynard 1994). Reflexive research is 'research on practice that treats research itself as a practice' (Schratz and Walker 1995, p. 13). As a means of making sense of this we will alert readers to some of the practical issues of being a researcher in a field setting to help theorize the inter- and intra-subjective processes in research.

Reflection theory and realism

A pervasive idea that motivates a good deal of description and illustration is one that has been termed 'reflection theory'. That is, the idea that description, especially illustrations and photography, can be an objective rendering of the object to be described. This view has an important place within some positivist and Marxist philosophies. But how 'accurate' are these reflections or, indeed, representations of 'reality'? Dissatisfied with the static descriptions of the mid-nineteenth century, scholars began to strive for ways of representing dynamic processes, which culminated in Eadward Muybridge's photographic studies of human and animal movements in the late nineteenth century. We shall look at how these early beginnings have informed the way contemporary researchers have attempted to describe and model dynamic processes that are characterized by movement, interaction and change and examine the meaning of systems theory and dialectics as models in health care.

Describing the world is not easy. Which world are we talking about? From which perspective is 'out there' reality being appraised or considered? Indeed, the apparent directness and actuality of some descriptions may itself be a carefully contrived persuasive device. The problems of realism, concerning our knowledge of objects in the world, pervade philosophy. Various questions are raised, such as the boundaries between reality as constructed through mind and language and that which is mind- and language-independent. This hot potato has yielded many interesting theories. For example, the Greek philosopher Plato considered our 'reality' to be a mere shadow play of universal or archetypal forms that exist independent of our world. And much later, the philosopher Berkeley suggested that objects need to be perceived by subjectivities to exist. Broadly speaking, realism opposes the kind of idealism proposed by Berkeley and others that what exists, exists only in the mind. Thus realism views objects as mind- and language-independent. At its most simplistic, this approach can promote an uncomplicated view of individual perception of objects, suggesting that all individuals would see any particular object in the same way, as having the same qualities, and so on. Yet we all know that we can be very wrong about our perception of the world – we may be subject to hallucinations at worst or illusions at best. A more sophisticated and modest realism determines that mind and language act as a bridge between 'out there' reality and our subjective experience. This perspective acknowledges that there is therefore potential for 'distortion' at an interpretative level, and thus salvages the idea that there might be some sort of reality out there, even if we can't see it directly.

When we use the term 'real' or say something is 'really there', it is not always clear what we mean. Are we referring to 'out there' objectivity or are we simply trying to convince others that our subjective appreciation of sensory input is what others might expect or experience. Yet it seems fairly commonplace that we can have substantial difficulties at times determining what is real or unreal and borne of fantasy. Much literature and many films play on the hesitation that exists between reality and fantasy.

As Potter comments, claims to realism often deliberately under-theorize the processes of apprehending nature and describing it:

> In realist discourse, where language is the mirror of nature, categorization is understood as a rather banal naming process; the right word is assigned to the thing that has the appropriate properties. In contrast, in the discourse of the construction yard that I have been elaborating, categorization is much more consequential. It is through categorization that the specific sense of something is constituted.
>
> (Potter 1996, p. 177)

Humberto Maturana commented that 'Any claim to objectivity is an absolute command for obedience' (Mendez *et al.* 1988). In postmodern theory, where all meanings are regarded as suitable targets for deconstruction, Potter (1996) begins to unpack 'facts' as things which are seemingly most difficult to refute and highlights how, like other forms of justification, they are meticulously crafted linguistic constructions that serve persuasive purposes and can therefore be deconstructed.

Often strange events seem to intrude upon the stability of the carefully contrived 'real' world. Psychosis and religious or 'supernatural' experiences problematize the realm of 'reality'. Who determines what is 'really' out there? Which subjectivity is accurate? The literary theorist Todorov (1973) writes of 'the fragility of the limit between matter and mind' where there can be 'multiplication of the personality; collapse of the limit between subject and object; the transformation of time and space' (p. 120). Inevitably, there is an interplay and interdependency between the real world and that which is unreal, created or fictive. People can hesitate or become uncertain about ambiguous events that may have either natural or unnatural/supernatural explanations. There is a boundary or threshold between the rational and irrational, between scientific and religious or mysterious realms that frequently challenges the notion of 'realism'. The notion of 'reality' or what is 'real', of course, is comforting. We can choose to avoid more disturbing notions that there are occluded regions to our experience which are not so homely or benign.

In an attempt to pin down 'out there' reality, photography seemed to have much to offer. From the rise of photography in the ninteenth century to the Visible Human Project in the late twentieth century, there have been rather sweeping assumptions about the descriptive power of imaging. But what do these photographers, illustrators and computer modellers think they can achieve?

Muybridge's photographic studies

As we know from Eadward Muybridge's photographs of humans and animals in motion, photography appeared to herald new and exciting possibilities for describing our world. Muybridge was a colourful character who started out as a landscape photographer. In 1874, suspecting that his son was not his, he shot dead his wife's lover, but was later acquitted of murder. His photography of movement was made famous through his solution to the controversy in horse racing circles as to whether a trotting horse ever had all four feet off the ground at any one point in time. He proved that they did, and his sequential photographs demonstrating this were published in the *Proceedings of the Royal Institution of Great Britain* in 1883. With his invention of the zoopraxiscope, Muybridge was able to create a moving image of successive photographic plates. Here were the beginnings of the motion picture!

In the case of qualitative research, the situation is even more complex. In addition to its attempts to provide descriptions of social life, it is often underpinned by a view of the world as socially constructed. This leads to a number of convoluted attempts to think about the researcher's role in creating the descriptions, under the banner of 'reflexivity', as we shall see.

Descriptive accounts of health care users

Description is a major part of the lives of health care clients or users. The very practice of health care is bound up with notions of description, as people give accounts of their own or their loved one's symptoms, and these are encoded into medical language, medico-nursing records and compressed into forms and standardized assessments. The kinds of frameworks that people use in these contexts can have far-reaching consequences for the lives of the people so described. Consider the case of people born with ambiguous genitalia, a condition that is believed to affect approximately one in 2000 babies (Blackless *et al.* 2000). For several decades, the response of doctors and to some extent the babies' parents has been to try to disambiguate the genitalia surgically. Generally, it is easier to remove 'excess' tissues to construct a female appearance. Parents sometimes feel that they're put under a good deal of pressure to have such an operation done to ensure a 'normal' life for their offspring. However, once the operation is performed, it does not necessarily result in better adjustment for the person later in life. In a study by Minto *et al.* (2003) of people who had undergone this kind of 'corrective' surgery, most did not report good outcomes in their subsequent sexual development. Minto *et al.* question the wisdom of this kind of surgery on the genitalia, even when it attempts to leave the major nerves and blood supplies intact. The point here is that perceptions and descriptions can be very powerful in terms of the course of action. Whether infant anatomies are seen as penises or clitorises, whether they are described as being somehow 'abnormal' or 'lacking', can have profound consequences. In this case, it is tempting to conclude, like Judith Butler (1990), that maybe if the present-day binary gender system were not so powerful these kinds of perceptions of people's bodies as somehow in need of intervention might not be so easily thought.

Autobiography and self-conceptualization

This sense of a person as a thing with a sex and a gender leads into another important consideration concerning the description of human beings and their lives. These biographies are often constructed in such a way as to impose a kind of coherence on the life in question. Everyday human interaction contains much description of who we are and what has happened to us. Furthermore, as we live we leave traces in the form of health records, official documents, employment records, bank details and so on. So there are multiple biographies for many of us. In a sense, drawing a leaf from the book of literary scholarship, each of these various accounts is to some extent 'fictionalized'. This fictionalization of an individual occurs in four important ways. First, the notion of self is a fluid one. As Olney (1980) states: 'Phenomenologists and existentialists have joined hands with depth psychologists in stressing an idea of self that defines itself from moment to moment amid the buzz and confusion of the external world and as security against the outside whirl' (pp. 23–4). If this is the case, we are forced, like Geoffrey Braithwaite in Julian Barnes's (1984) novel *Flaubert's Parrot*, to demand violently: 'How can we know anybody?' (p. 155). Furthermore, an individual's account of himself or herself is problematic. Conway (1990) highlights the reconstructive nature of autobiographical memory and asks: 'How wrong can an autobiographical memory be before we conclude that it is a fantasy?' (p. 2). He demonstrates that autobiographical memory is not a Xerox of our past experience. Disturbingly, it appears to recreate or fictionalize experiences or even wipe them from our consciousness. It may be that the self's life narrative is reconstituted from moment to moment. Autobiographical memories, Conway (1990) insists, 'Will never be wholly veridical but rather will (usually) be compatible with the beliefs and understanding of the rememberer and preserve only some of the main details of experienced events' (p. 11). Even Conway, however, seems reluctant to abandon altogether the notion that there is some sort of essential self underlying autobiographical memory. In psychology, the idea of a self as something that can indeed be represented, for example in a corporate biography (de Man 1984, p. 71), has been extremely persuasive.

Second, human activity takes place in dialogue. Some authors (e.g. Middleton and Edwards 1990; Edwards and Potter 1992) have reconceptualized memories as the collective creation of particular social situations. This suggests that the process of diagnostic encounters where patients perform their stories for clinicians is an unruly, 'dialogical' activity (Bakhtin 1984), which makes it difficult to extract a transparent account of the patient. Writing such a transparent account in the patient's records is an activity that we might characterize as monological and ultimately controlling.

Our memories are what we make them. This argument must be taken very seriously by anyone involved in clinical practice or research. Because we invent or fictionalize ourselves, Olney (1980) is right to highlight 'An anxiety about the self, an anxiety about the dimness and vulnerability of that entity that no one has ever seen or touched or tasted' (p. 23). Like the film-maker Bunuel, we can only speak of autobiographical memory as 'wholly mine – with my affirmations, my hesitations, my repetitions and lapses, my truth and my lies' (Conway 1990, p. 10). Like the English Romantic poet, John Clare, we might consider biography to be a total 'pack of lies' (Foss and Trick 1989).

Third, biographies are more rhetorical than 'real'. When autobiographical accounts are made into corporate biographies, fictional distance is significantly increased. In the written record, the patient becomes a constructed representation of the flesh-and-blood individual. A double fiction operates: the fictional representation of past events in autobiographical memory and the fiction of such representations constructed as text. As Elbaz (1988) indicates: 'Through the processes of mediation (by linguistic reality) and suspension (due to the text's lack of finality and completion), autobiography can only be a fiction. Indeed autobiography is fiction and fiction is autobiography: both are narrative arrangements of reality' (p. 1). The same argument applies to biography. Representations of an individual biographee by multiple biographers, amounting to a corporate biography, are necessarily an amalgam of narrative arrangements of reality.

Fourth, the impossibility of fixing the life story is foregrounded in literary critical accounts of biography. Literary critics have proposed that the importance of life-writing is 'not that it reveals reliable self-knowledge – it does not – but that it demonstrates in a striking way the impossibility of closure and of totalization (that is, the impossibility of coming into being) of all textual systems made up of tropological substitutions' (de Man 1984, p. 71). Where a figurative medium such as language is used, there is an inevitable inability to characterize something exhaustively in terms of what de Man calls a totalization. Taking up the ideas of Jaques Derrida, Michel Foucault, Roland Barthes and Jacques Lacan, Olney states that the autobiographical text

> Takes on a life of its own, and the self that was not really in existence in the beginning is in the end merely a matter of text and has nothing whatever to do with an authorising author. The self, then, is a fiction and so is the life, and behind the text of an autobiography lies the text of an 'autobiography': all that is left are characters on a page, and they can be 'deconstructed' to demonstrate the shadowiness of even their existence. Having dissolved the self into text and then out of text into thin air, several critics . . . have announced the end of autobiography.
>
> (Olney 1980, p. 22)

What corporate biographies achieve is the construction of an individual that 'deprives and disfigures to the precise extent that it restores' (de Man 1984, pp. 80–1). Jaques Derrida suggests that there is nothing beyond the text. Certainly it is difficult to exist as a patient outside health professional routines and story-telling, which are an amalgam of perspectives, judgements, opinions and embellishments regarding a patient's life and experiences funnelled into a narrative that replaces the real flesh-and-blood person.

People's own accounts of themselves may well be ambiguous or contradictory. In effect, they may be asking the fundamental question, 'Who am I?'. Again, writings by scholars of literature offer some insights. Sontag (1982) notes how Barthes's autobiography is a book of the dismantling of his own authority or what Thody (1977) has called an anti-biography. For Barthes: 'Who speaks is not who writes, and who writes is not who is' (Sontag 1982). The biographee, the subject of the biographer, cannot be reduced into a textual representation. People contain tensions, ambivalence and dissonance, which are difficult to capture in a unitary authoritative text.

Symbolic interactionism

Describing realities that exist in social settings such as hospitals is complex, because we are not the first travellers to have arrived in those places. As Becker (2001) notes when the observers arrive to study something – a community, a hospital or a primary care practice – they are not newcomers to an uninhabited landscape who can name its features as they like. Everything they look at is part of the experience of many other kinds of people. Some of the features, too, will have been not only named but laboriously constructed by the people one finds there, many of whom have their own ways of talking and writing about it. In addition, they will usually have specialized terms for the objects, events and people involved in that area of social life. From the point of view of Goffman (1961) and Becker (2001), those special words are never neutral objective signifiers but instead they express the perspective and situation of the people who use them. The natives are already there and everything significant to them in that terrain has been carved up, formulated and named, or even given many names.

Consider the example of illicit drugs. If we were to study the issue we might first of all note that there is a vast and ever-changing vocabulary, especially among people who use them, who may readily talk of being high, stoned, tripping, smacked or wasted, depending on their generation, geographical and social location and what they have ingested. The sheer volume of folk names for most common drugs defies enumeration here. The elite members of the setting, such as experts, medical and legal personnel, might place the folk terms in inverted commas and instead use the kinds of terms that appear in medical or legal discourse: opiates, cannabinoids, class A drugs and so on. The terms we use reflect moral and social judgements. There are a variety of moral connotations smuggled in with terms such as 'substance abuse', 'substance use' or 'recreational drug use'. 'Substance abuse' in particular implies that such activity is improper and, by extension, should be curtailed. Often, through use of terms like 'dependence', 'addiction' and 'habitual', the elite participants in the situation imply that drug use is undesirable, involuntary and harmful, whereas the language of users themselves implies that it is innocent, voluntary and harmless. Language, as the reader should be aware by now, is unlikely to be neutral.

The technical consequence for social or health scientists is that the phenomena they want to describe and generalize about are made up of concepts that smuggle in with them the moral attitudes of elite people and groups in the social setting, and the actions that have been taken towards them in consequence (Becker 2001). The result of that is a tremendous difficulty in finding anything to say about the phenomena, without subscribing to those same moral attitudes. If we are interested in describing the quality of life of people with schizophrenia, this may be scientifically important and it may lead to better and more humane consequences for people with that diagnosis in the future. However, it leaves many significant things about the situation unexamined and instead merely reproduces the categories we find there. For example, quality of life is something that was originally developed by researchers and medics, and has been developed further by respected bodies like the World Health Organization, such that it is readily researchable and measurable. Yet what would we find if we were to examine the area from scratch? Would researchers necessarily reconstruct the same kind of idea from the network of intersecting tales people tell about their lives?

To create a general construct like this, it means that a good deal of the lived content has had to be removed.

From a slightly more critical perspective, it is possible to talk about the results of being thought about as a kind of patient by using labelling theory. That is, what it feels like to be 'schizophrenic' or to have such a thing as a 'quality of life'. But this doesn't tell us anything about how people get that way, the underlying causes or possibilities for change, other than what is encoded in the scientific or lay accounts that are already there. The challenge is to break out of these categories and begin observing and thinking from scratch. Unless we do so, we will find that there is nothing new to discuss related to those matters that has not already been described by the people already there. And, as Becker (2001) concludes, you cannot do social science if you cannot find anything to generalize about.

There are important ethical issues involved in adopting the existing language and perspectives that the people in the study setting use towards the phenomena under study (Becker 2001). If we accept their descriptions, we accept all the assumptions about right and wrong embedded in their words and ideas. We might accept, in the case of drugs, the idea that addiction is some kind of disease, that it results in part from innate tendencies of the persons involved, and perhaps even that addicts are people who have 'lost control' of themselves and, therefore, cannot help themselves when it comes to crime or developing collateral problems such as 'personality disorder'.

The kinds of descriptions we adopt and the parallels we draw are important heuristic tools that allow analytic work to be done. In Goffman's (1961) account of mental hospitals, this kind of playful creative analogizing through language is used to particularly strong effect. The kinds of descriptions he uses are surprisingly dispassionate yet at the same time evocative. He defines what he calls 'establishments' as consisting of 'places such as rooms, suites of rooms, buildings or plants in which activity of a particular kind regularly goes on' (p. 7), and at once reminds the reader of things like offices, businesses, factories, prisons and consulting rooms, as well as perhaps households and leisure centres. It all sounds very 'neutral' or 'scientific'. Goffman classifies establishments in terms of their relationship to the lives of the individuals who go to make them up. Some institutions will not accept certain kinds of people at all. Many institutions have a rapidly changing population of customers, inmates or workers, while others, like families, change their personnel less frequently. The activities that institutions house may be very serious, while others are far more frivolous. In some, the coding used by the participants is keyed or reversed, such as in the nineteenth century when people talked of visiting a brothel as going to a 'respectable establishment'. Of these various establishments and institutions there are variations in terms of how encompassing the demands on the time and the lives of the inhabitants can be. A tennis club may demand relatively little – perhaps apart from an interest in tennis – but others such as a prison or hospital can demand far more.

In many institutions there may be evidence of disparities in status, prestige and in terms of what some members can get the others to do. In describing these disparities, Goffman is very coy about deploying terms that have negative connotations. Rather than, for example, 'domination', which might be negative, he talks about 'echelons' and 'echelon control'. This is used to describe the typical authority system of an institution such as a prison or a hospital. For example, '*any* member of the staff class has certain rights to discipline *any* member of the inmate class, thereby markedly increasing the probability of sanction' (Goffman 1961, p. 42). The terms are deceptively neutral, and Goffman has been careful to select words without immediate negative connotations in the way that a term like 'domination' would have. He simply describes one of several possible ways of organizing authority relations. For the observer, as Becker (2001) notes, it is far easier to find examples of 'echelon control' than of 'domination'. Echelon control is much more readily observable, because it is based on things that we can observe – who gives orders to whom. 'Domination' or 'power', however, include a (more debatable) implied judgement as to the moral desirability of the order-giving arrangement. In addition, Goffman identifies a number of other processes that go on as people enter institutions, especially what he calls total institutions, which impose some degree of isolation from the outside world on the inmates:

- 'role dispossession' to describe how new recruits are prevented from being who they were in the world they previously inhabited;

- 'trimming' and 'programming' to describe how 'the new arrival allows himself to be shaped and coded into an object that can be fed into the administrative machinery of the establishment, to be worked on smoothly by routine operations' (p. 16);

- 'identity kit' to indicate the paraphernalia people ordinarily have to indicate who they are but which is routinely denied inmates in total institutions;

- 'contaminative exposure' to indicate ways inmates are humiliated and mortified in public;

- 'looping' to indicate how an inmate's attempt to fight mortification led to more mortification;

- 'privilege system' to indicate the way ordinary rights that are withheld become privileges used to coerce conformity;

- 'secondary adjustments' to refer to 'practices that do not directly challenge staff but allow inmates to obtain forbidden satisfactions or to obtain permitted ones by forbidden means' (p. 54);

- a variety of 'personal adjustments', such as 'situational withdrawal', which (he notes) psychiatrists might call 'regression'.

This latter point emphasizes another important feature of the kinds of descriptions that Goffman provided. In them he tended to take the kinds of theories and knowledge that people used in these institutions as a kind of data too. The ways that people thought, spoke and wrote were raw material, the analysis of which would reveal something important about the basic character of the institutions where that language was used. In the case of mental hospitals, for example, he says:

> Mental hospitals stand out here because the staff pointedly establish themselves as specialists in the knowledge of human nature, who diagnose and prescribe on

the basis of this intelligence. Hence in the standard psychiatric textbooks there are chapters on 'psychodynamics' and 'psychopathology' which provide charmingly explicit formulations of the 'nature' of human nature.

(Goffman 1961, p. 89)

Goffman saw all these things as expressions of the kinds of institutions that he was studying. In his descriptions, he foregrounded the organization of everyday life in these establishments. In his statement on 'total institutions' in his book *Asylums*, he describes his project as follows:

I have defined total institutions denotatively by listing them and then have tried to suggest some of their common characteristics . . . the similarities obtrude so glaringly and persistently that we have a right to suspect that there are good functional reasons for these features being present and that it will be possible to fit these features together and grasp them by means of a functional explanation. When we have done this, I feel we will give less praise and blame to particular superintendents, commandants, wardens, and abbots, and tend more to understand the social problems and issues in total institutions by appealing to the underlying structural design common to them all.

(Goffman 1961, pp. 123–4)

In his descriptions of establishments and institutions, Goffman used language inventively to name things in ways that avoided conventional moral judgements and thereby helped to make adequate scientific descriptive work possible. Instead of either judgementally pointing out the 'inhuman practices' of mental hospitals or defending the staff as honest professionals doing the best they could with a difficult job, he showed how their activities made sense in context. He wrote about them so that it appeared that what they did was part of the necessary functioning of the organization. These features, moreover, were shared with other organizations – parallels could be seen between prisons, hospitals and religious organizations, for example. The resulting generalizations made possible a deeper understanding of these organizations and the people in them than either denouncing or defending them ever could. This, then, shows the importance of description in coming to an understanding of social phenomena.

Ethnography

Ethnography is a kind of fieldwork that seeks to form a detailed and comprehensive account of the point of view of individuals in any given everyday setting or social action. It is, quite literally, 'writing of culture' (Atkinson 1992). This may be done through participant observation or unstructured interviewing. As Hammersley and Atkinson (1983) write: 'The ethnographer participates overtly or covertly in people's daily lives for extended periods of time watching what happens, listening to what is said, asking questions. In fact collecting whatever data are available to throw light on issues with which he or she is concerned' (p. 2). The aim is to interpret and give meaning to events and individual actions. It seeks to extend commonsense knowledge of cultures and social phenomena in a systematic analysis, or if you like detailed 'folk description' (Agar 1986, p. 12).

Ethnographers tend to have a well-developed sense of the limitations of the use of observation and how they themselves become co-actors in any fieldwork, thus requiring a healthy regard for the potential for bias in any interpretations made. They aim to test any hypotheses or mini-theories about social action from real life, culture and context, ultimately searching out the most credible of a range of explanations.

As is often the case, this approach can be dismissed by those favouring a more scientific form of enquiry. This kind of attack usually points up the problem of subjectivity and rigour. Yet, this is partly to do with the continued warring that goes on between positivists and interpretivists, with the positivists often leading the debate with a question about validity. As Becker (1996) argues powerfully, this tactic is part and parcel of a false hierarchy in research, where the credible work of qualitative research is asked to answer for itself within a quantitative framework, instead of acknowledging ethnography as a highly reasonable approach to determine the meanings that structure social processes.

Ethnography can involve a number of variant approaches, not least because in the interpretive field different researchers will hold slightly different views about what it should achieve or, indeed, what can be achieved. For example, it can involve pinpointing aspects or patterns of social interaction or society itself, the status of cultural knowledge, or even analysis of communication and language.

Ethnographers aim to give a thick or complete description (Geertz 1973) of the social actions being analysed. Although this will always be selective in some way – that is, events or actions will be seen or recorded from one perspective or viewpoint as opposed to another – the ethnographer will usually try to maximize the number and range of 'soundings' taken. Thus, he or she may conduct a range of surveys, observations and unstructured interviews alongside a review of official records pertaining to the social action or setting being investigated. But the key issue will be 'getting up close' to the action and eliciting relevant data to the question at hand. Geertz has said that

> doing ethnography is like trying to read (in the sense of 'construct a reading of') a manuscript – foreign, faded, full of ellipses, incoherencies, suspicious emendations, and tendentious commentaries, but written not in conventionalized graphs of sound but in transient examples of shaped behaviour.
>
> (Geertz 1973, p. 10)

The ethnographer, seeking to describe what is going on in his or her purview or research setting, is confronted with layer upon layer of meaning. To make sense of the accumulated meanings that human action is bound up with, Geertz famously borrowed the term 'thick description' from Gilbert Ryle (1900–1976) (see Ryle 1990), who coined the terms thin and thick description. In Ryle's original example, he considered the movement of the eyelid – the contraction of the muscles necessary to bring it down across the eye and raise it again. A thin description merely described what's being done here. A thick description – which to Geertz is the very stuff of anthropology – involves identifying what the meaning of the movement is. It might be a twitch or a reflex action caused by a draught. On the other hand, it might be a wink, a meaningful gesture. The winker is communicating in a quite precise and special way: (1) deliberately, (2) to someone in particular, (3) to impart a particular message, (4) according to a socially established code, and (5) without cognizance of the rest of the company.

These are what Geertz (1973, p. 7) calls 'piled up structures of inference and implication', especially if some of these winks are done not just as gestures but as parodies, to mislead observers into thinking a conspiracy is going on or as rehearsals of subsequent winks. This, then, is the territory of 'thick description' where meaning, intention and context all play a role and are inferred by the observer. So too with health phenomena. They are susceptible to this kind of description, where the researcher examines the meaning and context. In some parts of India, for example, the smallpox goddess Shitala or Sitala is worshipped (Lopez 1995) and may be the mother goddess of an entire village. The temples to her are often decorated at the local spring festivals. Sitala is also associated with some other diseases such as cholera, tetanus and typhoid. This brief vignette enables us to see that there are spiritual dimensions to illness. Once we have spotted these in other cultures we can see how the apparently rather secular practices of health care in the West have spiritual aspects for those involved, and how the craft of scientific health care practitioners might resemble ritual, ceremony and liturgy. This, then, is one of the insights from ethnography.

But where did ethnography come from? Although often associated with the study of people in far-away countries, the rise of recognizably ethnographic methods can be found in the very heart of the British Empire. The rise of ethnography dates back to the nineteenth century and the large study that Henry Mayhew did on the poor of London, 'London Labour and the London Poor'. By the 1920s and 1930s, more and more scholars, particularly social anthropologists such as Malinowski, Boas and Mead, were interested in conducting observations of groups or masses of people in the kinds of locales that the European and American powers had been visiting and colonizing. This overall movement or approach to research gained ground with increased criticism of the limitations of positivistic, quantitative science and enquiry that has continued to the present day.

The value of ethnography to understanding health care is clear. Within any health care setting, or in relation to any professional group, ethnography can afford a deep or thick description of the larger organizations such as hospitals, community services and such like, or focus on much smaller settings such as wards or clinics and groups of practitioners. Through observations, interviews or analysis of documents such as care notes, patient histories and so on, the health care researcher will seek to gain a detailed and rich understanding of whichever interactive environment or setting they choose. The researcher enters their chosen 'field' of human activity, behaviour and culture, and collects data which they analyse, interpret and present in terms of patterns or themes. Such representations of health care 'realities', as Leininger (1994) notes, will need to be believable, confirmable through an audit trail of the evidence and be rooted in context. The researcher will need to establish that derived patterns or themes are recurrent over time, their description has reached saturation and that the findings are transferable to other contexts in similar conditions. Of course, some of Leininger's strictures are governed by an obsessive subservience to positivist methods, but deserve attention all the same.

To gain a closer look at ethnography in action, we will look at a few studies relevant to the field of health care. First, we focus on one of the classic studies in medical sociology, which we mentioned earlier.

Howard Becker's *Boys in White*

This famous study by Becker *et al.* (1961) illustrates how the world-view, means of representing and using knowledge and attitudes to patients, shift as people move from being novice to expert practitioners. The study investigated the development of medical students as they progressed through their academic and clinical learning. It sought to 'discover what medical school did to medical students other than giving them a technical education' (p. 17). Examining a rich variety of collective social action through participant observation and interviews, Becker and his colleagues were able to give a detailed account of the diverse and changing perspectives of the students as they became immersed in the 'drama of medicine' (p. 4). At first, the students in their white coats were 'full of enthusiasm, pride, and idealism about the medical profession', something they had dreamt of from childhood (p. 79). Yet, as the realities and politics of medical work encroached on these neophytes, their relationship to their work and, indeed, patients lost some of its shine. The ethnographic approach in this study helped the researchers get very close to the action. Even the students themselves were concerned that Becker, in his participant observer role, experience medical situations close up:

> A staff member demonstrated a patient with enlarged lymph nodes and had the fifteen members of the class take turns palpating these nodes. Several of the students, while waiting their turns, told me that I should get in line and feel the nodes too. One of them said, 'Go ahead. Get up there and feel those nodes. How are you going to know what happens to us unless you go through the same experiences?'
>
> (Becker *et al.* 1961, p. 249)

Becker took plenty of opportunities to 'get up there' in terms of mapping the progression of these students and changes in their actions. Some of his observations betrayed student attitudes that fell short of their idealistic beginnings. For example:

> A student I was spending some time with was required to do a blood count on a patient he regarded as not being sick at all. He drew a syringe full of blood and carried it out to the nurses' station. In front of the nurse, he held the syringe up to the light, looked at it, and handed it to her, saying, 'Here, you can have this now. I've already done my blood count and differential.' The nurse looked at him and laughed nervously. He said, 'Oh well, with somebody like her, what the hell difference does it make? She isn't likely to have any haematological trouble. We'll just fill it in with normal values. That will be all right.' While the nurse giggled, the student took the chart, opened it up to the page where lab results go and said,

'Let's see, her blood looked pretty good. I'll put down twelve grams of haemo-globin, that's about 77 per cent of normal.' He wrote down these figures and filled in imaginary figures for the other values to be reported. I said, 'Tell me, do people turn in lab results like this very often?' He said, 'Sure they do. What the hell, she hasn't got anything that needs a blood count. It's just a lot of damn fool scut work. I'll show that goddam Jones.' (Jones, the patient's doctor, was a member of staff this student particularly disliked, feeling that he, more than other staffmen, tried to 'keep the students in their place').

(Becker *et al.* 1961, pp. 264–5)

Again, the onset of less-than-ideal attitudes among the students was further illustrated in the following summary of a conversation:

Two students were discussing the kinds of practices they would have when they got out, and the way they would treat various diseases. One said, 'I'll tell you the way I would treat obesity. I would just tell them that I will give them a diet and if they follow this diet they will lose weight. If they don't want to follow the diet, then I will just tell them that I don't want to have anything more to do with them. It's all a matter of will power. I'd scare the hell out of them about all the diseases they could get from being overweight. If that didn't do it, I would just get rid of them.' The other student agreed.

(Becker *et al.* 1961, p. 317)

Finally, Becker reported elsewhere in the study:

I was talking with some of the students when a very pretty girl in a maternity smock walked by. White said, 'We never get any that look like that in GYN clinic [Gynaecology]. I don't know why. I sure wouldn't mind doing an examination on someone like her.' I said, 'What's this? I thought you guys had got over all that and just took it in your stride. You know, didn't bat an eyelash.' Barton said, 'When that happens, I'll be old and gray, believe me. I'm still young enough to enjoy looking at something like that.'

(Becker *et al.* 1961, p. 324)

These accounts present a rather different picture of medical students as they 'mature' into medical practitioners, which give cause for concern now as much as they did in the early 1960s. Becker and his colleagues are able to map this change in attitude with detailed ethnographic accounts of spoken transactions and behaviour. The 'boys in white', with their clinical coats, do not come out 'white' in the study. They appear to be socialized into, at times, rather dodgy attitudes to patients. One wonders if this has changed since Becker's study. But whatever the current situation, this study provides a useful and powerful insight into how ethnography can 'get behind the scenes' of health care dramas, and provide a rich account of the perceptions of those working in the various professions.

Phenomenology

In psychology, philosophy and sociology, there has been a good deal of interest in whether it is possible to describe the contents of consciousness. Is looking at the world within as easy as looking at the world outside? Why is it important to look at the subjective realm? We shall examine the approach taken by phenomenologists and discuss its relevance to research in health care.

Phenomenology, as practised by Husserl, Brentano and Heidegger, seeks to obtain an accurate description and understanding of lived human experience – that is, from the perspective of an individual's consciousness, directed or intended towards objects in the world (intentionality) – without being contaminated by assumptions about their 'objective reality'. It does this by 'bracketing' out the beliefs, attitudes and, indeed, prejudices of the researcher(s) that may unduly shape the description of whatever lived human experience is being accounted for. Examination of a person's subjective viewpoint or consciousness – something that is often discounted or taken for granted – may be extended to include others and how they interrelate (intersubjectivity). Whether the focus is on the subjective or inter-subjective realm, phenomenology seeks to provide a balanced account of lived experiences or the 'life world' of individuals. As a rather heterogeneous approach within an interpretivist tradition, phenomenology seeks to advance understanding of how consciousness and objective phenomena interact in the interpretation and, at times, construction of social life. Or, in other words, it examines the cognitive activity at the heart of human society. For example, if we were to study any given phenomenon in health care, we would be doing so by examining accounts of those experiencing it. We might investigate what is the lived, subjective experience of having a particular illness or condition, such as cancer or systematic lupus erythematosus. In addition, our descriptions as researchers may uncover different aspects of illness or disease that are novel or hitherto under-studied. Below we detail how a paradoxical illness experience can lead to new areas and concerns being opened up to scrutiny.

The pleasures of illness

How do professionals interpret a condition such as eczema? What is their thinking and interpretation of this condition, quite apart from their assumptions about what it must be like? If we look at the phenomenon of eczema from a professional or health care perspective, the condition may be perceived as bringing great distress, both physical and emotional, to an individual. However, this perception, largely rooted in an illness model of eczema, may miss how an individual may view their eczema as potentially pleasurable. Here is one of the author's (P.C.) own account of having eczema:

> As an eczema sufferer my condition is chronic partly because I really enjoy raking my flesh to the point of bleeding. I also like to see the product of this 'work', best of all against dark fabric or other similar backgrounds. Sometimes, I like to scratch my hands at night, in the dark, holding them above my head, when I can

feel my productivity gently falling like snow flakes on my face. If my feet are hot from being in boots all day, then the first scratch of the skin around my ankles can be quite exquisite. These are some of the pleasures of illness. My actions do not help my skin, but they do help me to accept my condition as something that contributes to my enjoyment just as it takes this away in distressing flare-ups and infection.

Now this sounds perverse, but it is worth remembering that the 'lived experience' of various illnesses or diseases are not always negative and can be uncovered by adopting a phenomenological approach. Such an approach can provide a different take on the health care world as seen through professional eyes.

This approach, then, can provide a deep or rich description of human experiences and the meanings that they generate that might otherwise go unnoticed. The researcher or investigator avoids directly shaping the findings and tries to ensure that his or her descriptions mirror closely the 'real-life' experience. Transcribed materials are treated carefully to ensure fidelity to that experience and, as noted above, the researcher 'brackets' out his or her own bias or influence upon the findings.

Of course, as with all approaches that are qualitative in manner, phenomenology depends on the articulation of the researcher and participant(s) and even a small range of investigations will demand a lot of time and effort. Again, because of the small numbers of participants that can be included in such intensive 'mining' of human meanings and experience, this approach will not promote the kind of generalizable findings that more scientific research celebrates. In addition to concerns that phenomenology may be so focused as to exclude broader contexts, including antecedents and consequences, this approach can be criticized as affording limited, time- and place-sensitive analyses.

Grounded theory

Grounded theory, which was developed by Glaser, Strauss, Corbin and others, is a framework for research that is heavily tilted towards induction. That is, from this perspective, researchers choose to see what is out there in any particular field or situation of human life without being directed by an overt theory or hypothesis. Indeed, such researchers are happy to let any theory or hypothesis emerge from the data they collect. This grounding of theory can be considered as an authentic, open means of achieving a comprehensive description of given situations or events prior to analytical closure through the formulation of a theory or set of theories.

The researcher examines individual cases and performs a synchronic collection and analysis of data, remaining open to various interpretations. The aim is to do this in such a way as to arrive at 'thick', comprehensive or rounded understanding of the meanings generated by individuals, situations or events. This 'thick' or deep understanding occurs when the researcher's enquiry has reached 'saturation' and no longer yields new information.

Grounded theory is not a loose or unsystematic approach. Done properly, with the use of ongoing memo writing and coding of data, the findings emerge and generate theories that are 'grounded' – that is, not distant from their real-life source. As the researcher collects data, he or she will continuously review it, and researchers can check, refine and develop their ideas and intuitions about their findings as the data are collected. The method has been used often and grounded theory investigations can be found in fields as diverse as tourism (Connell and Lowe 2001), death studies (Deves and Robinson 2002) and the experience of living with schizophrenia (Humberstone 2002). Indeed, putting the term 'grounded theory' into a search of any archive of electronic literature over the past few years would reveal an increasing proportion of material in health care research that uses this kind of methodology. However, despite its popularity, it is open to the charge that studies using it rarely produce robust theories. In most cases, such studies fall short of this, but instead provide a rich account of the real-life experiences of human interactants.

Summary

There are many more variants of qualitative methodology that take as their core the systematic description of social or subjective events. Our survey has been highly selective, but we hope to have illustrated several things. All of these approaches can be used to find out how people create and exchange meanings in their everyday lives, not least in health care interactions and settings. In a sense, they are a means to get up 'close and dirty' with human activity, behaviour and culture, and create new under-standing about these. Unlike quantitative approaches, they consider the constructed-ness of human society and how meanings are negotiated and built in relation to different settings. Of course, such approaches are not concerned with causality in the sense sought after by experimenters, and contest the scientific paradigm of the 'laboratory'. Instead, they tend to focus on functional explanations and on lived, natural experiences. Again, these qualitative approaches to knowledge acquisition do not always seek generalizable findings, or data that can be reconstituted in statistical terms, but provide 'deeper' informative accounts of the often messy business of human society and culture. In so doing, researchers employing such methods as ethnography, phenomenology and grounded theory try to be as rigorous and system-atic as possible, while addressing head-on the ambiguity in human social life. Here, they may well try to avoid being selective and excluding 'awkward' data, enhance validity by checking out their findings with other observers or coders and, indeed, other comparative studies.

Making the human condition visible: phrenology and the construction of physical maps of the mind

To illustrate a little more of the kinds of sciences which a focus on the visible and the factual leads us towards, let us consider phrenology. Here we can see what observation and an empirical approach can create. This might seem a paradoxical assertion because, in the conventional view, phrenology has been debunked as a kind of pseudo-science, a dead end, fit only for travelling circus shows. However, the enor-mous corpus of observation, which was variously anecdotal and quantitative, and from both the living and the dead, fitted in very well with the optimistic scientific spirit of the times. Moreover, far from having been debunked, it informed much twentieth-century thinking about cerebral structure, function and localization. Had it not been for phrenology, contemporary neurology could not have existed in its present form.

On the face of it, phrenology – the idea that one can read a person's character from the bumps on his or her head – is a classic tale of the rise and fall of a 'science'. It flourished for a century or so and is now considered to be 'discredited'. Yet a good many of its claims are reproduced in modern theories of the localization of function within the brain. This invites the question of why the original version is considered to be nonsense and the later version scientific. Surprisingly, scientific and non-scientific modes of thought can reach curiously similar conclusions, especially if the non-scientific one is under the impression that it is science. This is comparable to the way that alchemy can be seen as the precursor of chemistry, or how astrology might have prompted advances in astronomy, or how medieval scholasticism might have set the stage for early science. Though it has been abandoned, phrenology was once a central plank in the story of the new human sciences. It was here that the intersection between the body politic – which was being rendered visible through official statistics and social surveys – intersected with the physiological sciences of the human body. The sheer scope of this visibility encompassed not only social pathologies but human anatomy, and brought them into the same conceptual framework. In a sense, it was part of this drive towards unity between the natural and the newly emerging social sciences. The observations of head size and shape, then, were embedded within much larger-scale social, political and epistemological currents.

Like many of these strange historical conjunctures – few modern community pharmacists would consider themselves to be alchemists – today few people would consider themselves to believe in phrenology. It is difficult to imagine the massive impact this discipline had on thought across the whole spectrum of intellectual life in the nineteenth century. Phrenological ideas found their way into art, music and literature, as well as laying the ground for concepts and developments that are still a cherished part of today's scientific canon.

First, let us examine the ideas behind phrenology. It first made its appearance at the end of the eighteenth century. Despite the eighteenth-century Enlightenment being at its height, very little was known about the brain, and it was certainly not possible to do any more than speculate about how it worked. In this climate, a number of people were hard at work trying to find a physical basis for human character and abilities. Some of the groundwork was accomplished by Johann Lavater (1741–1801), a Swiss clergyman, who, in his book *Physiognomic Fragments* (1775–8), provides a method for reading a person's character from their face. His famous series of illustrations of 'heads of idiot women' is accompanied by detailed commentaries of what the form of the nose or the grin means, or what is signified by the lines on the forehead (Gilman 1982).

These ideas were revolutionized in 1796 by Franz Joseph Gall (1758–1828), a Viennese physician who pioneered a systematic attempt to relate the brain to the capabilities and character of humans. He proposed that the brain is the organ of the mind and that this organ is composed of a number of different faculties. If these individual faculties were especially powerful or well developed, the corresponding part of the brain is larger, and a corresponding lump can be found on the surface of the skull. The shape of the skull, then, according to Gall, was an index of a person's character. This character was a composite of a number of faculties, – 37 in all – elaborated by Gall and his collaborator Spurzheim. These included 'calculativeness', relating to the organ responsible for handling numbers, through to 'amativeness', relating to physical love, and 'approbativeness', concerned with seeking the approval of others. There were also faculties of 'inhabitiveness', an instinct prompting one to select a particular dwelling, and veneration, a tendency to adore God, venerate saints and respect others (Cooter 1984). Aside from these rather quaint faculties, there are a few more recognizable ones from the point of view of psychology. Verbal memory, language and conscientiousness would all be recognizable to the psychologist today.

In the early period, from 1796 to 1810, the practice of phrenology was restricted to Gall and Spurzheim, but thanks to a critical article in the *Edinburgh Review* magazine, and Spurzheim's rejoinder to this, the ideas behind phrenology began to reach a wider and more sympathetic audience. Phrenological societies were founded, beginning in Edinburgh in 1820, and the first issue of *The Phrenological Journal* appeared in 1823.

Phrenology found its way into literature. One of Britain's early phrenological enthusiasts, George Combe, published the very widely read *Elements of Phrenology* in 1834 and aspects of this crop up in plays, novels and popular culture. The novels of the Brontës are peppered with phrenological referents. In Charlotte Brontë's *Jane Eyre*, for example, the heroine examines Mr Rochester's face – 'Let me look at your face: turn to the moonlight . . . because I want to read your countenance' (Chapter 23) – before considering his marriage proposal. Charlotte Brontë's characters are not usually successful in their phrenological efforts. The interesting point is that these references are there at all. The notion of phrenology had a powerful effect on the intellectual community at the time. One of the founding fathers of social science, Herbert Spencer (1820–1903), was interested in phrenology and even created a device – the cephalometer – to facilitate the accurate, standardized measurement of the head.

The idea that one could infer the character of people from the shapes of their heads, allied to the powerful and influential ideas of Charles Darwin, produced an explosive mixture of ideas. The craniological work seeking to identify racial types was popular in the later Victorian period, where it was widely believed that the inferiority of certain peoples could be identified by the fact that their foreheads receded and their jaws jutted. Thus, it was believed that people of African descent were more closely allied to the lower primates. Shortly after the time of Gall, a Philadelphia doctor, Samuel Morton (1799–1851), started collecting skulls from different ethnic groups and measuring their volume. He was thereby able to create a kind of hierarchy of the races, with people of Western European or, as he put it, 'teutonic' character at the top with larger skulls, and Africans and native Australians at the bottom with the smallest. In Britain John Beddoe, founder of the British Anthropological Institute, published a book *The Races of Man* in 1862 (the key ideas of which were reproduced in his 1905 work), where he proposed an 'index of negressence' that enabled him to demonstrate quantitatively his view that the Irish had skulls similar to those of the Cro-Magnon prehistoric people and were a kind of 'Africanoid' white species. Thus, this particular legacy of phrenology has been aligned with politics, which has become increasingly unsavoury to the spirit of the twentieth century. The crude anthropological racisms of our intellectual forebears, chronicled by Steven J. Gould (1984) in his *Mismeasure of Man*, is uncomfortable for much of the present generation of anthropologists and psychologists.

However, the idea of psychological characteristics that one could see from the shapes of the face and the head found a strong supporter in the form of Cesare Lombroso (1835–1909) (e.g. Lombroso 1892). Throughout his active career, Lombroso became a professor of a number of disciplines, including psychiatry, forensic medicine and criminal anthropology, as well as running his own lunatic asylum. He is chiefly remembered for the notion that criminal types can be recognized from the shapes of their heads. He believed that criminality represented a more primitive stage in human evolution and criminals could be recognized by atavistic features. That is, the criminal would have characteristics such as a receding forehead or large jaw, reminiscent of an earlier stage in human evolution, or they might have other 'stigmata', perhaps by showing marked asymmetries in the face or body. Whereas the Lombrosian position in its strong form is today thought of as discredited, there is still a great deal in contemporary theories of crime that owes a debt to Professor Lombroso.

The atavistic argument, for example, is still present in contemporary models of emotion that see the limbic system as being a legacy from our past. Many scholars are still avidly looking at brain scans trying to detect differences in structure and function between the criminal and the law-abiding individual, especially where this involves a lack of activity or development in the frontal lobes. Family linkage studies attempt to detect genetic predispositions to crime. The search for personal characteristics of the criminal goes on too, in the form of researchers looking for – and discovering – that offenders tend to come from broken homes, have low self-esteem and poor school achievement. Crime, as a result of Professor Lombroso's intellectual revolution, is not something that anyone might do if they got the chance, but is something done by certain damaged individuals.

Gall has left his stamp on the human sciences even today. The idea of localization of function in the brain has survived the test of time and has led to a thriving branch of science seeking to locate the brain activity for a variety of functions. Language, vision, motor skills and short-term memory have all been isolated, at least according to introductory psychology textbooks. Some introductory books still present those latter-day variants of Gall's heads, Wilder Penfield's sensory homunculus and motor homunculus. These distorted images of the body allegedly represent the proportions of the cortex devoted to various parts of the body, with the lips and fingers enlarged in size. Of course, the fine grain of the research literature and individual case studies disclose a much more untidy picture, where some individuals are atypically lateralized or localized, or have demonstrated considerable plasticity, or may even be living relatively normal lives with very little brain at all. Gall's legacy is that we can gloss over this diversity with standardized maps of function, which if not the direct analogues of the china heads, at least come close in spirit.

One of Gall's lasting contributions to the study of the brain was the observation that the grey matter of the cerebral cortex was not as had been previously believed a kind of protective covering (cortex means bark), but was predominantly made up of cell bodies, hence its greyish appearance. Conversely, the white matter looked that way because it contained a higher proportion of nerve fibres with their fatty myelin sheaths. Moreover, the grey matter had to be important because it was nearest the skull and helped to provide the bumps. He made an inference that would be absurd to contemporary neuropsychology but, paradoxically, has important elements that have turned out to be durable.

Looking at heads and inferring characteristics, especially when it involved notions of atavism, has its roots in a much earlier notion, the Doctrine of Signatures, involving the belief that things that looked alike were believed to share characteristics in other respects too. The Elizabethan scholar and conjurer Dr John Dee, for example, believed that the Bedlington terrier was the most nervous kind of dog because it resembled a sheep. This sort of thinking pervaded the disciplines of psychiatric and criminological illustration (Gilman 1982). What we could see in the body of the madman or woman was, in Comte's sense, 'positive'. This was rendered even more literally present with the introduction of photography. The camera, it was said, never lies. The body in madness disclosed its secrets just as readily as any map of poverty or rate of suicide. This idea was central to what Showalter (1987) calls 'psychiatric Victorianism', where psychiatric luminaries such as Henry Maudsley were convinced that the signs of madness could be revealed in the physical features of their patients, their expressions, their gait or, indeed, the shape of their heads.

Allied to these developments in science of human diversity, there was a great deal of interest in the issue of crime. Again, this interest was accompanied by a conviction that this could all be made visible and hence manageable. As with sex, in the example earlier in this chapter, the medico-legal discovery of crime involved medics and scientists hard at work discovering the criminal – from their head shapes to their psychological profiles. The ambition was to construct an objective science of criminology whose facts – echoing Quetelet 50 years earlier – would speak for themselves. In both sex and crime, scientists were convinced that the secrets of the human condition would be yielded up to careful scientific scrutiny, and human deviance would have an ultimately biological explanation. We will analyse what led to this spirit in the human and health sciences, consider the implications for the philosophy of science and examine the broader implications of styles of thought, such as mentalism, individualism and reductionism, which are still present in the human sciences today. The idea, then, is that by taking a social phenomenon like crime, we can detect the origins of this in the minds and ultimately the bodies of criminals. Whereas the bumps on their heads are no longer of interest, the location of the causes of crime in the brains, or even the DNA of 'criminals' (Raine 1993), has become a fashionable quest. Now this latter kind of criminology is the sort of intellectual endeavour which has been made possible by the earlier sciences that focused on the genitalia of 'nymphomaniacs' or the heads of 'criminals'. As such, it has a reassuring and persuasive familiarity. Of course, modern criminal psychopathology has done a great deal to shake off the legacy of Dr Lombroso, and locate the 'causes' instead in patterns of brain activity revealed when scans of incarcerated criminals' brains are compared with those of medical students, for example. We could, perhaps proceed along the avenue of looking critically at the research, to see if it met some arbitrary criteria of 'good science'. This is relatively well rehearsed. Every introductory criminology textbook will tell you it is not good science. What we are trying to argue is something a little different. We're interested in how this came to be seen as a good idea. To understand that, you need to understand the 'history of the head'. It is this that has made the very idea of a physiology and genetics of crime possible. The positivistic spirit allowed the slippage between the social and the physical as these domains were merely different aspects of the same phenomenon and they could be studied with the same concepts and methods via these 'criminological displacements' (Pfol and Gordon 1986).

So far, we have seen how descriptions have a broader set of resonances with social and political concerns. The description of the shape and size of people's heads is, by itself, relatively meaningless. It becomes meaningful, and politically and socially important, as its implications are constructed and developed by practitioners and urged by policy makers.

To show how this sort of thing has implications for the study of how we look at nature and describe it in the present day, let us shift the frame and talk about social science once again. In this part of the chapter, we will look at a kind of phrenology of interaction. In conversation analysis, the analyst's intention is to provide as meticulous a rendering as possible of the lumps and bumps of conversational interaction. In doing this, there is considerable interest in the veracity of transcriptions as a vehicle for understanding the texture or the 'music' of social life.

The details of mundane interactions in health care – conversation analysis

Conversation analysis highlights the relationship between things that are descriptive and matters that are analytical. As a discipline, it starts from the same sorts of premises as phenomenology. As Alfred Schutz says:

> The world of nature, as explored by the natural scientist, does not 'mean' anything to the molecules, atoms and electrons. But the observational field of the social scientist – social reality – has a specific meaning and reference structure for the human beings living, acting and thinking within it.
>
> (Schutz 1962, p. 59)

As Drew *et al.* (2001) characterize it, conversation analysis is a method which focuses largely on the verbal communications that people recurrently use in interacting with one another. People are, in this view, attempting to produce meaningful action and to interpret the other's meaning. Again, this resembles phenomenology. In the view of Drew *et al.*, there are three key features to conversation analysis:

1 Any utterances are considered to be performing social actions, such as maintaining agreement between the participants, finding out the reasons for the present situation and securing the interactant's identity as a creditable person.
2 Utterances and actions are considered to be part of sequences of action, so that what one participant says and does is occasioned by what the others have just said and done. Conversation analysis thus focuses on dynamic processes of interaction from which sequences are built up.

3   These sequences appear to have stable patterns. How one participant acts and speaks can be shown to have regular, predictable consequences for how the other responds.

Social interactions are meaningful for the participants who produce them and they have a natural organization that can be discovered, and the analyst is interested in understanding the machinery, the rules and the structures that produce or constitute this orderliness. Thus it is assumed that there are particular strategic functions that conversational practices embody. The hesitations, the paralinguistic gurgles and the false starts do important interactional work just as much as the semantic content of the words. There are several basic assumptions involved in conversation analysis (from Psathas 1995, pp. 2–3):

1   Order is a produced orderliness.
2   Order is produced by the parties *in situ*; that is, it is situated and occasioned.
3   The parties orient to that order themselves; that is, this order is not an analyst's conception, not the result of some preformed or preformulated theoretical conceptions concerning what action should/must/ought to be based on generalizing or summarizing statements about what action generally/frequently/often is.
4   Order is repeatable and recurrent.
5   The discovery, description and analysis of that produced orderliness is the task of the analyst.
6   Issues of how frequently, how widely or how often particular phenomena occur are to be set aside in the interest of discovering, describing and analysing the structures, the machinery, the organized practices, the formal procedures, the ways in which order is produced.
7   Structures of social action, once so discerned, can be described and analysed in formal – that is, structural, organizational, logical, atopically contentless, consistent – and abstract terms.

As Harvey Sacks put it, there was 'order at all points'. Moreover, as far as conversation analysts are concerned, that's the only order there is. From the point of view of ethnomethodology and especially conversation analysis,

> the primordial site of social order is found in members' use of methodical practices to produce, make sense of and thereby render accountable, features of their local circumstances . . . The socially structured character of . . . any enterprise undertaken by members is thus not exterior or extrinsic to their everyday workings, but interior and intrinsic, residing in the local and particular detail of practical actions undertaken by members uniquely competent to do so.
> (Boden and Zimmerman 1991, pp. 6–7)

Conversation analysts do not use category systems that are preformed in advance of the actual observation of the interaction, and there is a great deal of interest in the local context of the utterance or exchange.

Moreover, conversation analysis has its own epistemology (theory of knowledge) in that it does not concern itself with matters that are outside the conversation:

No assumptions are made regarding the participants' motivations, intentions or purposes; nor about their ideas, thoughts or understandings; nor their moods, emotions or feelings, except insofar as these can demonstrably be shown to be matters that participants themselves are noticing, attending to or orienting to in the course of their interaction. Further, if and when this happens their doing so is done 'for all practical purposes, in and of that situated occasioned production. What is available to the hearer for such apprehendings is similarly available to the observer.'

(Psathas 1995, p. 47)

To illustrate what can be achieved with some of these kinds of descriptions and to show the reasoning strategies at work as researchers move from transcribed encounters to analytic work, let us look at some events in the health care journey, from the initial introduction to the giving of advice. In health care encounters, we can see by means of these kinds of approaches which rely on description how the social fabric is constructed by the interactants as they go along.

Getting started 'the "How are you?" sequence'

'How are you?' is a commonplace question with which to commence an interaction. However, in a health care context, it has a number of possible meanings, from a polite greeting to a request for an account of symptoms. Here is an example (from Drew *et al.* 2001, p. 62):

```
01   Dr:  Hi Missis Mo:ff[et,
02   Pt:  [Good morning
03   Dr:  Good morning
04   Dr:  How are you do:[ing
05   Pt:  [Fi:n]e,
06        (.)
07   Dr:  How are y[ou fe[eling
08   Pt:  [Much[(better)
09   Pt:  I feel good
10        (.)
11   Dr:  Okay. = so you're feeling
12        a little [bit better] with thuh
13   Pt:  [Mm hm,]
14   Dr:  three of the [Chlonadine?
15   Pt:  [Yes.
```

There are two occurrences of a 'how are you?' (HAY) question. One is in line 4 and is a common part of a greeting sequence. The second, in line 7, signals a frame shift to a biomedical frame of reference. Here the doctor is opening the biomedical frame – this might just as easily be done by 'What can I do for you today?', 'What brings you in today?', 'What seems to be the problem?' and so on. However, these three forms are the kinds of things one would use for a first time visit. By using 'how are you feeling?', the doctor is showing that she is aware that the patient has been in before with the same complaint. Thus, the forms – the phrenological lumps in the conversation if you will – are shown to be explicitly tailored to the matter in hand.

Going through the examination: the 'online commentary'

Another example of how a detailed description of the events concerned is used in a more multi-layered way comes from another study of face-to-face encounters in the clinical context. Here the clinicians and patients are described in some detail going through the routine of an examination by the analysts. The doctors are performing a kind of description and so are the analysts, in this case Heritage and Stivers (1999). There is thus a kind of 'double hermeneutic' of description. Let us consider two extracts from their paper. These concern what Heritage and Stivers call 'online commentaries'.

```
 1  Doc:   An:' we're gonna have you look s:traight ahea:d, =h
 2         (0.5)
 3  Doc:   J's gonna check your thyroid right no:w,
 4         (9.5)
 5  Doc:   .hh That feels normal?
 6         (0.8)
 7  Doc:   I don't feel any: lymph node: swelling, .hh inn your neck area
 8  Doc:   .hh Now what I'd like ya tuh do I wanchu tuh
 9         breathe with yer mouth open. = Nice slow deep breaths
                              (Heritage and Stivers 1999, p. 1502)
```

```
 1  Doc:   Can you open your mouth for me agai:n,
 2         (0.3)
 3         'at's it
 4         (0.7)
 5  Doc:   Little bit re:d (.) hm
 6         (1.6) ((moving sounds))
 7  Doc:   Alri::rght (h)
 8         ((more moving sounds))
 9         . . . . .
10         ((lines omitted))
11         . . . . .
12  Doc:   Ari:ght Michael. Can I loo:k >in your< ears
13         (0.3)
14  Mum:   This o:n[e:
15  Doc:        ['ank you
16         (0.9)
```

17	Doc:	'at's fi:ne, the other one?
18		(4.5)
19	Doc:	ktch okha:yh
20		(0.5)
21	Doc:	They're alri::ght (h). I mean there's just a li:(tt)le
22		redness in his throa:t an:d just a litt,le pinkness ther:e
23		which (.) means he's got one of tho:se co:lds that make them
24		cou:gh a lot .hh Because his chest is pe:rfectly all ri:ght
25		he ce:rtainly doesn't need (.) penicillin
26	Mum:	N:o[:
27	Doc:	['r anything like tha:t .hhh hh I think the coughing. . . .
		((continues))

(Heritage and Stivers 1999, p. 1506)

Now, as it stands here, this is the barest description of what happens in a medical encounter. There appears to be an ambition to render the ongoing interaction as literally as possible, down to the pauses and the paralinguistic noises. However, this description, with its complex punctuation, which makes it appear even more authentic, is recruited to a grander theoretical purpose. Heritage and Stivers (1999) use it to support an account of medical practice. Here they see the aim of the game as being the doctor's avoidance in issuing a prescription. That is, especially in the case of relatively mild respiratory problems, it is considered inappropriate to prescribe antibiotics. This description of interaction in the medical encounter, then, by downgrading the severity of the symptoms, makes the eventual refusal to prescribe an apparently logical conclusion. Thus the fact that there isn't a lymph node swelling, or that various areas of the small boy in the second extract are only a little bit pink or red, contrasts with other possible formulations of the problem, as involving severe inflammation or swelling, for example. Descriptions, then, are intelligible within a larger context. The doctors' descriptions of the problems in the cases above yield the kind of outcome that is desirable to the medical gaze. Moreover, the level of description provided by the analysts Heritage and Stivers is important in that it helps to bolster their thesis that important conversationally mediated work is being done in the encounter. It's not just about the biomedical story of disease, it involves how the parties work out what the problem is between them, in which negotiation the doctors' medical expertise is deployed in a kind of steering or management process.

Delivering the bad news: the perspective display series

To provide a clue about what this involves, let us consider the example of medical encounters in a study by Maynard (1991) of talk in clinics that specialize in disorders of childhood like autism and developmental disabilities. Children were assessed and then clinicians met the parents to discuss the nature of their child's problems and to provide recommendations for therapies and treatments and advice on dealing with specific difficulties. As clinicians introduced their findings and recommendations to the parents, they often asked parents for their perspective on the child and incorporated this into their report. These encounters Maynard called perspective display series (PDS), which involve: (1) the clinician's opinion, query or perspective display invitation; (2) the recipient's reply or assessment; (3) the clinician's report and assessment. Clinicians tend to fit their diagnostic news delivery to the occasioned display of the parents' perspective, especially by formulating agreement in such a way as to co-implicate the parents' perspective in the diagnostic presentation. The clinician's invitation (phase 1 above) could be marked or unmarked. Marked invitations looked something like the following examples, and involved a formulation of the problem as somehow being possessed by the child.

> (1.)
> (8.013)
> Dr. E.   What do you see? as his difficulty.
>   (1.2)
> Mrs. C. Mainly his uhm (1.2) the fact that he doesn't understand everythin (6.0) and also the fact that his speech (0.7) is very hard to understand what he's saying.
> (14.012 simplified)
> Dr. E.   What do you think is his problem
>   (3.0)
> Dr. E.   I think you know him better than all of us really. So that ya know this really has to be a (0.8) in some ways a (0.6) team effort to (4) understand what's (0.4) going o::n. .hh.
> Mrs. D. Well I know he has a- (0.6) a learning problem (1.2) in general. .hh and s:::peech problem an' a language problem (1.0) a behaviour problem. I know he has all o' that but still. hh at the back of my- my- my mind I feel that (0.4) he's t- ta some degree retardet.

An unmarked invitation does not propose a problem

> 10.002
> Dr. S.   Now- (0.6) uhh since (0.4) you've (0.1) been here and through this thing h:ow do you see R now
>   (0.4) Mrs C.
> Mrs. C. I guess i (0.2) see him better since he here
> 9.001
> Dr. S.   Now that you've- we've been through all this I just wanted to know from you::::. (0.4) how you see J at
>   this time.
>   (2.2)
> Mrs. C. The same
>   (0.7)
> Dr. S.   Which is?
>   (0.5)
> Mrs. C. Uhm she can't talk . . .

Let us consider another example which involves the refusal of a marked invitation by the parent:

22.007
04 Dr. N: It's obvious that uh- you- understand a fair amount (0.2)
05   about what Charles' problem i[s
06 Mrs. G: [y]is. (yeh).

16 Dr. N: S::o at this point there is a certain amount of
17   confusion.
18   (0.2)
19 Mrs. G: Mm hmm
20   (0.3)
21 Dr. N: In your mind probably as to what the problem really
22   is?
23 Mrs. G: Mm
24 Dr. N: .hh and we haven't really had a chance to hear from
25   you at all as to (0.7) what you
26   f[eel the situation.
27 Mrs. G: [well I don't think] there's anything wrong with him.

Marked and unmarked invitations differ in terms of what follows in the sequence. Marked invitations are 'suggestions or proposals that require acceptance'. If parents disagree that the problem resides in the child, the interactive work of modifying that disagreement has to be accomplished and the parents' positions modified in ways which sustain the clinician's claim to expertise. The unmarked invitation's alignment between parents' and clinicians' views is sought but in a different way. It enables parents to provide indications that something is wrong, which the clinician can then elaborate on so that their diagnoses appear more confirmatory than presumptive. 'A result of strategically employing these various procedures . . . is to maximise the potential for presenting clinical assessments as agreeing with recipient's perspectives or in a publicly affirmative and non conflicting manner' (Maynard 1991, p. 87).

Giving advice – 'displaced didacticism'

A further feature of talk between health professionals and clients which we have discovered in our own research is the way that professionals tend to use a variety of rhetorical devices to lend authority to what they say by reference to other sources of information. To show how the sources of information are deployed in the discourse of the nurse advisers, let us examine a sequence of discourse from a study of our own into interactions occurring in the UK's telephone health advisory service, NHS Direct. Here the caller is concerned with whether it is possible to drink alcohol while taking antibiotics:

HA: Here you're there now you're just interested in how much alcohol would be safe to drink with Metronidazole.
FP: Yeah, yeah.
HA: Okay now I've had a look at two sources of information for you. One of them is the British Medical Association [BMA] their new guide to medicine and drugs.

> FP: Eh ha.
>
> HA: Now under the alcohol chapter it does suggest that you should avoid it really it said taking with this medication may cause flushing, nausea, vomiting, abdominal pain or headache and I also checked it on the British National Formulary [BNF], which is a drug interaction checker.
>
> FP: Yeah.
>
> HA: And they also said that you'd get a reaction there as well eh so you need to have to be aware if you were to drink then it's probable.
>
> FP: Right.
>
> HA: They'll react badly together and sort of give you those symptoms.
>
> FP: Right.
>
> HA: And it doesn't really say if there is a safe limit, it's just to avoid altogether really.

In this sequence, we can see the sources of authority combined to provide a synergistic prohibition. The individual contributions from the various sources of authority are themselves modalized by the terms used to describe their claims. The BMA guide 'suggests', whereas the BNF says it is 'probable' – both terms are usually used to mitigate the strength of a claim – yet the overall cumulative weight of the recommendations is to 'avoid it altogether'. Indeed, a third source of authority is added later in the interaction:

> HA: You know you could always check with another pharmacist . . .

But the degree of closure imposed by 'altogether' implies that the result of further enquiries would yield the same answer and that they would be redundant. These sorts of events, where authority for a course of action is demonstrated yet only modestly owned by the speaker, are a kind of 'displaced didacticism' or instruction.

Summing up: describing medical encounters

Thus, in this case, a description of what goes on, in terms of the turns taken in the conversation and the words spoken, can yield insights about what is happening socially in the health care encounter. That is, this sort of approach with its detailed attention to the structure and content of interaction tells us about social aspects of medicine in a non-reductive manner and allows the kinds of account of the territory that add something new, in the manner encouraged by Becker, which we mentioned earlier. These descriptions, even after a careful and detailed process of transcription, are only partial. Perhaps, rather like when photography replaced artists' impressions and stenographic accounts of heath care phenomena in the nineteenth century, we might soon see more digital recordings of interaction in electronic presentations. Once more, we are on the cusp of a revolution in description.

Describing as resistance: the degradation ceremony

How we describe things has important medical, political and social consequences too. Earlier, we described Goffman's and Becker's technique of deliberately describing morally suspect behaviour and activities in terms that were non-judgemental, so as to yield new insights about them. Thus, although the moral tone is deliberately deadpan and understated, this can be most effective in highlighting problematic aspects of a practice and leading to reform. Another technique that can highlight new aspects of the phenomena it seeks to describe involves dealing with an apparently innocent procedure as if it were morally outrageous. That is, the sorts of rituals that Goffman identified as being part of the introduction of new members to some institutions could be described in very different terms. Around the same time that Goffman was writing, his contemporary, Harold Garfinkel, was developing his idea of a 'degradation ceremony'. Garfinkel (1956) delineated the ideal typical 'degradation ceremony', which was calculated to publicly degrade the target of the ceremony. This formulation involves seeing degradation as the lowering of a subjectively important attribute such as honour or status. The *Oxford English Dictionary* defines degradation as 'lowering in honour, estimation, social position, etc.'. Garfinkel used degradation to refer to ceremonies which aimed at 'the destruction of one social object and the constitution of another . . . The other person becomes in the eyes of his condemners literally a different and *new* person' (p. 421). Goffman's (1963) later work, *Stigma*, also focuses on perceptions of status (pp. 4–5). This might well be obvious in the case of ceremonies to expel a person from the military or to impose a sentence on a defendant in a legal case. However, as Murray (2000) points out, some procedures which are ostensibly for the efficient running of an institution or for law enforcement can be seen as a kind of degradation too. Strip searches, for example,

> call up a cultural prohibition against public nakedness that goes back to the book of *Genesis*; drug testing challenges traditions that urination is a private affair; and finger-imaging conjures up an image of criminality. In these situations, some of the targets are likely to interpret the procedure as an assault on their dignity.
>
> (Murray 2000, p. 40)

As Murray goes on to suggest, one could say, for example, that a psychiatrist's diagnosis of schizophrenia is degrading even if the patient concurs with the psychiatrist's assurances that the label should not be seen as degrading. This situation recollects the Gramscian issue of hegemony, in that Gramsci saw ruling class ideology as so deeply internalized that the subordinates accept the claim of superordinates that the rituals are not degrading. This approach lets one speak of 'latent degradation', which is a useful concept, as illustrated by Spradley's (1970) analysis of how 'making the bucket' (being arrested for public intoxication) was cited by skid row alcoholics as the experience that convinced them that they were 'bums'. This particular labelling effect may be unintentional on the part of the police officers involved, but is perhaps part of a grander social process of marginalizing disadvantaged groups. The police may routinely or even casually pick up drunks, yet the meaning of this for the arrestees and for society as a whole may be to degrade the person concerned. Thus Garfinkel's and Spradley's work shows us the new meanings which can be achieved when we look at the small-scale actions through the lens of larger social processes.

This formulation of degradation rituals that we have considered so far has been fruitful, but there are also more subtle and also effective degradation ceremonies. Murray (2000) coins the term 'deniable degradation'. Here, the ceremony's official purpose is bureaucratic or instrumental; however, the latent symbolic message may be degrading. Officials can deny there is any degrading or labelling while still achieving degradation in practice. Murray uses the example of an electronic fingerprinting technique, which has been used on US welfare recipients ostensibly in an attempt to prevent them making multiple claims. Officials tended to deny the potential degradation contained in the procedures. As Murray quotes from a TV programme broadcast at the time:

> Interviewer: Of course, some of the critics of finger-imaging say that a lot of the refusal to go through it is just because, well these people may very well be entitled to benefits but they don't want to be put through what seems it's a central booking experience.

> Official: Well, of course, Bob, they come up with all these weak-kneed excuses, but the people who really need public assistance put their finger on [the] laser. It takes a second and a half to do it. It's not like getting your flu shot where you get a little after pain, and so, that's all nonsense. Those are stupid comments.
>
> (Murray 2000, p. 47)

Thus, taken at face value, these statements indicate that digital finger-imaging is not degrading for welfare recipients. It is a purely instrumental policy, designed to weed out fraudulent claims. However, the resistance to this procedure seemed to coalesce about a number of different themes, for example the way it seems to identify poverty and welfare dependency as deviance, fraud as deviance and fingerprinting as a kind of criminalization. It is, however, deniable degradation because the officials responsible for the policy are able to claim it is simply an efficient way of identifying people.

In terms of how we describe the features of social life, then, this example highlights how frames of reference can shift. To what extent is it possible to see some of the procedures of health care being degradation ceremonies. For example, is questioning people about their recreational drug habits a subtle kind of degradation, even though this information might be medically desirable. Likewise, the persistence of procedures such as episiotomy – which, as we have seen in the previous chapter, might have more to do with their popularity among the health care professions – might be considered as a degradation ceremony. These are two kinds of procedures that clients might resent and feel are invasive, yet the health care professionals concerned would probably not see them as problematic and certainly not as degrading to clients. To describe something as a degradation ceremony, then, does not necessarily make any strong assumptions about the nature of the participants' subjective feelings. As Foucault says about analysis of social action:

> [I]t should refrain from posing the labyrinthine and unanswerable question: 'Who then has the power and what has he in mind? What is the aim of someone who possesses power?' . . . Let us not, therefore, ask why certain people want to

dominate, what they seek, what is their overall strategy. Let us ask, instead, how things work at the level of on-going discourse.

(Foucault 1980, p. 97)

That is, in health care contexts, in describing things, we should not necessarily accept the subjective self-report statements about the phenomena in question. As we have seen from Becker's insights above, that is merely to reproduce the wisdom of the locals. To make sense of things, we have to describe them in new ways that expose the moral and epistemological baggage of the descriptions that are already in place.

Therefore, by way of conclusion for this chapter, let us return to one of the ideas with which we started, the way that descriptions are things for doing social business as well as – or perhaps instead of – being reflections of what happens outside. In that sense, we have hoped to call into question the commonly held modernist notion put forward by Bishop Butler that 'everything is what it is and not another thing'. Instead, it is hoped that the reader will be inspired to look closely at the things that purport to be descriptions, facts or objective knowledge in the health care disciplines and begin to be able to see descriptions as things that are pre-eminently human creations. Like Potter (1996), it is difficult to see factual descriptions as separable from the rhetorical processes that make us social beings. The descriptions of events or objects might be in social play to resolve legal proceedings, scientific debates, health care dilemmas or domestic arguments. However, we would be well advised to ask how the 'facts' were created as descriptions and how they are used. Potter (1996) draws our attention to the way that descriptions used in academic disciplines are often expressive of a particular rhetorical practice of 'working up representations to portray "out-thereness"'. The objects described are presented to the reader or viewer as if they had no connection to the authors writing about them. The bare bones of description, no matter how morally and politically denatured, often have something to do with the authors' interests. The authors' choice of these phenomena of study and the probability that they would be willing to accept Nobel prizes for writing about these facts, all conspire to haunt their descriptions. In Potter's view, descriptions and factual accounts should be understood as influential ways of producing forms of knowing that meet the rhetorical standards of the communities of speakers in which they will be shared.

References

Agar, M. (1986) *Speaking of Ethnography.* Qualitative Research Methods Series No. 2. London: Sage.

Atkinson, P. (1992) *Understanding Ethnographic Texts.* Qualitative Research Methods Series No. 25. London: Sage.

Bakhtin, M.M. (1984) *Problems of Dostoevsky's Poetics.* Manchester: Manchester University Press.

Barnes, J. (1984) *Flaubert's Parrot.* London: Cape.

Becker, H.S. (1957) *The Boys in White.* New York: Transaction Books.

Becker, H.S. (1993) How I learned what a crock was, *Journal of Contemporary Ethnography,* 22(1): 28–35.

Becker, H.S. (1996) The epistemology of qualitative research, in R. Jessor, A. Colby and

R. Schweder (eds) *Ethnography and Human Development*. Chicago, IL: University of Chicago Press.

Becker, H.S. (2001) La politique de la representations: Erving Goffman et les institutions totales, in C. Amourous and A. Blanc (eds) *Erving Goffman et les institutions totales*. Paris: L'Harmatton.

Becker, H.S., Geer, B., Hughes, E.C. and Strauss, A.L. (1961) *Boys in White: Student Culture in Medical School*. Chicago, IL: University of Chicago Press.

Blackless, M., Charuvastra, A., Derryck, A. *et al.* (2000) How sexually dimorphic are we? Review and synthesis, *American Journal of Human Biology*, 12: 151–66.

Boden, D. and Zimmerman, D.H. (1991) *Talk and Social Structure: Studies in Ethnomethodology and Conversation Analysis*. Cambridge: Polity Press.

Butler, J. (1990) *Gender Trouble*. London: Routledge.

Connell, J. and Lowe, A. (2001) Generating grounded theory from qualitative data: the application of inductive methods in tourism and hospitality, *International Journal of Tourism Research*, 3(2): 165–8.

Conway, M.A. (1990) *Autobiographical Memory: An Introduction*. Milton Keynes: Open University Press.

Cooter, R. (1984) *The Cultural Meaning of Popular Science: Phrenology and the Organising of Consent in Nineteenth Century Britain*. Cambridge: Cambridge University Press.

de Man, P. (1984) Autobiography as de-facement, in *The Rhetoric of Romanticism*. New York: Columbia University Press.

Deves, E. and Robinson, K.M. (2002) The making of a grounded theory: after death communication, *Death Studies*, 26(3): 241–53.

Drew, P., Chatwin, J. and Collins, S. (2001) Conversation analysis: a method for research into interactions between patients and health care professionals, *Health Expectations*, 4: 58–70.

Edwards, D. and Potter, J. (1992) *Discursive Psychology*. London: Sage.

Elbaz, R. (1988) *The Changing Nature of Self: A Critical Study of the Autobiographical Discourse*. London: Croom Helm.

Foss, A. and Trick, K. (1989) *St. Andrews Hospital Northampton: The First 150 Years*. Cambridge: Cambridge University Press.

Foucault, M. (1980) *Power/Knowledge: Selected Interviews and Other Writings*, New York: Pantheon.

Garfinkel, H. (1956) Conditions of successful degradation ceremonies, *American Journal of Sociology*, 61: 420–4.

Geertz, C. (1973) *The Interpretation of Cultures*. New York: Basic Books.

Gilman, S.L. (1982) *Seeing the Insane: A Cultural History of Madness and Art in the Western World*. New York: Wiley.

Goffman, E. (1961) *Asylums*. New York: Anchor.

Goffman, E. (1963) *Stigma*. Englewood Cliffs, NJ: Prentice-Hall.

Hall, J. and Stevens, E. (1991) Rigor in feminist research, *Advances in Nursing Science*, 13: 16–29.

Hammersley, M. and Atkinson, P. (1983) *Ethnography: Principles in Practice*. London: Tavistock.

Heritage, J. and Stivers, T. (1999) Online commentary in acute medical visits: a method of shaping patient expectations, *Social Science and Medicine*, 49: 1501–17.

Humberstone, V. (2002) The experiences of people with schizophrenia living in supported accommodation: a qualitative study using grounded theory methodology, *Australian and New Zealand Journal of Psychiatry*, 36(3): 367–73.

Leininger, M. (1994) Evaluation criteria and critique of qualitative research studies, in J.M. Morse (ed.) *Critical Issues in Qualitative Research Methods*. Thousand Oaks, CA: Sage.

Lombroso, C. (1892) *Les applications d'anthropologie criminelle*. Paris: Author.

Lopez, D.S. (1995) *Religions of India in Practice*. Princeton, NJ: Princeton University Press.

Maynard, D. (1991) The perspective display series and the delivery of diagnostic news, in D. Boden and D.H. Zimmerman (eds) *Talk and Social Structure*. Cambridge: Polity Press.

Maynard, D. (1994) Methods, practice and epistemology: the debate about feminism and research, in M. Maynard and J. Purvis (eds) *Researching Women's Lives from a Feminist Perspective*. London: Taylor & Francis.

Mendez, C., Coddu, F. and Maturana, H. (1988) The bringing forth of pathology, *Irish Journal of Psychology*, 9: 144–72.

Middleton, D. and Edwards, D. (1990) *Collective Remembering*. London: Sage.

Minto, C.L., Liao, L.M., Woodhouse, C.R.J., Ransley, P.G. and Creighton, S.M. (2003) The effect of clitoral surgery on sexual outcome in individuals who have intersex conditions with ambiguous genitalia: a cross sectional study, *Lancet*, 351(9365): 1252–7.

Murray, H. (2000) Deniable degradation: the finger imaging of welfare recipients, *Sociological Forum*, 15(1): 39–63.

Muybridge, E. (1883) The attitudes of animals in motion, illustrated with the zoopraxiscope, *Proceedings of the Royal Institution of Great Britain*, X(1): No. 75.

Northway, R. (2000) Disability, nursing research and the importance of reflexivity, *Journal of Advanced Nursing*, 32(2): 391–7.

Olney, J. (1980) Autobiography and the cultural movement: a thematic, historical and bibliographical introduction, in *Autobiography: Essays Theoretical and Critical*. Princeton, NJ: Princeton University Press.

Pfol, S. and Gordon, A. (1986) Criminological displacements, *Social Problems*, 33(6): S94–S113.

Potter, J. (1996) *Representing Reality*. London: Sage.

Psathas, G. (1995) *Conversation Analysis: The Study of Talk in Interaction*. London: Sage.

Raine, A. (1993) *The Psychopathology of Crime: Criminal Behaviour as a Clinical Disorder*. San Diego, CA: University of California Press.

Ryle, G. (1990) *Collected Papers, Vol. 1: Critical Essays*. Bristol: Thoemmes.

Schratz, M. and Walker, R. (1995) *Research on Social Change: New Opportunities for Qualitative Research*. London: Routledge.

Schutz, A. (1962) *The Problem of Social Reality*. The Hague: Martinus Nijhoff.

Showalter, E. (1987) *The Female Malady*. London: Virago.

Sontag, S. (ed.) (1982) *A Barthes Reader*. London: Jonathan Cape.

Spradley, J.P. (1970) *You Owe Yourself a Drunk: An Ethnography of Urban Nomads*. Boston, MA: Little, Brown & Co.

Thody, P. (1977) *Roland Barthes: A Conservative Estimate*. London: Macmillan.

Todorov, T. (1973) *The Fantastic: A Structural Approach and a Literary Genre* (translated by Richard Howard). Cleveland: Press of the Case Western Reserve University.

Waterman, H. (1998) Embracing ambiguities and valuing ourselves: issues of validity in action research, *Journal of Advanced Nursing*, 28: 101–5.

9

The post-modernist challenge

In this chapter, we shall sum up and extend some of the issues that have been raised in earlier chapters regarding the scepticism that has been expressed about either nature or the possibility of knowing it. The assumptions of positivistic and realist science have been challenged most strongly over the past three decades by postmodernism, which has problematized the assumption in both qualitative and quantitative work that we are discovering a reality which is 'out there'. Researchers of a postmodern bent seldom agree with the conventional wisdom in the field they are studying and see the techniques and beliefs of the scientist to be just as much social science data as the patients and their so-called diseases. The sense of reality, according to this perspective, is itself a human construction and we must look to language to see how human beings construct their realities.

The field of postmodernism is large and unruly and contains texts of the utmost difficulty by founding fathers such as Derrida (1977), Lyotard (1984) and Deleuze and Guattari (1984), to name but a few of the usual suspects. On the other hand, it is possible to find material in the health care and social sciences that adopts a self-consciously postmodernist stance which is much more user-friendly.

The postmodernist assault on the health and social sciences proceeds on a number of interrelated levels. There are some who are trying to conduct research that embodies postmodernist principles – this often takes the form of qualitative investigations emphasizing language, experience and social processes. On the other hand, there are others who wrestle with the founding texts of the field and attempt to critique, revise and extend the thinking itself.

The styles of thinking, writing and research that have been popularized under the banner of postmodernism have been controversial. Critical social scientists, especially those adopting a Marxist or realist approach, have been concerned that an emphasis on postmodernism has deflected attention away from material conditions of life and inequalities. Equally, others with a more conventionally scientific cast of mind have been concerned that what they see to be the progress towards scientific mastery of the universe is being undermined and the intellectual waters are being muddied.

To give an idea of this in more practical terms, consider the case of James Randi, a conjurer by trade, who has made a name for himself as a polemical sceptic. He challenges claims by anyone who purports to have discovered paranormal phenomena and endeavours to show that these events can best be explained in terms of conventional science or by trickery. Claims such as that by Jaques Benveniste to have discovered 'water with memory', which could form the basis of homeopathic medicine, are gleefully debunked in such a way, by reference to methodological flaws and credulous interpretations (Randi 1992). Randi, then, can be seen as the voice of enlightenment science. He has famously offered a prize of $1 million to anyone who can convincingly demonstrate any of the strange phenomena he investigates. Whereas it makes good polemical television, in a sense this doesn't tell us very much over and above a school science education. Yet despite such scepticism, strongly and colourfully expressed, there does not seem to be any abatement in the popularity of alternative therapies, spiritual belief systems and the desire for communion with supernatural phenomena. So where does this leave us in the quest for understanding the state of society or the state of health care?

It is a common misinterpretation of the postmodernist position that it is somehow soft on sloppy thinking. That it validates the epistemology of the charlatan and undermines the integrity of the scientist. It is claimed that if social constructionism were true, then we would have flying carpet passenger services as well as commercial airlines (Atkins 2003). This is a rather facile point. What we are able to do with the benefit of postmodern means of thinking is appreciate that there are a variety of ways in which events may be interpreted. The Wright brothers flew without any formal theory of aerodynamics as we would recognize it today. Further back in time the Mongolfier brothers flew, clad in elaborate wigs and frock coats and intoxicated on red wine so as to better survive the sudden landings. If they had a theory of gases, it was probably not one which we would recognize today. It would most likely be based on long forgotten ideas about phlogiston rather than modern kinetic models of air as a mixture of molecules of nitrogen, oxygen and carbon dioxide. In the same way, attempting to demonstrate that people who see auras cannot read them accurately under scientifically rigorous, blind conditions can only tell us so much. The process of seeing auras, for example, was never designed to work in such laboratory conditions and even though we might show its apparent failure fairly readily, again this tells us little. What we need to understand is what this all means to the practitioners and how they construe the world so as to get social business done. It is this feature that makes postmodern variants of social science useful for making sense of health care. In a sense, it urges us to bracket our presuppositions and explore the social world in the participants' own terms. To follow the example above, we need to know what people think they're doing when they see, 'read' or communicate about one another's auras. Moreover, like any good system of knowledge, they will very likely have technologies for controlling and cultivating the texture and colour of a person's aura, as well as a set of theories linking it to other aspects of well-being. Whether we agree with these or not, they are important aspects of that particular belief system.

In this sense, a postmodern social or health scientist is doing the same sort of work as a phenomenologist. Indeed, it is possible to go even further back to the earlier work of thinkers like Piaget who famously developed a typology of children's ways of thinking at different stages in childhood. The trouble with conventional measures of children's thinking like intelligence tests he felt was that they do not tell us much about how children succeed in getting to the wrong answer. Child reasoning in his view was not simply a less accurate version of the adult variety, it was qualitatively different.

In this way, the postmodern challenge in health care research is to take some of the implications of this sort of approach a bit further. We might also see echoes of the 'strong programme's' symmetry thesis in the social study of science. Whether beliefs are true or false is a matter for the seekers after knowledge themselves. To the researcher they are all equally interesting. To the postmodernist researcher, moreover, every aspect of what can be seen, heard, touched or smelt in a health care setting is important. The ceremonies of giving and receiving care, the 'liturgy of the clinic', is just as important as the members' pharmacological theories about what the medications do.

Postmodernism has foregrounded the way that knowledge may be intimately related to power structures and that mainstream knowledge marginalizes the viewpoints of disempowered social groups. In the variants of postmodern thinking that take their cue from Michel Foucault, knowledge is seen in terms of historical processes and the exercise of power. The development of psychiatry as a medical speciality has not happened because maladies of the mind are somehow naturally part of the purview of medicine, in this view. It has happened as a result of a long process of historical struggle as doctors sought to expand their territory. The same could be said for the medicalization of sex. It is not naturally or inherently medical but a series of historical, political and scientific manoeuvres over the past 300 or 400 years have made it so. Much postmodernist thinking, then, has drawn upon – but is not coterminous with – earlier critiques of heath care provision from feminist, Marxist and anti-racist scholars, yet in its attempt to be inclusive, some would argue it has lost the political edge of these earlier positions and fails in its account of material inequality. The regress into phenomenologically based considerations of people's thinking, experience and local social orders has made it difficult to think clearly about oppression and inequality. However, postmodernism also opens up the possibility of thinking about the operation of power in new ways. Let us try to illustrate what we mean. One way of thinking about this is by analogy with gardening. Put crudely, the conceptions of power in much historical materialist critical thinking sees the exercise of power as being a bit like weed-killer. It oppresses, distorts, denies our potential and reduces us as human beings. Within postmodern conceptions of power, it is much more like topiary, in that it encourages social institutions and people to grow in particular ways. In this vein, maybe, as Parker et al. (1995) note, the crucial feature of health care systems is not whether they 'cure' people, but whether they are successful in attaching pathological identities to vulnerable people. Thus developing an identity as a 'schizophrenic' or 'substance abuser' may not result in a 'cure' – quite the contrary – but it provides an identity for the person so named and an explanation as to why the attempted interventions fail. As Rose (1990) has documented, the flourishing of psychology and psychiatry over the past century and a half have given us new ways to think about ourselves and one another.

Another way of thinking about knowledge from a postmodern perspective that we have found useful with students is to think of it like railways. The rise of science, like the contemporaneous rise of rail transport, allowed the exploration and exploitation of new territories and resources. Both railways and science have facilitated universal standards of business, timekeeping and social practice. Yet both also transform the territory they are built through, allowing new patterns of exploitation, living arrangements and human geographies. Postmodernism provides some clues as to how we might think about the relationship between knowledge and the societies which produce it and within which it has meaning.

From our point of view, the postmodernist movement, if it can be called such, has implications for how we think about research in health care. That is, it calls into question the assumption that science is progressive and that knowledge flourishes with the growth of research. It also foregrounds the possibility that research which works and produces clinically useful knowledge in one place will not do so in others. The most far-reaching implication of postmodernism for the philosophy of science and the conduct of enquiry is its radical anti-foundationalism. That is, reality is not something which is 'out there' in any simple sense. In terms of its implications for research, consider, for example, ethnomethodology and conversation analysis. These approaches invite us to consider whether and how people build physical and social realities in their conversations and social interaction patterns. They are concerned with the method that ordinary people ('ethnos') use to navigate their way through social life. In other words, like postmodernism, these approaches adhere to an anti-foundationalist approach and take seriously the strategies people use to convince others of the truth of their 'reality'. As Schegloff (1997) urges, the Archimedian point of leverage should be sought in the interaction itself. In deciding what is relevant or what is happening, the analyst should, in Schegloff's view, look at the people to whom it matters most – the interactants themselves. If you think you see inequalities at work in a setting, look to see whether the participants themselves are talking about inequalities or showing clear signs of dominance or deference. From this point of view, if one were to look at people in health settings, one might wish to consider how interactants work together to construct notions of health, illness and disability and apply them to the particular case in question. For example, in the previous chapter, Maynard's (1991) studies of the process of giving and receiving diagnostic news have shown how the reality of a patient's problems results from a complex dance whereby the patient's, professionals' and relatives' views are brought into alignment. Thus, practitioners and clients are very much practical philosophers as they go about their health care tasks of being ill and providing treatment. This offers the possibility that different interactional dances could yield very different accounts of clients and their problems and is a potentially challenging and destabilizing perspective within health care. Rather than just being an academic exercise, it might be possible for this approach to be used to help practitioners imagine how their own realities are constrained by the terminology they use and the interactions they participate in.

One implication of taking postmodern ideas seriously in health care research is to recognize the sheer diversity of views, beliefs and practices that health care encompasses. The interactions that practitioners, clients and researchers participate in may involve very different perspectives and world-views on the part of the various members (Green and Britten 1998). Qualitative studies performed under the umbrella of postmodernism often take the interaction itself as a focus of research. This marks them as distinct from research in a more positivistic mould, which often pre-defines what the factors under study will be. This focus on interaction highlights the diversity of viewpoints in clinical encounters. Katon and Kleinman (1981) viewed consultations between doctors and patients as the synthesis of conflicting explanatory systems about health and illness. This potential conflict required careful negotiation to achieve a satisfactory outcome. The clinical consultation may be a meeting between very different views of reality (Mishler 1984). Qualitative researchers, often working from within a postmodern – or at least a relativistic – perspective, have shown the importance of taking these competing perspectives and explanatory systems at face value. Green and Britten (1998) give the example of studies of asthma sufferers in the context of their adherence to recommended medication regimes. Although the official medical 'reality' is that asthma medication reduces morbidity and mortality, and can benefit users, qualitative studies disclose a very different 'reality' for patients themselves. First, some patients have negative views about the medications, believing them to be 'unnatural' substances that diminish the body's own ability to fight disease and cause dependency (Britten 1994). Doctors, on the other hand, make the common-sensical assumption that patients consult them because they are seeking medication (Hull and Marshall 1987). This is borne out in studies of patients with asthma by Osman *et al.* (1993), which show that patients worry about becoming physically and psychologically dependent on bronchodilators, and worry about the long-term effects of inhaling corticosteroids (Hewett 1994). Now from a medical point of view one might wish to dismiss these concerns or reassure patients. However, as Green and Britten (1998) note, regarding patients' realities as ignorant or misguided and attempting to persuade them of the value of a biomedical approach have limited value in increasing adherence. Green and Britten urge the need to recognize and incorporate patients' perspectives to ensure a better treatment outcome experience. One might even go further and ask how it is that patients and professionals decide whether a particular outcome is desirable, or whether an experience is an outcome or merely coincidental. In a sense, the very terms themselves are up for grabs.

Within philosophy itself, the interest in postmodernism goes back a little earlier than its sudden arrival in the health care disciplines. Some of the first flurry of interest can be traced to the publication in English of the works of Jaques Derrida (e.g. 1977). He pursued the fascination with language even further. His contention was that words, sentences and language itself have no fixed meaning and the relationship between language and the world is indeterminate. The slogan 'there is nothing outside the text' is attributed to him. He has also pointed to the internal contradictions in texts themselves, and the inadequacy of what he calls 'logocentrism', the idea that words express things in the mind, or describe things in nature. His view that language cannot express ideas and concepts in the mind is closely bound up with his critique of phenomenology, inasmuch as language cannot express consciousness in any simple sense. This suggestion that language is somehow all we have is also found in the work of the psychoanalyst Jaques Lacan (1977), who contended that our psychic contents, especially our unconscious, are structured in and through language. In particular, it is not a language which transparently reflects either reality or our thoughts, for it is subject to a whole variety of processes of condensation and displacement as theorized by Freud, as well as being highly metaphoric and metonymic and imbued with patriarchal ideology. In a sense, then, consciousness, and indeed the self, are kinds of allegorical stories. Or possibly they are multiple, allegorical stories.

The possibility that there are multiple stories about nature, rather than a single reliable epistemology, has, as we have seen, been a central plank in postmodern theory. For example, Lyotard (1984) has contended that the twentieth century saw the collapse of what he calls 'grand narratives', the hopeful stories that we are making progress, proceeding towards enlightenment, or towards the betterment of the human condition. This was the story behind positivism, but also Marxism, psychoanalysis and most of the nineteenth-century schemes for the improvement of our circumstances. Instead, Lyotard argues that we have a multiplicity of competing language-games and it is impossible to judge any one of these in terms of any other. It is therefore not possible, in this view, to perform critique, to enlighten or to achieve rational consensus. This story is reminiscent of the Tower of Babel, such that the grand projects to improve the lot of humanity have disintegrated into competing interest groups spouting incommensurable languages.

Postmodernism, then, represents a far-reaching paradigm shift in which 'reality has been replaced with simulation, rationality by multivocality, monolithic organization by fragmentation, and grand theories by plans' (Spitzer 1998, p. 164). Post-modernism is associated with a scepticism bordering on incredulity towards the so-called grand narratives and an abandonment of the search for a stable reality on which to anchor our claims to knowledge. Instead, in this view, the world is constituted by 'differance' (Derrida 1978; Lyotard 1984; Sarup 1988; Boyne 1992; Fox 1993; Gurevitz 1997; Spitzer 1998).

The suggestion that knowledge is a form of power and that regimes of truth are made to work through a range of coercive practices has also been rediscovered, from Bacon and Nietzsche, and has been expressed most strongly in the work of Michel Foucault (e.g. 1965). Foucault was interested in how knowledge itself was not a neutral servant of humanity but tended to constitute the 'subject' – the individual – in particular ways. The 'knowledge' of nymphomania and masturbatory insanity helps to constitute the individuals who allegedly suffer from what we now admit to be highly questionable, if not humorous maladies. One could perhaps say the same in our own time about the knowledge of 'sex addiction' or 'co-dependency'. The idea that we have access only to representations, through language or imagery, and never the 'real thing' is elaborated in some detail by Baudrillard (1990). He would appreciate the irony that the term 'real thing' has been hijacked as a Coca-Cola advertising slogan. He argued that the 1991 Gulf War 'never happened' because it took place largely on television (Baudrillard 1995). All we have access to is endless simulation, a hyperreal world where simulations become more lifelike and vibrant than the lacklustre realities they have left behind. Father Christmas was usually depicted in grey clothing until 1931 when he appeared in a red and white outfit as part of a winter advertising campaign run by Coca-Cola. The advertising-enhanced version soon outstripped the older incarnation. The hyperreal supervenes over the real. In health, the currently fashionable drive to 'detox' the body has very little to do with sober scientific research on the optimum concentration of certain chemicals in the tissues, and there is often neither funding nor personnel to conduct such research anyway. The momentum of the cultural phenomenon is to do with whether it sounds like it could be scientific. The analysis of these phenomena is more readily accomplished if we look not so much at the biochemistry or earnest scientific 'protocol statements' about nature, but grasp the hyperreal surface directly.

Language, simulation and representation have always been central to the theory and practice of a good deal of health care, much of which is transacted through language: in day-to-day verbal and written communications involving staff, patients and relatives; in counselling; in patient records and care planning. Recently, the demand for health care practitioners to communicate effectively both in speech and writing has become more urgent. Health care practice must now satisfy a wide audience of clients, purchasers, professional bodies and the law. However, while there has been a good deal of research on doctor–patient interaction, scholars have only recently begun to focus on language in nursing, occupational therapy, physiotherapy and other professions allied to medicine. Work on clinical encounters has only occasionally focused on pharmacists, audiologists, speech therapists or dentists. Because this fundamental concern has not been sufficiently emphasized, language has been used frequently by health care professionals themselves as if it were somehow a transparent means of communicating. This naivety has been revealed in a lack of awareness of the way in which words impact upon care and has left practitioners sometimes ill-equipped to deal with challenges to define exactly what they mean by the language they use.

For anyone to define what exactly they mean by the language they use is, of course, no easy matter. A huge academic industry has grown up around the question of language, trying to establish what language does, how it can achieve meaning, whether it mirrors or creates reality, to what extent human beings and their cultures are constructed by language, how powerful it is, how ideological it is. Disciplines as diverse as philosophy, linguistics and anthropology, literary criticism, psychology and sociology, have tackled the problem of language and meaning.

An increased scepticism about accepted values and a greater willingness to question what has gone before has also characterized the spirit of postmodernism, which can be seen in almost every aspect of life. Although great emphasis is placed on the importance of evidence-based heath care and reflective practice, these very notions are problematic. Ideas about what constitutes evidence and practice itself may be controversial. There is a multitude of ways in which nursing activities may be understood, described, justified or disseminated. Often, a variety of ideas will be in competition with each other and not result in any clear-cut pathways for care.

This kind of problem surrounds a general debate about the nature of meaning and language which is at the core of the whole discourse or condition of postmodernism. To recapitulate, postmodernism, like the ideas and philosophies it seeks to describe, is difficult to define. In part, it is to do with increasing scepticism of about the ability of 'grand narratives' to explain and improve the human condition. In health care, there is a growing feeling that much of what is done in the name of treatment may be ineffective, expensive and sometimes harmful. The grand narratives that accounted for human life have been eroded to the point that we are no longer sure about what it means to be human and how to live our lives. This is liberating for some while threatening to others. Postmodernism, then, broadly concerns the rootlessness of late twentieth-century life, the fragmentation of institutions and the wild pro-liferation of the media.

In the UK, it could be argued that what has happened to the health service with its fragmentation into purchasers, providers and fund-holders and the loss of a coherent institutional framework is a prime example of a postmodernist world. More generally, we now live in a world of hyper-communication; information technology churns out vast amounts of texts and images so that stable meanings are difficult to detect. Paradox and uncertainty rule.

Within the postmodernist world-view, emphasis is placed on discourse or 'language in use' as the substance of social life. Reality becomes something that is constructed by language. Thinkers such as Jaques Derrida have cast considerable doubt over the possibility of a resolution to the issues around meaning and language. Although postmodernism prioritizes language as a major feature of social life, its insistence that meanings are only local, provisional and controversial and that our methods of enquiry are value-laden mean that it is difficult to make any definite statements about the world.

Postmodernism itself has resisted definition: whether postmodernism represents a sharp break from modernity or simply a late stage in that historical development has been debated. In a sense, the question 'what is postmodernism?' is a profoundly modernist question. It may well not be possible to answer it from within postmodernism itself. Debates have focused on three overlapping terrains: the *experience* of contemporary reality (subjectivity and identity); the *representation* of the contemporary (in the arts, architecture, the media, advertising and consumer goods); and the *analysis* of the contemporary (the state of knowledge in postmodern society) (Scannell *et al.* 1992, p. 2). Yet even amid this uncertainty, there are some features that cut across most postmodernist claims: 'Postmodernism mistrusts all modernist claims to ground an understanding of the contemporary social world in scientific rationality' (Scannell *et al.* 1992, p. 3). The relationship between modernism and postmodernism is often central to the definition of the latter. It is almost as if postmodernism is defined by what it lacks rather than what it contains:

> Modernism acknowledged the fragmentary, transient, dislocated character of the social world but tried to overcome it, to retrieve a lost unity, whereas postmodernism is content to accept and celebrate a de-centred political, economic and cultural global environment. It rejects deep structures, any notion of an underlying, determining reality. It accepts a world of appearances, a surface reality without depth.
>
> (Scannell *et al.* 1992, p. 3)

Thus, in health care, a modernist ambition might be to try to find out what the patient's real problem is and to do this by the use of stethoscopes, blood tests, CAT scans and diagnostic interviews. The idea is that however incoherent the patient's symptoms, there must be some unitary underlying pathology that can be discovered by the skilled clinician. From a postmodernist perspective, the patient's worry about who will feed her cat is as much a feature of the illness experience as the swelling, fracture or blood test results.

Postmodernism lends its weight, then, to a growing tradition of scepticism about health care. As Lewis (2000) reminds us, in the West medicine benefited from tremendous popular support in the first three-quarters of the twentieth century. But, increasingly, this support is evolving into a chorus of criticisms. Over the past quarter of a century, health care providers have been rebuked. Edmund Pellegrino, writing nearly a quarter of a century ago, criticized health care specialists for a long list of shortcomings, including: overspecialization; technicism; overprofessionalism; insensitivity to personal and sociocultural values; too narrow a construal of the doctor's role; too much 'curing' rather than 'caring'; not enough emphasis on prevention, patient participation and patient education; too much economic incentive; a 'trade school' mentality; overmedicalization of everyday life; inhumane treatment of medical students; overwork by house staff; and deficiencies in verbal and non-verbal communication (Pellegrino 1979). To this list identified by Pellegrino, Lewis (2000) adds the current debates and disaffections around the issues in health economics where critics have pointed to increasing costs yet profound inequalities in access.

In Lewis's view, the situation is even more acute in mental health care. In the USA, and to some extent in the UK, psychiatry suffers from all of these problems and more. Psychiatry is the only specialty which has a protest movement ('antipsychiatry', 'mad pride' and so on) organized against it. People who might once have been treated in clinics are now increasingly found struggling in prisons, shelters or in the streets. As Lewis puts it, 'Psychiatrists are having more and more of their procedures denied, psychiatric hospitals are closing, research money is dwindling (except for the problematic funds coming from pharmaceuticals), and fewer and fewer residents are pursuing psychiatry as a career choice' (Lewis 2000, p. 72). Yet, in spite of its clearly beleaguered status, psychiatry continues to organize its core knowledge structures with few significant changes aside from a drift towards an even greater reliance on neuroscience, biochemistry and genetics as sources of explanation for the disorders it tries to deal with.

If we take postmodernist thinking at face value, there are disturbing implications for the practice of health care (Clarke 1996). If it is impossible for researchers and practitioners to reach a satisfactory understanding of what they do, if reality is indeed indeterminate, how do they know that they're doing any good? How can researchers be sure that the data they have so painstakingly gathered will not become hopelessly outdated in a short time? There is, nonetheless, something to be salvaged from the postmodernist assault on convention. It can sensitize us to the fact that there may be conflicting opinions about illness, unexplored dimensions and different layers of reality. What doctors know is different from what nurses know and differs again from the patient's experience. Postmodernism allows us to grasp this diverse picture without feeling the need to establish 'the truth'.

In a sense, some health care disciplines were drifting in this direction long before the term postmodernism was in common currency. Nursing began to define itself as a discipline that was primarily concerned with interpersonal and communicative issues a full half century ago with Peplau's famous book (Peplau 1952). This interpersonal dimension has been underscored in the work of other nurse scholars. Virginia Henderson consolidated nursing's role as an interpersonal process when she wrote: 'The unique function of the nurse is to assist the individual, sick or well, in the performance of those activities contributing to health, or its recovery (or to a peaceful death) that he would perform unaided if he had the necessary strength or will' (Henderson 1966, p. 15).

Here, the modernist project, with its technically skilled individuals focusing their powers on the individual is clearly visible. Yet at the same time, the emphasis on interpersonal processes is also beginning to subvert the focus on the more archetypal modernist matters of science. This dilemma, between the modernist focus on the individual and the postmodern concern with specificity and local activities can be seen in the present day too. Dougan (1995) puts it thus: 'the philosophy of nursing in the 1990s is firmly rooted in recognising people as individuals with specific wants and needs' (p. 63). There are a number of different strands in this form of thinking. On the one hand, there are tendencies which are profoundly modernist – for example, the idea of wants and needs reinforces the Cartesian notion of the individual who is captain of his or her own ship and can thus be persuaded to take responsibility for his or her own health through social psychological techniques designed to manipulate their 'attitudes' or 'health beliefs'. On the other hand, the individuality and specificity of the process of nursing and the disarticulation of the process of nursing from enlightenment project science. As the structure of health care changes and health care delivery is reorganized, the postmodern condition may involve nurses in more holistic care for their clients and might involve a reorganization of care at a local level so as to empower clients (Lister 1997, p. 42). Indeed, nurses may be able to become even more client-focused in that spaces may be opened up for new approaches to care that have hitherto been marginalized, such as complementary therapies. On the other hand, the relative instability, constant reorganization and the break-up of nationally organized systems of care into competing organic units may force health care into a situation which emphasizes market forces at the expense of client care. The model of health care delivery appears to involve a larger number of small, organic organizations competing for trade. As Lister (1997) and Morgan (1986) note, this is curiously reminiscent of a kind of social Darwinism and an implicit endorsement of market forces. In this way, it seems to subscribe to the idea that competition is inevitable and that the capitalist system is a natural and implacable fact.

Such diversity in the forms of provision for health care and the diversity in meanings that can be assigned to language adds up to a 'strain' on the use of language. Health care practitioners need to be aware of this strain; the words they speak or write may convey meanings they did not anticipate or desire. While carers and researchers, like everyone else, can never guarantee the meanings of their spoken or written words, this diversity means that there is a vastly increased scope for misinterpretation and this requires a constant vigilance or self-surveillance when considering the meanings of one's own or other people's spoken and written texts. The strain on meaning in language, combined with the power of language to construct the world in which we live, makes it more important than ever for practitioners to monitor health care language as it affects the lives of others.

Postmodernism also tackles the style and substance of writing in the health sciences and attempts to reformulate it in a way that brings in a wider variety of issues than are conventionally included in academic writing. Here is Nicholas Fox, who produced a good deal of writing in the early 1990s based on his experiences as a participant observer in a hospital, describing what he was trying to do in his book *The Social Meaning of Surgery*:

> I was conscious of how visual were the events that I wished to record. Along with the smell – a sense often omitted from ethnography – the visual does not necessarily translate easily into a written record, and I have often imagined the kind of visual ethnography of surgery which I should like to produce – something between 'Your Life in Their Hands' and a piece of 'new journalism'. Certainly, both kinds of media are evocative, and I share Tyler's sentiment (1986) that ethnography should have evocation as its task.
>
> (Fox 1992, p. ix)

In a similar vein, here are Lather and Smithies talking about their work on AIDS:

> This is organized as layers of various kinds of information, shifts in register, turns of different faces toward the reader, in order to provide a glimpse of the vast and intricate network of the complexities of cultural information about AIDS in which we are all caught. Although this book is not so much planned confusion as it might at first appear, it is, at some level, about what we see as a breakdown of clear interpretation and confidence in the ability/warrant to tell such stories in uncomplicated, non-messy ways.
>
> (Lather and Smithies 1997, p. xvi)

These are both manifesto statements of researchers trying to explore the possibility of new styles of writing in health care scholarship. As Abma (2002) notes, a great many scholars in the qualitative and postmodern traditions have observed the shortcomings of conventional writing and have taken the risk of presenting their findings in non-traditional ways. A great many qualitative researchers are experimenting with hitherto unexplored forms of narrative representation for their work. For example, workers have explored literary forms that include poetry (Richardson 1993; Glesne 1997), (auto)biography (hooks 1990; Barone 1997; Denzin 1999; Ellis and Bocher 2000), *testimonio* (Beverley 2000), ethno-drama and fiction (Pfohl 1992) and theatre plays (Falk and Perron 1995). There are also examples of people promoting and exploring the use of non-literary forms, including photo essays (Lapidus 1996), video (Abma 1998), music (Kivnick 1996), theatre (Mienczakowski 1995) and dance performances (Blumenfeld-Jones 1995). As Abma (2002) notes, like Fox, these writings and performances aim to be evocative so as to draw the audience in. This perhaps will enable audience members to experience the topic from a variety of perspectives and to be 'touched at an emotional level' (Abma 2002, p. 6). The figurative styles of expression deployed by these authors can readily be distinguished from the more sober, narrowly descriptive, toneless language of conventional social science writing. Although the insistence on traditional research writing has been stronger in the health disciplines than in education and the humanities (Norris 1997, p. 90), qualitative health researchers have also been drawn to explore these new forms of representation to present their findings.

Language in action

Despite the pervading sense that meaning in language is problematical, many theorists have tried to arrive at plausible interpretations of what words can do and mean. The Speech Act Theory of Austin (1962), Searle (1969) and Grice (1975) has been useful in this regard – examining how actions are performed through speech. Recent developments in conversation analysis and discourse analysis show up some fundamental problems in medico-nursing knowledge. From a conversation-analytic perspective, speakers are not simply conversing about a world that is external to them, but are mutually constructing it. Discourse analysis draws attention to the way in which repertoires of health care language produce the sense that carers are talking about a world that is external to their patients.

In much analysis of the nature of language, there is a tendency for the written text to be considered more important than the spoken word. For example, in grammar, what we call the 'parts of speech' are usually based on the language as it is written. In health care situations, too, the fact that written records are permanent and that they are very important if legal issues arise or patients complain mean that they are often given a higher status than what has been said. The written language of health care can be analysed in reports, care plans and patients' notes and it is easy to see how verbal communications between doctors, nurses, students, social workers and other staff are informed by the linguistic structure of written records.

It is not, perhaps, immediately apparent that what practitioners say in spoken or written texts are also actions. But actions they are. When a health care professional, for example, orders a patient to stop doing something, the effect of the words may well be that the patient does indeed stop. Here the words 'Stop that!' can be seen to have a similar power to the act of physically stopping someone from doing something. Equally, the way that health professionals judge a person in written and spoken text may well act against the person in a very obvious way. Staff may communicate that a client is 'manipulative' and this negative tag then affects how that client feels about himself if it is said directly to him, or the way in which others respond to him if such a meaning is conveyed in spoken or written reports to others. Such negative communicative acts are far from the ideal of promoting well-being. Since health care staff perform a variety of speech acts in their daily work, it is clearly important to examine them critically.

Telling stories about distress – from modernism to postmodernism

Health professionals make sense of the world in which they work by drawing on the resources of meaning with which their culture and trainings provide them. This is not surprising, as the scientific story we learn about the practice of health care has a sense of coherence and optimism. Since the eighteenth century, sometimes known as the Age of Reason, the belief that the world will yield its secrets to scientific enquiry has been extremely popular in Europe and the United States (Hollinger 1994). This belief is associated with the view that rational, systematic means of acquiring knowledge are the best, and that knowledge should be based on scientifically derived facts.

The distinction between modernism and postmodernism can be seen at work here. Modernism is the perspective still taken by most textbooks of psychology, psychiatry and nursing, which carefully avoid what the authors consider to be myths, superstitions or metaphysics. Modernism is associated with what has been called an 'up the mountain' theory of science, which proclaims that we know far more now than we ever did in the past, and that practice and treatment are getting better as time goes on. The naivety and cruelty of medicine and nursing in the past are contrasted with the enlightened, humane and caring approach of the present day. The modernist point of view (e.g. Ritzer 1992) is often sustained by some grand narrative as to the nature of the material world, such as that human consciousness can ultimately be explained in terms of brain chemistry. Michel Foucault (1975) has argued that, from its inception, 'The science of man . . . was medically based' (p. 36). The education of health professionals is pervaded with such assumptions.

Allied to this outlook is the notion that individuals are the authors of their own ideas, speech or writing. From Descartes' assertion, 'I think; therefore, I am', to contemporary concern with individuals' thoughts, emotions and actions, the idea of authorship or responsibility has been essential to the sciences and humanities.

Postmodernism takes a very different stance. Postmodernists do not find the world to be ordered and coherent and consider grand narratives doomed to failure. Postmodernism is a loose collection of philosophies which emphasize difference rather than unity, fragmentation rather than integration, and the minority or unusual point of view rather than the majority or mainstream viewpoint. Postmodern thinkers are often concerned with language: 'Language is now necessarily the central consideration in all attempts to know, act and live' (Lemert 1990, p. 234). Lemert (1990) and Ritzer (1992) explain that scientific theories are texts – we usually encounter them in written form. Lyotard (1984) argues that 'Scientific knowledge is a form of discourse' (p. 3). And the empirical reality to which scientific theories apply is often textual as well. In nursing, care plans, patient records, the wider body of theory and research on which practice is based, all are texts. Almost every part of health care, certainly as it is performed by people directly involved with clients, is mediated through language. Clarke (1996) argues that a postmodernist perspective requires nurses to 'connect with the devolved needs/wants of patients, in respect of their autonomy and medication, and cease pursuing abstract, doctrinaire ideals' (p. 261).

In his book *The Precession of Simulacra*, Baudrillard suggests an underlying sense of melancholy inherent in postmodern experience that is the result of inhabiting a world of ambivalence. He writes of 'a liquidation of all referentials' (Baudrillard 1983, p. 4), the result of a proliferation of images that replace previous notions of truth with an ever-changing world of simulation (Clayton 2002). This melancholy is marked by the way we feel about the world: 'Our age is characterised by invisible latent threats working quietly in the air we breathe and the bodies we inhabit' (Mansfield 2000, pp. 169–70).

Postmodernism encourages a greater sensitivity to the local concerns of patients. For many years, nursing education was a matter of learning about hygiene and practising techniques and memorizing procedures, the grand narratives of biomedical models of health. More recently, nursing thinking has come to emphasize more strongly the caring role of nurses and the importance of nurses reflecting critically on their practice. This might be described as the beginnings of a postmodern conscious-ness among nurses.

The importance of texts in health care has been increasingly recognized as scholars strive to understand the nursing process. As Cheek and Rudge (1994) say, 'nursing and nursing practice can be considered to represent a reality which is text-ually mediated' (p. 15). The turn to texts in nursing scholarship is also associated with a scepticism of 'grand narratives' – Darbyshire (1994) warns us off sets of abstract principles in making sense of health care practice. The postmodern concern with minority points of view has led some to ask why conventional health care research ignores the 40 million Americans without health care (Allen 1995).

Postmodernism itself contains some interesting paradoxes too. On the one hand, it is associated with a tendency to overthrow stable notions of the self, with the notion of *cogito ergo sum* instead reminding us that selves are contrived, constructed and liable to be shattered as our circumstances change. On the other hand, the question of authorship is also central in postmodern scholarship because the author of a text is seen as crucial. A scientific paper, for example, cannot, in the postmodern view, be seen as a transparent window on reality, but will instead be seen as reflecting the interests and cultural location of the researchers and authors. There are a number of pieces of contemporary scholarship that attempt to look at the professional discourses of the helping professions in this way. The entities, concepts and findings that have been so painstakingly elicited from tragic clinical experiences and through meticulous observation and research are increasingly called into question. The questioning is not necessarily aimed at the integrity or honesty of the clinicians and researchers. Rather, it is directed at the very foundation of the categories and concepts themselves.

To take an example of this, consider a contemporary category that has arguably been constructed in this way: attention deficit hyperactivity disorder. As Laurence and McCallum (1998) ask, to what extent is this category being developed to aid the management of troublesome children? Perhaps psychiatry is engaged in a attempt at 'the production and maintenance of social normality and competence' (Rose 1996). Laurence and McCallum (1998) go on to say, 'the possibility of thinking and acting on modern categories of child arose from governmental attempts to know and under-stand the disruptive individual by means of techniques of calculability which carved out a new space – the space "inside the child's head" – for the operation of power'. That is, even when we can find youngsters to appear on television to attest to the benefits the drug Ritalin has brought them, and how it has enabled them to conquer their 'illness', this does not necessarily tell us very much about the nature of the problem. It may just as easily reflect the fact that the drug companies are funding the support group to which their parents belong (Breggin 2000). It might well be through social manoeuvres that the idea of a person's healthy core becomes detached from the parts of themselves which appear to be undesirable. Concept formulations, then, might be involved in supporting the moral order, such that we can identify parts of ourselves which are alien and which must be conquered, while the failures in our social institutions can be attributed to the actions of a few bad apples with medical pathologies.

However, once we look at the conceptual diversity that exists in some fields, it is a little difficult to sustain this idea of concepts being somehow constructed with a certain set of governmental interests in mind. Some areas of health care do have such a fragmented field of activities and concerns, with a large number of individuals with few ideas in common yet all of whom are more or less engaged in the same practices. People often don't share concepts, even though they appear to be involved in the same system of suffering and healing. For example, Lee-Treweek (2002) examines complementary medicine and considers how the clients and the professionals involved may have rather different understandings of what is going on in the therapy itself. As Lee-Treweek discovered, many of the clients attending a cranial osteopath had theories of the treatment that departed from the manifest position of the discipline itself. For example, they said things like 'is he not putting out signals and getting the blood flowing?' (Lee-Treweek 2002, p. 60). Some of the clients were even more vague about what was going on: 'I have to say I don't know the name of what he does I think it's cranial cranio something. But I think it's like acupressure which is putting your fingers in specific points to release tension . . . the main thing is to balance out your body so you're not pulling off to one side and your muscles aren't pulling you over' (Lee-Treweek 2002, pp. 62–3). That is, the clients were using and grouping concept formulations together in a way that seemed to them to be sensible, deploying analogies between the cranial osteopathy treatment and acupressure; ideas about getting blood moving around the body, fluid intake and toxins were used by clients, but not in a way that corresponded with the 'official version' of events. Cranial osteopathy, as it was originally conceived by William Garner Sutherland in the late nineteenth century, relies on the idea that there are minute movements in the plates of the skull and that any restriction of these 'breathing' movements would lead to physical, psychological and emotional problems (Sutherland Society 2001). Even more interesting, from our point of view, is that while osteopathy is often thought of as a complementary or perhaps holistic therapy, the practitioner in Lee-Treweek's study did not think of himself as performing holistic therapy, though perhaps his clients thought he was.

This example could no doubt be multiplied if we studied a number of different topic areas. The point is that there are a number of incommensurable concept formulations in the healing encounter and they do not necessarily have to come into alignment for there to be a sense of benefit to the client. Indeed, maybe it is the incommensurability of concept formulations that enables everyone to proceed as if all was well. If people actually knew about the concepts that the other members held, then the veneer of accord might be ruptured.

The veneer of accord that contemporary critical and postmodern scholars seek to rupture can be seen in some of the guiding assumptions of health care too. Whereas it has often been taken for granted that a 'positive attitude' is desirable for clients of the caring professions, there are some who sound a note of caution about this. Held (2002) notes that according to both popular and professional indicators, the push for the positive attitude in America is on the rise. She considers this popular culture *Zeitgeist* and notes that it appears in psychotherapeutic disciplines as diverse as 'positive psychology' and so-called 'postmodern therapy'. Held sees both of these as resting on a foundation of optimism and positive thinking despite their opposing views about a proper philosophy of science. She notes that cross-cultural evidence does not necessarily support the North American assumption that a positive attitude is necessary for a sense of well-being. She also notes findings in health psychology, clinical and counselling psychology, and organizational studies that undermine the assumption that accentuating the positive and eliminating the negative is necessarily beneficial in terms of physical and mental health. Held calls this assumption the 'tyranny of the positive attitude'. Moreover, this invites the possibility that the unprecedented pressure to accentuate the positive could itself contribute to some forms of unhappiness. This possibility of entertaining paradox is also a feature of postmodernist thinking. Striving for consistency is a characteristic of modernist discourse, whereas the postmodern tendency is to observe and celebrate the 'play' within the structures.

The postmodern tendency to explore contradictions and divergences can lead us to examine hitherto under-exploited crevices and schisms in the fabric of experience. For example, there are some curious tensions in how we think about health and disease. Take the case of Caesarean sections in giving birth. In some parts of the world, the incidence of this operation is much higher than others. In Western Europe, Australia and North America, where rates are very high, there is a good deal of concern about whether the operations are strictly necessary. There is also a concern that this represents a kind of medicalization of childbirth on the part of the health care professions and that control is being taken away from women themselves. Studies such as that by Fenwick *et al.* (2003) disclose unpleasant feelings on the part of women who have had a Caesarean, such as those who feel that the fact they have had a Caesarean means that they are inadequate or that the experience of birth has been taken away from them.

On the other hand, studies in other parts of the world reveal a different meaning for the operation. For example, Béhague (2002) examined the meaning of Caesarean operations in Brazil and explored the reasons for women's preferences for Caesarean section births in Pelotas. She argues that women strategize and appropriate both medical knowledge and the technology of Caesarean sections as a creative form of responding to the economic, cultural and ideological system in which they find themselves. In a sense, demanding a Caesarean is also about demanding a better deal from the health care system. It is not surprising, then, that women are demanding the operation in ever larger numbers. Béhague (2002) argues that, for some women, the effort to medicalize the birth process represents a practical solution to problems found within the medical system itself. Thus, a procedure which some enlightened practitioners are seeking to reduce in the 'West' is gaining in popularity in other parts of the world because of what it signifies about one's lifestyle and as a way of increasing the medical attention one gets in conditions of medical scarcity. Postmodern approaches to the study of health care and society would delight in exploring such disparities and curiosities.

A further feature of postmodernism that deserves comment is how it allows us to think in new ways about familiar phenomena in such a way as to defamiliarize it and make it strange. This enables fresh insights to be gained. To illustrate this, let us forget for a moment that illness is somehow undesirable and think about the ways in which it is perhaps enjoyable. To deal with this, we can draw our theoretical position from Bakhtinian literary theory and encompass the interplay of different, apparently contradictory strands of illness experience within a dialectical model. This will help us establish a niche for these enigmatic and under-explored issues. Increasingly, as a growing corpus of personal accounts testifies, it is becoming clear that a variety of experiences of enlightenment, transfiguration or aesthetic production can be detected in illness experience. Narrations of the experience of illness do not always describe it as unremittingly painful and may contain moments of comfort, positive transformation and even pleasure.

Whereas it may seem paradoxical to assert that illness may be pleasurable, it is clear that this is not a new idea to students of the area. A close reading of many of the classic texts of medical sociology and psychology reveals that pleasures are lurking just beneath the surface of illness. Talcott Parsons' (1951) concept of the sick role involved a legitimate release from the workaday obligations of the person's other roles and an opportunity, if not an obligation, to seek out nurturing and restorative experiences with health professionals. Gerhardt (1989) commented that the sick role is a kind of 'niche in the social system where the incapacitated may withdraw while attempting to mend their fences, with the help of the medical profession' (p. 15). Being a good patient may even be about putting on a token show of healthiness – bearing up well or being brave, for example. In another classic from the 1950s, Isobel Menzies Lyth (1988), in a psychoanalytically flavoured evocation of hospital life, saw the libido at work eroticizing the encounters between staff and patients.

Recent texts on the body and illness also repay an examination. Apparently for some authors there exists what Gillian Rose (1995) calls a state of 'accentuated being' afforded by illness. In academic life, illness experience that at an everyday level may be painful, debilitating or humiliating is a source of much storytelling (Frank 1995). As Arthur Frank (1997) puts it, there is an 'awesomeness' to accounts of the experience of illness which perhaps modifies how the experience itself is encoded and communicated. There is thus a dialectical interplay between pain and its amelioration. Our mention of the work of Bakhtin in this context is not capricious; he is apposite because he not only had much to say on dialogues and dialectics, but also about the grotesque and subversive aspects of the body. For Bakhtin (1973, 1981, 1984a,b), the grotesque body is a central feature of a topsy-turvy world which interrogates our familiar, stable world and questions its authoritarian monism. The grotesque body offers a symbolic subversion of the 'real' world and questions the cultural authority of official versions of the world with various alternative carnivalesque postulations. The phenomenon of carnival was central to Bakhtin's thought, for it was at these festivals throughout Europe in the Middle Ages and the Renaissance that the hierarchies of authority were temporarily challenged and inverted and the gross, profane and scatological aspects of the human condition were celebrated. Likewise, the grotesque, suffering body creates a 'gap' in the fabric of society and makes the 'body' less certain, homely or defined (Holquist and Clark 1984). The vulgarity of the grotesque body lies in its openness to the world. Illness, assault and modification tend to disrupt the body's envelope, puncture it, slit it, redefine its shape and its secretions (Pitts 1988). This *liminality*, or state of transition between health and illness, invites new sensations, experiences and identities. Biomedical accounts that stress the physiological aspects of disease can never exhaustively specify what the experience will be. Despite the discourses which emphasize the dire, desolate and agonizing aspects of illness, there are nevertheless possibilities for retrieving benefits, advantages and even pleasures from the experience. Furthermore, as Bakhtin (1986) would emphasize, 'I must find myself in another by finding another in myself' (p. 63). This highlights how these experiences themselves can be seen as interconnected with the social context where they are occasioned, constructed, interpreted, cared for and healed.

Although pain and illness anchor us in our bodies, they also highlight the way that symptoms are not just obdurately there; they are often performed. Clearly, this can be seen in the great medical demonstrations of the late nineteenth century where prominent specialists displayed their patients' symptoms and cures before an audience. Most famously, Jean Martin Charcot demonstrated his cases of hysteria (Showalter 1987), but we can find less celebrated cases where an appropriate display of symptoms yields an identifiable payoff. In the present, community nurses speak of 'social ulcers' – that is, where isolated elderly clients cultivate their wounds so as to facilitate contact with the nurse (Carnegie 1994; Nesselroth and Gahtan 2000).

On the one hand, the display of illness and disability marks one as a person who is defined through the body (Seymour 1998); on the other, Bakhtin reminds us that the grotesque attributes of the body – which may well emerge in sickness – make identity ambiguous, multiple and marginal and it is to these possibilities for novel, sociohistorical productions of bodily experience to which we now turn. Central to grotesque realism is the principle of degradation, 'the lowering of all that is high, spiritual, ideal, abstract . . . to the material level, to the sphere of earth and body in their indissoluble unity' (Seymour 1998, pp. 19–20).

Western medicine has tended to focus on the biologically based causal mechanisms of illness. Moreover, it has tended to proceed on the assumption that the systems and organs of the body can be treated in relative isolation. The successful 'transplant' – the jewel in the crown of scientific medicine – is predicated on the notion that many of the body's parts are interchangeable between certain individuals. Generally, a further assumption is that the technologies of health care are separate and morally neutral entities that humans can use to shape their experience of the world for the better. These ideas have been problematized by postmodernism.

There are contradictory tendencies in medicine. At the same time as there is a growing interest in evidence-based practice, with the assumption that there can be a universal standard of evidence, there is the so-called postmodernization of general practitioners (Clayton 2002). This describes an increasing tendency on the part of practitioners not to rely on formal, scientifically derived knowledge, but on 'clinical legitimacy', whereby treatments are selected that appear to work for that particular patient. Thus, we see GPs referring their patients to complementary therapists, for example. There are also powerful voices calling for a renewed vision of medicine as an art of healing rather than a science, for example, while others (e.g. Eastwood 2000) strengthen their call for a greater reliance on science. Hence, even in the era of evidence-based practice, there are signs that not everyone is singing from the same song sheet.

Within postmodern approaches to health and illness, the familiar divisions between mind and body, culture and nature are blurred. It becomes possible to see diseases as somehow more profoundly linked with culture. Helman (1994) makes the point when he describes culture-bound disorders, where particular organs are preferential for particular cultures. In France, there is the *crise de foie* (liver), whereas in Iran it is *narahatiye qalb* or heart distress. Britain prefers disorders of the bowel and, as Clayton (2002) argues, the organ of choice for women in Australia would be the breast. She speculates whether breast cancer is the manifestation of a society's obsession with stereotypical femininity. These links between culture and disease go beyond the familiar modernist medical concern between, say, smoking and lung cancer or diet and heart disease. Here, disease is seen as a kind of manifestation of culture.

Indeed, postmodernism invites us to be sceptical of the very symptoms we see in patients. Baudrillard (1983) says: 'For if any symptom can be "produced", and can no longer be accepted as a fact of nature, then every illness may be considered simulatable and simulated, and medicine loses its meaning since it only knows how to treat "true" illnesses by their objective causes' (p. 5). Clayton (2002) goes on to say: 'If subjectivity is in a continual state of flux, the body and mind are unstable referents. Therefore, the body as a site of experiential metamorphic production is worthy of further investigation' (p. 840). Thus, the meanings of symptoms and signs of the kind that previous generations of practitioners have been taught to recognize as a particular kind of disease may not be sufficient to make sense of the maladies of the twenty-first century. The past decade has seen a burgeoning of different kinds of health problem centred on immunity or some kind of ill-defined relationship between mind and body such as chronic fatigue syndrome, attention deficit hyperactivity disorder, depression or dissociative disorders. The grand illnesses of the past – tuberculosis, diphtheria, scarlet fever and the like – have been eclipsed by more complex syndromes with far less obvious aetiology.

As this chapter draws to a close, it is perhaps appropriate to ask what a post-modern approach to health care might look like. In this we are guided by the comments of Derrida (2001) about the humanities of tomorrow and a further commentary by Peters (2002) about the applicability of these to health care, in particular nursing. Derrida provides a list of seven programmatic statements as to how he would like to see the humanities disciplines developing, and it is to these we turn to see what implications postmodernism has for health care.

> 1) These new humanities would treat the history of man [*sic*], the idea, the figure, the notion of 'what is proper to man' . . . The most urgent guiding thread here would be the problematization . . . of those powerful judicial performatives that have given shape to this modern history of this humanity of man . . . on the other hand, the Declaration of the Rights of Man – and of course woman . . . and on the other hand, the concept of crimes against humanity, which since the end of the Second World War has modified the geopolitical field of international law . . .

> 2) These new humanities would treat, in the same style, the history of democracy and the idea of sovereignty. The deconstruction of this concept of sovereignty would touch not only on international law, the limits of the nation state, and of its supposed sovereignty, but also on the use made of them in judicio-political discourses concerning the relationship between what is called man and woman.

> 3) These new humanities would treat, in the same style, our history of 'professing', of the 'profession', and of the professoriat, a history articulated with that of the premises or presuppositions . . . of work and of the worldwide-ised

confession, there where it goes beyond the sovereignty of the Head of State, the nation state or even of the 'people' in a democracy. An immense problem: how to disassociate democracy from citizenship, from the nation state and from the theological idea of sovereignty, even the sovereignty of the people?

(Derrida 2001, pp. 241–4)

Let us pause for a moment and consider some of the implications of these statements for the health care disciplines. The concerns about government, jurisprudence and sovereignty here have, as Peters (2002) reminds us, a direct relevance to health care in the UK at least. Debates about refugees, asylum seekers and immigration have implications for how health is managed in the UK, and the increasing role of private sector finance in the health service invites concerns about the protection of the public sphere and the encroachment of market values into health care. Peters (2002) notes also that scholars of health care may well find it productive to investigate the 'government of health', in relation to citizen rights and democracy, emphasizing political, historical and philosophical aspects. Moreover, we may wish to be concerned with the question of to what extent is health a right of the citizen and to what extent this is related to democracy. In addition, it might be appropriate to ask which medical and commercial interests have most to gain from the privatization process. Moreover, how will the increasing introduction of market forces into health affect the relationship between patients and professionals? The concern over global health problems such as HIV or the scare over severe acute respiratory syndrome (SARS) in 2003 highlight the fact that there are health care issues that transcend national or sovereign boundaries. How do we conceptualize and study the differences between the 'health rich' and the 'health poor' in the globalized health market? Peters adds a further question: 'To what extent in the era of globalization is the government of health passing from the state to the multinational corporation?' (Peters 2002, p. 56). Furthermore, we might ask about the effects of all this privatization of health care on the research process, the kinds of tests which are done, the drugs which are approved and the commercial interests at stake in health care research.

Returning to Derrida's programme, let us consider some more of his vision of the new humanities and the questions they raised for health care:

4) These new humanities would treat, in the same style, the history of literature. Not only what is commonly called the history of literatures or literature themselves, with the great question of its canons . . . but the history of the concept of literature, of the modern institution named literature, of its links with fiction and the performative force of the 'as if', of the concept of oeuvre, author, signature, national language, of its link with the right to say or not to say everything that founds both democracy and the idea of the unconditional sovereignty claimed by the university and within it by what is called . . . the humanities.

5) These new humanities would treat, in the same style, the history of profession, the profession of faith, professionalization, and the professoriat. The guiding thread could be, today, what is happening when the profession of faith of the professor, gives rise to a singular oeuvres, to other strategies of the 'as if' that are

events and that affect the very limits of the academic field or of the humanities. We are indeed witnessing the end of a certain figure of the professor and of his or her supposed authority, but I believe as now should be obvious, in a certain necessity of the professoriat.

6) These new humanities would thus finally treat, in the same style, but in the course of a formidable reversal, both critical and deconstructive, the history of the 'as if' and especially the history of this precious distinction between performative acts and constantive acts that seems to have been indispensable to us until now.

7) To the seventh point, which is not the seventh day, I finally arrive now. Or rather, I let perhaps arrive at the end, now, the very thing that, by arriving, by taking place, revolutionises, overturns and puts to rout the very authority that is attached, in the university, in the humanities: (i) to knowledge (or at least constantive language); (ii) to the profession or to the profession of faith (or at least to its model of performative language); (iii) to the mise en oeuvre, the putting to work, at least to the performative putting to work of the 'as if'.

(Derrida 2001, pp. 241–4)

In addition to these kinds of ambitions about the humanities of tomorrow, Derrida paints a picture of what he calls the university of the future, which he says must be unconditionally free in both formulating questions and in the right to say publicly what is required by investigating, knowing and thinking. It needs, in his view, to be free from the commercial and political pressures that inhabit a good deal of academic life at present. He sees the ideals as a place of critical (deconstructive) resistance against the ideas of the powerful and the dogmatic interest groups within society. This resistance, this civil disobedience, is best expressed, in his view, through these new humanities that he outlined in the seven points above. These humanities are specified in a rather quaint manner, redolent of classical or Enlightenment ideas about academic freedom. The crucial difference, he sees, is that these studies must be deconstructed beforehand. Derrida's model of the new humanities is a profession of faith (*profession du foi*) of someone who performs the profession of professor. The question he asks is: what does it mean to profess (*professer*)? To reply to this question, Derrida tentatively accepts Austin's division of speech acts into constantive and performative, where constantive language is about things that are true and perfomative language is concerned with the performance itself. In Derrida's model, profession should not be constantive, but performative, because it is a work (*oeuvre*) itself, hence not in a final form.

However, according to Derrida, it is also necessary to ask the question of what is work (*travail*). The starting thought is: 'How the end of work was at the beginning of the world'. The term 'the end of work' is taken from the title of Rifkin's (1995) book *The End of Work*, and is connected with 'mondialation' (Derrida prefers this term to 'globalization'). Derrida's reading of Rifkin's book leads him to suppose that there has been a new revolution, 'moving us to the edge of a workerless world'. He claims that technological upheaval has occurred not only through cyberspace, microcomputing, cellular telephones and robotics, but by layoffs of millions of workers, including 'underpaid part-timers' at universities.

Let us pause for a moment and think about how some of this relates to the position in health care: the deskilling and deprofessionalization of many care tasks and the increasing reliance on voluntary and charitable labour to perform the more labour-intensive tasks of care; the loss of transport to clinics for elderly and infirm people, the difficulty in obtaining respite care and the waiting lists for many commonly required services are aspects of this. Discussion of the professoriat, and the issue of professing knowledge, is particularly apposite in health care too, for as Peters (2002) reminds us, the development of courses in nursing, physiotherapy, occupational therapy and audiology in universities means that there are new cadres of academics growing and developing careers in these professions. Equally, some of the traditional professions such as medicine have come under increasing suspicion. Peters sees one of the important tasks at stake here to be the development of a methodological self-reflection to theorize the relations of power in the teaching and practice of health care.

Derrida's keenness to break down the distinction between matters which are constantive (i.e. they make claims to the true, correct or verifiable depiction of existing states of affairs) and those which are performative (i.e. concerned with performance, presentation and doing) has implications for health care research and health care practice. If we cannot readily make the distinction between truth and doing, this means that there must be much greater attention to how health care is done in practice. Scholars such as Nicholas Fox (1993) and Marc Berg (1999) have provided sensitive, reflexive evocations of the use of technology in illness, suffering and care. When we perform operations upon patients, and store their data in electronic systems, this may have important implications for how we think about them. Whereas we cannot fully address these questions here, perhaps Derrida's most important claim is that to understand health care we need to make sense of the philosophy, politics and history behind it.

Derrida is also keen to suggest ways of thinking in universities and in the new humanities. As far as he is concerned, the university must be performative and this performativity must be 'as if' (*als ob*). This 'as if' is not an invitation to a fiction of possible futures. Instead, it takes into consideration the hypothetical or provisional nature of deconstruction. The humanities, he says, will have to study and analyse the concepts that they themselves introduced in their own historical construction. That is, Derridean philosophy invites us to become more fully reflexive, and understand how our own tools are involved in making the history of our disciplines and in creating our findings.

References

Abma, T.A. (1998) *The Art of Being Responsive to Differences*. Video presented to the AREA Annual Conference, San Diego, CA, April.

Abma, T.A. (2002) Emerging narrative forms of knowledge representation in the health sciences: two texts in a postmodern context, *Qualitative Health Research*, 12(1): 5–27.

Allen, D.G. (1995) Hermeneutics: philosophical traditions and nursing practice research, *Nursing Science Quarterly*, 8(4): 174–82.

Atkins, P. (2003) *Galileo's Finger: Ten Great Ideas of Science*. Buckingham: Open University Press.

Austin, J.L. (1962) *How To Do Things with Words*. Oxford: Clarendon Press.

Bakhtin, M.M. (writing as V.N. Voloshinov) (1973) *Marxism and the Philosophy of Language* (translated by L. Matejka and J.R. Titunik). New York: Seminar Press.

Bakhtin, M.M. (1981) *The Dialogic Imagination* (translated by C. Emerson and M. Holquist). Austin, TX: University of Texas Press.

Bakhtin, M.M. (1984a) *Rabelais and His World* (translated by H. Iswolsky). Cambridge, MA: MIT Press.

Bakhtin, M.M. (1984b) *Problems of Dostoyevsky's Poetics* (translated by C. Emerson). Minneapolis, MN: University of Minnesota Press.

Bakhtin, M.M. (1986) The problem of speech genres, in C. Emerson and M. Holquist (eds) *Speech Genres and Other Late Essays* (translated by V.W. McGee). Austin, TX: University of Texas Press.

Barone, T.E. (1997). Among the chosen: a collaborative educational (auto)biography, *Qualitative Inquiry*, 3(2): 222–36.

Baudrillard, J. (1983) The Precession of Simulacra, in J. Fleming and S. Lotringer (eds) *Simulations* (translated by P. Foss, P. Patton and P. Beitchman). New York: Columbia University Press.

Baudrillard, J. (1990) *Fatal Strategies: Crystal Revenge*. London Pluto/Semiotexte.

Baudrillard, J. (1995) *The Gulf War Did Not Take Place*. Sydney, NSW: Power Publications.

Béhague, D.P. (2002) Beyond the simple economics of Caesarean section birthing: women's resistance to social inequality, *Culture, Medicine and Psychiatry*, 26(4): 473–507.

Berg, M. (1999) Patient care information systems and health care work: a sociotechnical approach, *International Journal of Medical Informatics*, 55: 87–101.

Beverley, J. (2000). Testimonio, subalternity, and narrative authority, in N.K. Denzin and Y.S. Lincoln (eds) *Handbook of Qualitative Research*. Thousand Oaks, CA: Sage.

Blumenfeld-Jones, D.S. (1995) Dance as a mode of representation, *Qualitative Inquiry*, 1(14): 391–401.

Boyne, R. (1992) *Foucault and Derrida*. London: Unwin Hyman.

Breggin, P. (2000) *Reclaiming Our Children: A Healing Solution for a Nation in Crisis*. Cambridge, MA: Perseus Books.

Britten, N. (1994) Patients' ideas about medicines: a qualitative study in a general practice population, *British Journal of General Practice*, 44: 465–8.

Carnegie, A. (1994) Leg ulcer care in the community, *Journal of Wound Care*, 8(4): 157–8.

Cheek, J. and Rudge, T. (1994) Nursing as textually mediated reality, *Nursing Inquiry*, 1(1): 15–22.

Clarke, L. (1996) The last post? Defending nursing against the postmodernist maze, *Journal of Psychiatric and Mental Health Nursing*, 3: 257–65.

Clayton, B. (2002) Rethinking postmodern maladies, *Current Sociology*, 50(6): 839–51.

Darbyshire, P. (1994) Reality bites: the theory and practice of nursing narratives, *Nursing Times*, 90(40): 31–3.

Deleuze, G. and Guattari, F. (1984) *Anti-Oedipus: Capitalism and Schizophrenia* (translated by R. Hurley, M. Seem and H.R. Lane). London: Athlone.

Denzin, N.K. (1999) Two-stepping in the '90s, *Qualitative Inquiry*, 5(4): 568–72.

Derrida, J. (1977) *Of Grammatology* (translated by G.C. Spivak). Baltimore, MD: Johns Hopkins University Press.

Derrida, J. (1978) *Writing and Differance*. London: Routledge.

Derrida, J. (2001) The future of the professions or the unconditional university (thanks to the 'humanities', what could take place tomorrow), in L. Simmons and H. Worth (eds) *Derrida Downunder*. Palmerston North, NZ: Dunmore Press.

Dougan, H.A.S. (1995) The role of the nurse, in P.I. Peattie and S. Walker (eds) *Understanding Nursing Care*, 4th edn. Edinburgh: Churchill Livingstone.

Eastwood, H. (2000) Complementary therapies: the appeal to general practitioners, *Medical Journal of Australia*, 173: 95–8.

Ellis, C. and Bocher, A.P. (2000) Authoethnography, personal narrative, reflexivity: researcher as subject, in N.K. Denzin and Y.S. Lincoln (eds) *Handbook of Qualitative Research*. Thousand Oaks, CA: Sage.

Falk, L. and Perron, M. (1995) The conversion of Père Version, in C.H. Gray (ed.) *The Cyborg Handbook*. New York: Routledge.

Fenwick, J., Gamble, J. and Mawson, J. (2003) Women's experiences of caesarean section and vaginal birth after caesarean: a Birthrites initiative, *International Journal of Nursing Practice*, 9: 10–17.

Foucault, M. (1965) *Madness and Civilisation*. New York: Random House.

Foucault, M. (1975) *The Birth of the Clinic: An Archaeology of Medical Perception*. New York: Vintage.

Fox, N.J. (1992) *The Social Meaning of Surgery*. Philadelphia, PA: Open University Press.

Fox, N.J. (1993) *Postmodernism, Sociology and Health*. Toronto: University of Toronto Press.

Frank, A. (1995) *The Wounded Storyteller: Body, Illness and Ethics*. Chicago, IL: University of Chicago Press.

Frank, A. (1997) Narrative witness to bodies: a response to Alan Radley, *Body and Society*, 3(3): 103–9.

Gerhardt, U. (1989) *Ideas about Illness: An Intellectual and Political History of Medical Sociology*. London: Macmillan.

Glesne, G. (1997) That rare feeling: re-presenting research through poetic transcription, *Qualitative Inquiry*, 3(2): 202–21.

Green, J. and Britten, N. (1998) Qualitative research and evidence based medicine, *British Medical Journal*, 316: 1230–2.

Grice, H.P. (1975) Logic and conversation, in P. Cole and J.P. Morgan (eds) *Syntax and Semantics 3: Speech Acts*. New York: Academic Press.

Gurevitz, D. (1997) *Postmodernism, Culture and Literature at the End of the 20th Century*. Tel Aviv: Dvir.

Held, B.S. (2002) The tyranny of the positive attitude in America: observations and speculations, *International Journal of Clinical Psychology*, 58(9): 965–91.

Helman, C.G. (1994) *Culture, Health and Illness*. Oxford: Butterworth Heinemann.

Henderson, V. (1966) *The Nature of Nursing*. London: Collier Macmillan.

Hewett, G. (1994) *'Just a Part of Me': Men's Reflections on Chronic Asthma*. Occasional Papers in Sociology and Social Policy. London: South Bank University.

Hollinger, R. (1994) *Postmodernism and the Social Sciences*. London: Sage.

Holquist, M. and Clark, K. (1984) *Mikhail Bakhtin*. Cambridge, MA: Harvard University Press.

hooks, b. (1990) *Yearning: Race, Gender, and Cultural Politics*. Boston, MA: South End.

Hull, F.M. and Marshall, T. (1987) Sources of information about new drugs and attitudes towards drug prescribing: an international study of differences between primary care physicians, *Family Practitioner*, 4: 123–8.

Katon, W. and Kleinman, A. (1981) Doctor–patient negotiation and other social science strategies in patient care, in L. Eisenberg and A. Kleinman (eds) *The Relevance of Social Science to Medicine*. Dordrecht: Reidel.

Kivnick, H.Q. (1996) Remembering and being remembered: the reciprocity of psychological legacy, *Generations: Journal of the American Society on Aging*, 20(3): 49–53.

Lacan, J. (1977) *Écrits* (translated by A. Sheridan). London: Tavistock.

Lapidus, I.M. (1996) Photo essay, *Women's Studies*, 25: 363–70.

Lather, P. and Smithies, C. (1997) *Troubling the Angels: Women Living with HIV/AIDS*, Boulder, CO: Westview.

Laurence, J. and McCallum, D. (1998) The myth or reality of attention deficit hyperactivity disorder: a genealogical approach, *Discourse: Studies in the Cultural Politics of Education*, 19(2): 183–200.

Lee-Treweek, G. (2002) Trust in complementary medicine: the case of cranial osteopathy, *Sociological Review*, 50(1): 48–68.

Lemert, C. (1990) The uses of French structuralisms in sociology, in G. Ritzer (ed.) *Frontiers of Social Theory: The New Syntheses*. New York: Columbia University Press.

Lewis, B. (2000) Psychiatry and postmodern theory, *Journal of Medical Humanities*, 21(2): 71–84.

Lister, P. (1997) The art of nursing in a postmodern context, *Journal of Advanced Nursing*, 25: 38–44.

Lyotard, J.-F. (1984) *The Postmodern Condition: A Report on Knowledge* (translated by G. Bennington and B. Massumi). Manchester: Manchester University Press.

Mansfield, N. (2000) *Subjectivity: Theories of the Self from Freud to Haraway*. St Leonards, NSW: Allen & Unwin.

Maynard, D. (1991) The perspective display series and the delivery of diagnostic news, in D. Boden and D.H. Zimmerman (eds) *Talk and Social Structure*. Cambridge: Polity Press.

Menzies Lyth, I. (1988) *Containing Anxiety in Institutions: Selected Essays*, Vol. 1. London: Free Association Books.

Mienczakowski, J.E. (1995) The theatre of ethnography: the reconstruction of ethnography into theatre with an emancipatory potential, *Qualitative Inquiry*, 1: 360–75.

Mishler, E.G. (1984) *The Discourse of Medicine: Dialectics of Medical Interviews*. Norwood, NJ: Ablex.

Morgan, G. (1986) *Images of Organisation*. London: Sage.

Nesselroth, S.M. and Gahtan, V. (2000) Management of pressure ulcers in the home care setting, *Home Healthcare Consultant*, 7(4): 34–42.

Norris, J.R. (1997) Meaning through form: alternative modes of knowledge representation, in J.M. Morse (ed.) *Completing a Qualitative Project: Details and Dialogue*. Thousand Oaks, CA: Sage.

Osman, L.M., Russell, I.T., Friend, J.A.R., Legge, J.S. and Douglas, J.G. (1993) Predicting patient attitudes to asthma medication, *Thorax*, 48: 827–30.

Parker, I., Georgaca, E., Harper, D., McLaughlin, T. and Stowell-Smith, M. (1995) *Deconstructing Psychopathology*, London: Sage.

Parsons, T. (1951) *The Social System*. London: Routledge & Kegan Paul.

Pellegrino, E. (1979) *Humanism and the Physician*. Knoxville, TN: University of Tennessee Press.

Peplau, H.E. (1952) *Interpersonal Relations in Nursing*. New York: G.P. Putnam.

Peters, M. (2002) Derrida and the tasks for the new humanities: postmodern nursing and the culture wars, *Nursing Philosophy*, 3: 47–57.

Pfohl, S. (1992) *Death at the Parasite Cafe: Social Science (Fiction) and the Postmodern*. Basingstoke: Macmillan.

Pitts, V.L. (1988) Reclaiming the female body: embodied identity work, resistance and the grotesque, *Body and Society*, 4(3): 67–84.

Randi, J. (1992) *Conjuring*. New York: St. Martin's Press.

Richardson, L. (1993) Poetics, dramatics and transgressive validity: the case of the skipped line, *The Sociological Quarterly*, 34(4): 695–710.

Rifkin, J. (1995) *The End of Work: The Decline of the Global Labor Force and the Dawn of the Post-Market Era*. New York: J.P. Tarcher.

Ritzer, G. (1992) *Sociological Theory*. New York: McGraw-Hill.

Rose, G. (1995) *Love's Work*. London: Chatto & Windus.

Rose, N. (1990) *Governing the Soul: The Shaping of the Private Self*. London: Routledge.

Rose, N. (1996) Psychiatry as political science: advanced liberalism and the administration of risk, *History of Human Sciences*, 9(2): 1–23.

Sarup, M. (1988) *An Introduction to Post-Structuralism and Post-Modernism*. Hemel Hempstead: Harvester Wheatsheaf,

Scannell, P., Schlesinger, P. and Sparks, C. (eds) (1992) *Culture and Power: A Media, Culture and Society Reader*. London: Sage.

Searle, J. (1969) *Speech Acts: An Essay in the Philosophy of Language*. London: Cambridge University Press.

Schegloff, E.A. (1997) Whose text? Whose context?, *Discourse and Society*, 8(2): 165–88.

Seymour, W. (1998) *Remaking the Body: Rehabilitation and Change*. London: Routledge.

Showalter, E. (1987) *The Female Malady*. London: Virago.

Spitzer, A. (1998) Nursing in the health care system of the postmodern world: crossroads, paradoxes and complexity, *Journal of Advanced Nursing*, 28(1): 164–71.

Sutherland Society (2001) Cranial osteopathy (http://www.cranial.org.uk).

10

Philosophy and research design in practice

Introduction

This chapter considers how we might conceptualize knowledge in health care and how researchers might go about the knowledge generation process. Rather than simply rehearse a set of methodological guidelines about how research might be better done if researchers were aware of philosophical issues, we will attempt to show how different kinds of epistemologies and approaches to knowledge exist in different branches of the health care disciplines. There are a variety of growths in the health care garden, many of which co-exist comfortably, yet which appear to be structured in dominance according to issues such as prestige, status, fashion and finances. In addition, different health care disciplines have conceptualized the kinds of knowledge they are based on differently. In contrast to the enthusiasm for randomized controlled clinical trials in medicine, nursing has a well-known typology originated by Carper (1978) that divides knowledge into empirical, ethical, personal and aesthetic knowledge; the notion of socio-political knowledge was added by White (1995). We will discuss how different conceptions of knowledge, different values and different positions in the socio-political framework might yield different kinds of research questions and might predispose actors towards differing research methods. The knowledge desired by a community mental health nurse seeing an isolated elderly client may be different from that desired by a drug company, or a lecturer on a health studies programme.

It is also perhaps important to consider how knowledge is represented by practitioners, yet as we shall see, expertise has been extremely difficult to characterize. Generally, more tacit knowledge is deployed by expert practitioners, and we will examine how this might lead to the formulation of research questions and strategies for interrogating existing research knowledge. We shall also consider what practical implications there are in adopting a philosophical turn of mind for health care researchers and practitioners. We shall show how this offers powerful intellectual tools for making sense of the medical and social world, evaluating theories, research designs and methods and even critically appraising completed studies.

There are a variety of practical and financial issues in promoting and implementing research, and the policies adopted by research councils, government bodies and industry will be crucial in determining the kinds of knowledge which emerge from the research community. These foci of concern may have an impact on the kind of philosophy of science we adopt in trying to make sense of research. On the way to becoming practitioners and researchers, students will thus need to acquire a sense of why and how research and knowledge are paid for and how economic considerations may inform the choice of research topic, research personnel and even, perhaps, the outcome of research in the industrialized economies of the West. Some of the issues described in this book so far might be useful to help understand this process.

Ways of knowing: nursing and beyond

The idea that there are different levels or 'ways of knowing' has a long pedigree in nursing. For the past 50 years or so, nursing scholars have tried to define what it is that nursing does, and how this relates to the kind of knowledge derived and used by nurses in their everyday practice. Peplau's (1952) generative work sought to redefine nursing as a primarily interpersonal discipline and, more recently, a famous taxonomy of 'ways of knowing in nursing' was developed (Carper 1978). This framework, where knowledge is seen as involving four kinds of 'knowing', has been influential in nursing for nearly a quarter of a century at the time of writing: these are empirical, ethical, aesthetic and personal knowledge. This point in the development of the profession represented a move away from its positivistic roots. Let us describe these four kinds of knowledge in more detail.

Empirical knowledge corresponds to the legitimized, scientific version of what the world consists of and how it can be operated upon. Like many conventional accounts of science that we have encountered in this volume, it is aimed at developing general laws, principles and theories so as to explain, describe and predict phenomena in nursing. It might involve the usual suspects in the education of health professionals – anatomy, physiology and pharmacology – as well as the growing body of scientific knowledge in general. In the present day, it might correspond to the kinds of scientifically derived knowledge, rich in quantification and double-blind randomized controlled designs, which go to make up the canon of evidence-based practice as it is currently conceived.

Ethical or *moral knowledge* concerns ethical issues in nursing and focuses on issues of duty and responsibility. This involves knowledge of codes of conduct and the ability to distinguish ethical issues and appreciate the moral dimensions of an issue. This way of knowing comprises the understanding and the ability to apply moral and ethical frameworks to complex situations requiring moral insight and judgement. It encompasses valuing, clarifying and advocacy on behalf of the client, while acknowledging that they have the human freedom, will and knowledge to make decisions on their own behalf. This may also involve awareness of the way that some moral dilemmas cannot easily be solved. It might, moreover, be possible to subsume political and spiritual knowledge under this heading, as well as knowledge concerning the larger-scale contribution to human welfare made by a health care intervention.

Personal knowledge involves self-understanding and is 'concerned with the knowing, encountering, and actualizing the concrete, individual self' (Carper 1978, p. 18). In this view, knowing oneself makes it possible to use the self therapeutically. Personal knowledge involves the capacity to 'access one's own feeling life – one's range of emotions: the capacity instantly to effect discriminations among the feelings and, eventually, to label them, to enmesh them in symbolic codes, e.g. language, touch, writing to draw upon them as a means of understanding and guiding one's behaviour' (Gardner 1983, p. 239).

Johns (1995a) describes the *aesthetic way of knowing* as the 'intuitive grasp of and response to a clinical situation' (p. 228). Aesthetics also includes the expressive aspect of nursing and comprises knowledge gained through the 'subjective acquaintance' of direct experience and becomes visible in the craft skills through which the nurse uses self on behalf of the individual (Carper 1978, p. 16). Aesthetic knowing involves the synthesis and expression of all of the patterns of nursing knowledge and, of necessity, will be unique to each nurse. It also necessitates the recognition of unique details and particulars rather than the universal, and is based around integration, synthesis, perception, intuition, creativity and empathy. Aesthetic knowing requires a process of engagement, interpretation and envisioning. This may even appear in the informal language of health care. A friend of one of the authors (B.B.) described how in wound care a wound might look 'sweet'. On exploration of this term, it appeared that this was to do with how likely the wound was to heal satisfactorily. It might appear smaller from day to day, less 'sloughy' and less red around the edges. It might have new granulations around the edge closing in. A 'sweet' wound, however, might still look gruesome to the uninitiated.

This typology of ways of knowing has been enhanced by the addition of a fifth kind. White (1995) argues that socio-political knowledge merits a category of its own. This relates to the context of nursing and addresses the context of the people involved, including the nurse and the client, as well as the profession. This involves both society's understanding of nursing and nursing's understanding of society and its politics. Socio-political knowing includes a focus on whose views are being heard and whose are being silenced. In practice, it involves exposing, exploring, transforming, transposing and critically analysing.

The identification of these forms of knowledge by Carper and White has led to a considerable degree of reflection in nursing on the kinds of knowledge that nurses use and the way that knowledge informs practice. The dominance of medicine in health care studies has perhaps resulted in it having a rather static view of its science, philosophy and practice, as if the knowledge from the laboratory and the clinical trial were unproblematically translatable to consulting room. This has not developed to anything like the same extent in nursing, where, despite the proliferation of models and protocols, the field has been characterized by much greater diversity and a greater hunger for ideas from other disciplines. This tendency is not unique to nursing. It may be possible to detect it in occupational therapy, too, especially as this has recently moved to being a more academically based subject and has carved out roles for itself in counselling, therapeutic and forensic contexts. In addition, the training curricula of a variety of professions allied to medicine are in the process of being modified so as to include more social, interpersonal and communication-related concerns. These changes in the organization of education and training cannot help but shift the knowledge bases and world-views of the professions concerned.

This tendency to focus on the interpersonal aspects of the health care encounter is often found hand in hand with a more interpretive stance in relation to the issue of how we make sense of what takes place in health care. Lathlean and Vaughan (1994) argue that this 'interpretative school' of scholarship in nursing has provided the profession with considerable insight into the nature of its practice. The 'interpretative school' is usually dated from the pioneering work of Benner (1984) and Benner and Wrubel (1989), but in some ways its origins go back much further, possibly even to Florence Nightingale herself. She was especially concerned with the 'moral qualities' of the nurse, which, in a rather quaint nineteenth-century idiom, may well have been addressing similar issues to those concerned today with the interpretive and interpersonal aspects of nursing.

Nursing, then, is a useful example because it illustrates the epistemological drift that has overtaken some of the health care professions. This drift away from positivism – or at least what its detractors believe positivism to be – has confronted health care scholars with the need to place their understanding of what they do on other footings. In tandem with this epistemological drift, then, it is possible to detect commitments on the part of nursing scholars that emphasize issues which are profoundly philosophical. In addition to the layers of knowledge or ways of knowing outlined by Carper above, some equally puzzling dilemmas remain to be negotiated. In illustrating this we will remain with the example of nursing because that is the one that has been most fully theorized, but the remarks may well apply to other health care disciplines.

One difficult thing to learn in the process of becoming a health care practitioner is that health care – at least according to some of its theorists – is not essentially concerned with tasks but with judgement. To simply learn how to do tasks is to only learn enabling skills (Benner 1982). Nursing, for instance, is believed to be a context-bound activity and one can only learn to be an interpretative nurse by entering into the world of the client. This, then, confronts the practitioner or researcher with a need to develop expertise as a phenomenologist. To be both an effective practitioner and an effective researcher it is desirable to be able to imagine what the world looks like from the point of view of the client and to understand how interpersonal processes have a role to play in facilitating the growth of understanding in particular ways. This area of expertise is different from, and sometimes sits uneasily with, the technical rationality of what Carper calls empirical knowing. However, in some cases, the kind of knowledge that derives from experience and understanding can have an equally valuable role to play in clinical contexts.

Layers of knowledge, layers of experience and new social objects

Let us illustrate this with the example of violence and the use of restraint in mental health contexts. This is a notoriously fraught area and was the subject of a study by Bonner et al. (2002), who interviewed both staff and clients who had been involved in incidents of this kind. In describing the run up to these incidents, clients often described some sort of failed communication prior to the outburst. For example: 'I got very angry because they wouldn't listen to what I was trying to tell them. Telling them that I needed help, wanted to hurt myself . . . it was horrible, I never want it to happen again' (Bonner et al. 2002, p. 468). Once incidents had taken place, there was sometimes a good deal of bitterness about how the event had been handled. 'I didn't feel like a human being, I felt like I was just a number, I thought they were going to kill me' (p. 468). The incidents also left their mark on the staff. 'It's the frustration of not meeting her needs, although I try' (p. 469). And, after a particularly noteworthy incident in which a patient armed with a weapon had mounted an attack on staff, one nurse recounted the following story:

> I was terrified. I've never been so scared in all my life. The incident happened at 13.30. I didn't sit down until 16.20. I had wet myself because I was so terrified and I couldn't go home to change my trousers. The duty senior nurse wouldn't let me go because she said that she couldn't find a free trained member of staff throughout the entire hospital. I didn't want to tell her or anybody else that I'd wet myself so I had to stay in my wet trousers until the end of the shift.
>
> (Bonner et al. 2002, p. 469)

In addition, both patients and nurses disclosed that the events had brought back memories of earlier traumatic or violent incidents, such as being raped.

From the point of view of practical applications, although this study was small in scale and included only six incidents, it has yielded a number of implications for research and practice. Staff and patients expressed the importance of adequate debriefing – being able to talk through the incident afterwards was especially appreciated by patients who had been restrained. It also highlights the practical benefits of being able to spot the signs of an impending incident before it happens, especially given that patients claimed to have made it clear that they were going to become angry. In addition to these practical benefits that come from attempts to understand, there are some more philosophically oriented issues that this raised. For example, the way that everyday events are opportunities to do some sort of investigation, no matter how difficult they may be. As Hans Gerth and C. Wright Mills (1964) observed in *Character and Social Structure*, 'Problems of the nature of human nature are raised most urgently when the life-routines of a society are disturbed, when men are alienated from their social roles in such a way as to open themselves up for new insight' (p. xiii). These disjunctures in social reality tell us something important about the kind of world we are embedded in as researchers, patients and practitioners. Individual thoughts, feelings and experiences gain their meaning from the parts they play in larger-scale social wholes. Moreover, this kind of incident and the research that has been done on it shows how the close observation of regrettable everyday events can yield new insights into the nature of trauma. Bonner et al. (2002) note that their research has yielded a unique observation about the nature of trauma. The experience of restraint incidents in the hospital involved a traumatic re-experiencing of previous violent events for some of their patients and, more intriguingly, also for some of the staff. This shows how, with an eye for detail, the observation of mundane phenomena can open up new lines of enquiry. Once we have a theory, no matter how incompletely formed, we can use it to identify other observations of a similar kind. As Karl Popper ([1935] 1959) noted, theory is 'the net which we throw out in order to catch the world – to rationalize, explain, and dominate it' (p. 26).

Even where there is some agreement between staff and patients as to what is important and what matters, there can still be some important discrepancies. Holden and Smart (1999) were interested in what 'adds value' to the experience of being an 'emergency room' patient. They found that whereas issues such as waiting time, symptom relief, a caring and kind attitude on the part of staff and a diagnosis were all important to both staff and patients, waiting time was most important to patients but least important to staff. Thus, even when there was some agreement on the issues, there was a mismatch between patients' priorities and the perceptions of staff. The authors say that this justifies the use of waiting times as a performance indicator for emergency medicine. In this sense, then, a piece of research as ordinary as this can lead to policy changes in health care. Here, although the research itself is worthwhile, it is not methodologically or theoretically ambitious.

In the two examples above, we have discussed the entities 'patient' and 'staff' as if it was possible to tell the difference between the two, and as if these formed neatly bounded classes of people, as they clearly do in many classic studies of institutional life, for example by Goffman (1961). In terms of what is going on nowadays, of course, these very categories are blurring. Informally, we have noted that patients do jobs for each other on hospital wards that might once have been done by nurses. More officially, the present policy framework in the UK involves users being involved in service planning, research, needs assessment and in a helping role for one another as advocates. In any case, the use of the very term patient is being eclipsed by terms like 'user' or 'consumer'. This then prompts the possibility of reflection on what the social actors in health care are. Aspis (1997) reported some users who wanted to be called 'students' rather than clients. In addition, this kind of relationship creates new collective social objects as people get together to support each other (Aspis 1997). In addition, as consumers are encouraged to be more active in negotiating and organizing their care, new kinds of social body are unfolded. The new entrepreneurial patient, consumer, user or 'student' may well also find new ways of complaining about services that do not measure up to their new expectations. They may, as Abbott et al. (2001) discovered, be disappointed about the lack of information provided, they may be unclear about how their needs had been assessed and be unhappy about the lack of regular contact with health or social services personnel. So there are new sources of dissatisfaction and failure as well as new successes to be measured.

In addition, relatively new areas of concern have opened up. One example is the issue of disability and sexuality, where over the past few years increasing concern has been expressed by both carers and service users themselves. People with learning difficulties in particular have moved from a position where intimate relationships were treated with an unhappy mixture of disapproval and sterilization. Having intimate relationships while being disabled is complicated by the fact that people with disabilities often find themselves policed by caregivers and excluded from the range of informal and formal processes by which non-disabled people are socialized into intimate relationships and sexuality (Davies 2000). In addition, as Davies points out, once people with disabilities begin to see themselves as gay, lesbian, bisexual or transgendered, the whole situation becomes even more complex.

In the face of all this creation and recreation of people and identities, it is particularly useful to have a philosophically informed cast of mind as we examine these new issues and movements. As researchers and practitioners in health care, we have a dual role both as observers and participants. The likelihood is that sooner or later we, too, will have health problems or disabilities that will involve us in being a client, patient or user. Philosophy does not necessarily give us a set of guidelines for understanding the world, but by confronting the different ideas and perspectives from thinkers, researchers, sufferers, healers and philosophers, we can perhaps make some headway.

Representing knowledge and becoming expert

Knowledge and how it is represented have been continuous themes throughout this book. We have attempted to address the diverse ways in which health professionals conceptualize the world. However, so far our account has been based largely on their written, drawn or photographed traces, what they write in textbooks or technical journals, and what is encoded in policy documents. In addition to this, it is also possible that practice itself, especially skilled practice, draws on different domains of knowledge and different ways of representing expertise which we have scarcely begun to characterize. To get a grip on this it is necessary to consider the processes involved in intuition and tacit knowledge. The intuitive aspects of skilled practice in health care are particularly difficult to study because they have been reduced in relevance under the technical rationality of the biomedical model. Yet health professionals, especially when they are experienced, may well use intuitive skills frequently. These skills enable practitioners to 'understand, to speak, and to cope skilfully with our everyday environment' (Dreyfus and Dreyfus 1985, p. xx). Because it is largely tacit, intuition is a nebulous form of knowledge that has not been studied extensively, as it cannot be explained or observed easily (Johns 1995b). In making sense of intuition, researchers have often turned to the work of Edmund Husserl (1859–1938), the originator of the phenomenological movement in Germany, who sought to interpret the inner spiritual and cognitive understandings of humans. In Husserl's formulation, the term 'intuiting' was central to phenomenology. Here, intuition involves 'logical insight based on careful consideration of representative examples: it is not second sight or inspiration' (Wilkes 1991, p. 233). Rew (1988, p. 150) identifies it as a 'higher form of vision'.

To place the notion of intuition into a framework that locates the kinds of skills found in health care, let us examine the work of Benner. Benner (1992) describes the progression of skill development in nursing, but it could equally well apply to other health professionals. It is proposed that skill levels develop from that of novice, to an advanced beginner stage, to a competent stage, to a proficient stage, to an expert stage. This typology was based on a model of skills acquisition developed by Dreyfus and Dreyfus, who believed that artificial intelligence, for example computer programs, was limited when it came to 'commonsense understanding' (Paterson 1991, p. 7). In Benner's account, as nurses acquire skills their thinking moves from reliance on abstract rules to reliance on past concrete experiences. As it does so, it undergoes a shift from rule-based analysis to intuition. The practitioners' perception changes from perceiving parts of a situation to the whole situation (Benner 1992). Dreyfus and Dreyfus (1985) suggest that novices use overly simple heuristic rules, while experts internalize their knowledge. This implies that domain experts are less able to explain their behaviour than novices. Warelow (1997, p. 1022) adds that when nurses become experts and practise using intuition, their 'theory, practice and experienced wisdom . . .' work in harmony.

Dreyfus (1979) outlined six key aspects of intuition, which it is possible to identify. These are normally listed as if they were a kind of progression from the simplest to the more complicated, yet it is clear that they depend on one another and are closely interrelated. The first is pattern recognition, where relationships between a group of features within a particular context are perceived as a recognizable pattern. The second key aspect of intuitive judgement is similarity recognition, where the observer detects features which the situation or the person has with others. The third key aspect of intuition is commonsense understanding, which involves knowledge of the culture and language, and some sort of tacit grasp of what happens and what matters. The fourth aspect of intuition is skilled know-how, which is where one's body can carry out the task without consciously thinking, called 'embodied intelligence' by Paterson (1991, p.14). Some refer to this as 'brain-stem memory'. It seems that we are in automatic pilot, yet we are not performing mindlessly or mechanically. The fifth aspect of intuition is a sense of salience, which is where some features stand out in a situation as being more important than others. Finally, deliberative nationality involves comparing current situations with situations in the past, while considering the different perspectives and interpretations of the situations.

This progression of knowledge and practice – from the explicit procedural and technical knowledge acquired by the novice to the invisible exercise of skill on the part of the advanced practitioner – has meant that the sorts of knowledge representation involved in this kind of advanced practice have remained elusive. Indeed, many theorists have described it in somewhat mystical terms. Darling (1995, p. 16) describes intuition as 'the power of gaining knowledge without rational thought'. This notion of understanding that somehow occurs before or without reasoning appears to be widespread among writers on the subject. Schraeder and Fischer (1986) also say intuition is 'the immediate knowing of something without the conscious use of reason' (p. 161).

The sense of ineffability about the skilled practitioner's intuition and expertise is widely touted as being a key feature. The awareness involved in intuition is immediate and is a 'knowing in action' (Lumby 1991, p. 467). It is believed to be common to all people to the extent that it is 'a universal characteristic of human thought' (Rew 1988, p. 150). It is often expressed as a feeling or knowing and, despite the commonplace distinction that is drawn between reason and intuition, it is not necessarily in conflict with analytical reasoning. Schraeder and Fischer (1986) agree with Carl Jung that 'intuition is another dimension of knowing and is not in opposition to deductive or inductive reasoning' (p. 1). Indeed, intuition and analytical reasoning often work together (Benner and Tanner 1987).

Part of the appeal of these quasi-mystical accounts lies in the difficulty of specifying exactly what it is that experts do as they apply their obscurely represented knowledge so as to solve new practice problems creatively. Artificial intelligence theorists have struggled for many years with the problem of representing expertise in such a way as to enable it to be run on a computer. This is taken to suggest that there are parts of the creative process which defy automation. Moreover, some theorists, notably Dreyfus and Dreyfus (1985), warn of the mediocrity that arises from replacing too much of the human thought process with automation. The rule-governed, programmable variety will never be as good as the intuitive version, it is argued. As Dreyfus and Dreyfus (1985) have argued in their classic critiques of traditional approaches to artificial intelligence, experts have a well-tuned sense of relevance that saves them from having to consider irrelevant aspects of the situation at hand. Computer chess-playing programs, for example, almost invariably proceed by considering a large number of moves, whereas the human chess expert – pretty evenly matched with a computer these days – tends to see patterns and possibilities in the game.

This, then, invites the problem of how people represent knowledge, which is one we have thought about periodically throughout this book. A reflective and scholarly stance on the part of readers will enable them to consider what kinds of knowledge are present in a given situation and think about how they are represented – is the knowledge implicit or explicit, traditional or postmodern, public or secret? This kind of literacy with knowledge, concepts and world-views is increasingly important in the current climate in health care with the vogue on both sides of the Atlantic for some form of evidence-based practice and the growing expectation that practitioners will be research literate. The kind of philosophical awareness that we have been illustrating and advocating throughout this book is one step on the way towards being able to make one's way through this new set of demands and apply philosophy in practical contexts.

The climate researchers encounter during their careers will also depend on the kinds of philosophies they adopt. At present, qualitative and interpretive researchers complain that they are disadvantaged when funding for research is dispensed and that the purse strings are loosened for those with a track record of quantitative research. An alignment with the more powerful interests in a given situation will very likely yield a different kind of experience than attempting to plough a less prestigious furrow. Thus, the old cliché 'That's a great idea, boss' may well apply in research and clinical practice as well.

The study of folk concepts: social representations

One way to fine-tune the thinking tools we have at our disposal is to look at those of other people and borrow from them. We have just discussed how difficult it is to characterize expertise, so to some extent this possibility doesn't look hopeful. However, there are a number of ways to study how thinking is done in everyday contexts. To illustrate this, let us look at one influential approach, namely that of social representations theory. Looking at concept formulations in their natural habitats as people go about their everyday tasks of making sense of the world, being ill or performing acts of healing, has frequently been used in the study of 'social representations'. Again, let us take a detour into the social sciences to see what the progenitors of this approach have been able to achieve in terms of examining the concepts that exist in everyday sense-making. The idea of social representations was originated in the 1950s by Moscovici (1976) to explain how a good deal of terminology from psychoanalysis had found its way into everyday culture in France. This tendency of everyday conversation to include terms from psychology and psychotherapy was also noted in California by Rosen (1977), in his book *Psychobabble*. In France in the 1950s,

Moscovici's original study used sources of data such as surveys, as well as church publications and women's magazines. There was a good deal of evidence that terms like 'repression' had become part of everyday vocabulary – people were using psychoanalysis to think about themselves and each other without appearing to do anything theoretical at all. This version of psychoanalysis, however, was a simplified one. Some terms like 'libido' had not found their way into the popular lexicon. The 'social representation' of psychoanalysis, then, is the simplified shared representation that is drawn on by ordinary people in everyday circumstances.

Thus Moscovici developed his own account of social representations, which included the following features: 'social representations are cognitive systems with a logic and language of their own . . . They do not represent simply "opinions about", "images of" or "attitudes towards" but "theories" or "branches of knowledge" in their own right, for the discovery and organisation of reality' (Moscovici 1973, p. xii). In addition,

> social representations concern the contents of everyday thinking and the stock of ideas that gives coherence to our religious beliefs, political ideas and the connections we create as spontaneously as we breathe. They make it possible for us to classify persons and objects, to compare and explain behaviours and to objectify them as parts of our social setting. While representations are often to be located in the minds of men and women, they can just as often be found 'in the world', and as such examined separately.
>
> (Moscovici 1988, p. 214)

Furthermore, Moscovici has claimed that social representations can also be described as

> systems of values, ideas and practices with a twofold function: first to establish an order which will enable individuals to orient themselves in their material and social world and to master it; and secondly to take place among the members of a community by providing them with a code for social exchange and a code for naming and classifying unambiguously the various aspects of their worlds and their individual and group history.
>
> (Moscovici 1973, p. xii)

Moscovici (1984, 1988) believed that human beings create a 'thinking society' within which social life is constructed and reconstructed. Representations have a changing, dynamic nature – 'social life in the making'. They are created, sustained and reconstructed by individuals and groups in everyday interaction.

> they lead a life of their own, circulate, merge, attract and repel each other, and give birth to new representations, while old ones die out . . . being shared by all and strengthened by tradition, it constitutes a social reality *sui generis*. The more its origin is forgotten, and its conventional nature ignored, the more fossilized it becomes. That which is ideal gradually becomes materialized.
>
> (Moscovici 1984, p. 13)

According to Moscovici, thinking is done in terms of two processes, anchoring and objectification. *Anchoring* occurs where a new or unfamiliar object is rendered familiar by means of comparing it with a prototype or model that is familiar and culturally accessible. If we decide the new stimuli are similar to the representation we already have, then we will attribute other characteristics of the prototype to them. The object can be readjusted so as to fit in with the prototype. 'The ascendancy of the test case is due . . . to its concreteness, to a kind of vividness which leaves such a deep imprint in our memory that we are able to use it thereafter as a "model" against which we measure individual cases and any image that even remotely resembles it' (Moscovici 1984, p. 32). In other words, giving things names assigns them a place in the societal identity matrix. For example in the UK, the 'model' of disability might be the widely used wheelchair symbol, or the 'model' terminal illness might be cancer or AIDS. These are the sorts of images or ideas that are most readily called to mind when the concept is mentioned.

Objectification is the process by which abstract and unfamiliar ideas are transformed into concrete and 'objective' commonsense reality. As Moscovici (1984) stated, 'To objectify is to discover the iconic quality of an imprecise idea or being, to reproduce a concept in an image' (p. 38). Thus, as a result of the popular appropriation of psychoanalysis, people might believe they have egos, complexes and neuroses. This process of objectification may involve:

1   *Personification.* For example, in the case of psychoanalysis, it might be personified perhaps by Freud. This can be seen at work in other health care disciplines, too, where operations, procedures, instruments and parts of the body come to be known by their originators' names. Fallopian tubes may be grasped with Spencer Wells forceps, for example.

2   *Figuration* occurs where an abstract notion is identified with a metaphorical image. For example, when Moscovici and Hewstone (1983) asked about people's ideas of the European Community, responses came in terms of butter mountains and wine lakes.

3   *Ontologization.* This is where abstract entities and hypothetical constructs are treated as if they were material entities. In health care, we can see this at work where suffering participants come to see their illness as having a real existence, or where healers or sufferers come to define their distress in terms of something that sounds concrete and scientific. Diffuse facial and jawbone pains, once defined as trigeminal neuralgia, take on a much more real quality and, arguably, are more easily dealt with. Furthermore, once it is proposed that the sufferer have an operation to coat the offending nerve in teflon, to prevent it being irritated by surrounding blood vessels, the idea takes on yet another kind of ontologization as something susceptible to technological intervention and possibly cure.

Thus, the general drift of this kind of theorizing is that people will very often be thinking in terms of concrete phenomena, rather than more abstract ones, as a result of these processes of personification, figuration and ontologization.

A number of topics relating to health and illness have been investigated through the framework of social representations theory. Let us review a few examples of this variety of research, as it has something to tell us about the way that concept formulations of health and illness, ideas of the body and their conceptual folkways are constructed, formulated and deployed in everyday explanation.

Our first example of a domain of thinking about the body that has been studied with a view to discerning the social representations involved is the idea of left and right hemispheric specialization in the brain (Moscovici and Hewstone 1983). The pioneering work of Roger Sperry (1913–1994) on 'split brain' patients, for which he earned the Nobel Prize, had placed these issues on the scientific and popular agenda. However, what is equally interesting is how these ideas found their way into everyday language. Here, laypeople can talk readily about which of the hemispheres does what, for example the idea of language in the left, with intuition, emotion and subjective functions allegedly being located in the right. This 'cerebral dualism' is sometimes used in popular parlance to explain a number of other 'dilemmatic' cultural themes, for example femininity versus masculinity, reason versus intuition, even the epithets 'left brained' and 'right brained' used to describe reasoning, strategies for problem solving and styles of living. These concept formulations, then, have a life far in excess of their original formulation in neurology and may appear in a variety of popular discourses about such things as stress, lifestyle and gender. In a sense, the liveliness of the concept formulations occurs because they have long since been liberated from Sperry's laboratory and can take their place in the popular lexicon.

A second example concerns mental health and the idea of madness. This is an especially interesting one because mental ill-health has proved to be especially enigmatic and, despite the efforts of biologically oriented researchers, there are relatively few reliable pegs on which to hang the phenomena in question. In her book *Madness and Social Representations*, Jodelet (1991) describes how people thought about mental illness in a small French community, Ainay-Le-Chateau, where care in the community dates back to the early years of the twentieth century and mentally ill people are housed with 'foster families' as 'lodgers'. As she interviewed people about what they thought 'madness' was about, they would often begin with 'mental illness, I don't know about that' (p. 149). Yet they would also be able to say a great deal about the lodgers and their problems. In particular, the interviewees were often concerned with issues of dirt and contamination. However, in talking about their lodgers' dirtiness, informants also expressed a good deal of loyalty towards them:

> dirtiness seemed to siphon off the major part of the negativity of insanity and is a less disturbing manifestation of the illness than others. Ultimately it is reassuring. One then begins to understand the foster parent who declared, 'a bad lodger is a dirty lodger' and then told us of her oldest one, 'He's been with me for twenty-seven years. He's not bad at all. I'm not frightened of him'. Of course, 'He's dirty I could kill him sometimes. Every day he goes in his trousers'. To have to wash a pair of trousers every day for twenty-seven years! But 'He's not wicked. That's what I'm afraid of I would hate to change. I would prefer to put up with it'. Dirtiness which is due to illness is unthreatening. That alone makes it worth

putting up with, whatever unpleasantness that entails, provided that it does not exceed a limit of revulsion which appears to be quite high.

(Jodelet 1991, pp. 143–4)

Dirtiness, then, could be used to justify the lodger having separate meals from the rest of the family – it was not through prejudice or fear but matters of taste and hygiene.

In the same way, their professed lack of knowledge about mental illness is a strategy for managing the potential threat posed by mental illness: 'It was as if by becoming the object of an explicit knowledge or formulation the power of mental illness to generate anxiety would be released' (Jodelet 1991, p. 150).

The concepts in use here appear to facilitate a particular conceptual and practical way of dealing with the phenomenon. The determined reluctance to formally conceptualize the phenomenon in question is itself a kind of strategy to manage the issue. The absence of concept formulations which explicitly address the symptoms of mental disorder may in itself be an interesting research phenomenon. Sometimes the absence of concepts, or the deflection of the issue by other concept formulations that address different aspects, might, paradoxically, yield a more functional way of dealing with the issue.

However, there are several examples of issues relating to mental health being described much more explicitly by the participants in research designed to elicit the everyday concept formulations of the phenomena. For example, to investigate the 'social representations' of madness in India, Wagner et al. (1999) provided their participants with a brief hypothetical description of a young person who had started behaving strangely and asked participants a series of questions about what they thought the problem might be and what they might do if a member of their own family behaved in this way, whether they would consult a traditional healer or a psychiatrist and if so what would be done. The participants tended to explain the events in terms of (1) family norms and adjustment, (2) ideas of heredity and its moral threat to the family, as well as (3) ideas of ghost or spirit possession:

1   Family issues included such explanations as 'any of his demands was not fulfilled, internally suffocated he wants something, some desire was suppressed inside this can also be a cause' (R33, F) (p. 425). Or, speaking of a case he knew of, another respondent said, 'Yes, there was a famous story about him. Some girl had cheated him in love. He was a fertilizer engineer and the girl's love for him was based on sex. After that her father did not agree to the marriage. He left his job and became mad' (R18, M) (p. 426).

2   The idea of family issues was also prominent in the second theme, but in a slightly different way as this related to notions of heredity and contagion: 'I know such families which have a mentally ill person [among them] and the behaviour of the villagers towards them [families] is not good. People say that he is mad. The second thing is that in villages there is a concept, that if there is one who is mentally ill in a family, the other members will also be mentally ill for sure, because there is a big contribution of the family in making a person mentally ill' (R15, M) (p. 427).

3   The third theme, of ghost and spirit possession, was curious in several ways. Few interviewees admitted to believing in this themselves, though many others said that it is a commonplace belief in their neighbourhood. 'I can only say that there is some invisible power, a ghost possessed him, which was treated by sacred words. Sacred words have power' (R22, M).

'*Interviewer*: Sir, do you think that those people who are possessed by a ghost cannot be treated by a psychiatrist?

Respondent: No they cannot treat this, only the traditional healer can treat them. These things are out of his [the psychiatrist's] reach' (R22, M) (pp. 430–1).

Thus, concept formulations and social representations are often concerned with the kinds of tools for thinking which participants might use themselves, but they are also concerned with what other people might think; perhaps, as in this case, people who are seen as less advanced and somehow more superstitious. The conceptual machinery is all present and in working order but it is as if the participants do not quite fully endorse it. Thus, sometimes people can appear to be aware of a variety of different possible formulations which might explain events. This theme of diversity and flexibility in terms of the way people might deploy concepts is an important one and we shall return to this later. As well as being able to display this flexibility, it may be that people are aware of the persuasive consequences of adopting one concept formulation rather than another, and of thinking in terms of concrete examples from their own experience or from that of people in their neighbourhood.

There are a number of aspects of the health and illness theme that have been investigated to examine the kinds of concepts and representations which people hold. In a classic study. Herzlich (1973) conducted a series of interviews to determine how middle-class people in France thought of health and illness. Again, there were a number of common themes detectable in the results:

1   The urban way of life was thought to be responsible for a number of complaints, for example because it resulted in fatigue and nervous tension. Food in cities was not considered to be trustworthy either.

2   Illness came from the external environment, whereas the individual was the source of health and healing. In this respect, the social representation of health was rather like the vitalistic notions of the eighteenth and early nineteenth century we mentioned earlier.

3   The individual and his or her relationship with illness was structured around a number of binary oppositions such as internal versus external, healthy versus unhealthy, urban versus rural, natural versus unnatural, individual versus society. For example, in the present day, food advertising often represents rural environments, crops and livestock, rather than the factory setting in which many foodstuffs are manufactured.

4   In Herzlich's study, illnesses themselves were not classified along the same lines as within medicine, but were constructed along lines that were concerned with severity, with whether or not it was painful, the duration of the illness and the nature of its onset.

Whereas this sketch of social representations and some of the work that has been done to elicit the representations groups of people are using to interpret the field of health and illness might seem persuasive, as befits a book with a philosophical bent, we should point out some problems with the idea and the research on which it is based.

First, as Potter and Edwards (1999) argue, social representations theory is primarily about perception and cognition and does not have much to say about action. Potter and Edwards argue that action is central to people's lives and involves the 'enormous range of practical, technical and interpersonal tasks that people perform while living their relationships, doing their jobs, and engaging in various cultural domains' (p. 448). Thus, social representations theory leaves out a substantial amount of human activity and practice.

Second, in social representations theory, the notion of representation is crucial, but these representations are rather passive entities. On the other hand, Potter and Edwards argue that representations in everyday discourse are often highly contrived and constructed entities, as people build their representations through language to persuade, assign blame, elicit agreement and so forth. Language, in other words, is about doing social business, in a way that Wittgenstein would have appreciated, rather than simply representing things. This is partly why we have chosen the term concept formulation, because we wish to alert the reader to the way that conceptualizing things is an active, strategic process and may involve selecting and promoting courses of action too.

Third, social representations theory foregrounds communication, but it does not address the actual communicative process in very much detail. Moscovici disparages conversation as 'babble'. In practice, it is very difficult to examine, say, the transcript of a conversation and see where the messages relating to a particular representation are and how they are being transferred. The representations have a kind of ghostly presence behind the transcript of an interview or a naturally occurring conversation and this prompts sceptics such as Potter and Edwards to ask whether they are instead impositions on the part of the researcher.

Fourth, the emphasis on cognition in social representations theory has made it attractive to social psychologists, because it assumes that people are information processors, storers and retrievers, just like cognitive psychology and philosophy of mind from the 1960s to the present. However, Potter and Edwards say that maybe there is more to cognition than this image of people as information processors allows. Perhaps cognition might instead be going on in conversational interaction as people formulate thoughts, memories, feelings and intuitions – and maybe even concepts – jointly through interpersonal processes. It may not be the case that cognitions neatly live inside someone's head in any simple sense.

So, to assess what this all means for making sense of health care research, health care practice and how to think about these issues, we shall pause to assess what can be learned from this approach. For example, we might deduce that arguments work best if they are ontologized and exemplified with things that the people concerned find easy to visualize or think of as entities. It also tells us, if we step back slightly, that this is a way of making sense of thinking processes themselves. Whereas it has largely been used with everyday concepts, it could also be used with more esoteric concepts in health care and could even go some way towards addressing the problem of studying expertise that we identified above.

Lay theories and everyday explanations

A related strand of work which aims to elicit the kinds of concepts that people hold concerning health and illness is that of 'lay theories'. As the name suggests, this involves a systematic investigation of the sorts of folk theories which are likely to be held by the layperson. This area of work has been contributed largely by Adrian Furnham and colleagues (e.g. Furnham 1988; Furnham and Cheng 2000; Furnham and Murao 2000; Furnham *et al.* 2001), but a number of other researchers have entered the fray to discover the cognitive structure of everyday concepts, beliefs, theories and explanations.

To give a flavour of this kind of research as it impacts on concepts relevant to health, let us consider a paper by Mercado-Martinez and Ramos-Herrera (2002) concerning lay beliefs about diabetes in Mexico. Among their sample of Mexican diabetics, it was clear that their theories about how their condition had started did not correspond with current medical thinking. Participants tended to attribute their condition to social and emotional circumstances linked to life events and experiences, with men tending to focus on work and social circumstances outside the home, while women tended to mention family life and their domestic settings. This was rather different to the kinds of explanations for diabetes reported in the English-speaking world, where people's explanations tend to incorporate more contemporary bio-medical thinking. According to Garro (1995) and Kay (1979), Anglophone sufferers were likely to attribute diabetes to food, diet heredity and stress. Moreover, in South America, people have been noted to believe that diabetes is a result of an episode of fright (*susto*) (Rubel *et al.* 1992). Although Mercado-Martinez and Ramos-Herrera's (2002) participants did not specifically mention the idea of fright, they were in many cases concerned that drinking while in an intense emotional state – anger, surprise, fear or suffering – had brought on diabetes.

From investigations such as this, it is claimed by some critics of the health care system that it would be beneficial if health care providers were to move away from an authoritative role as providers of information and knowledge and instead search for a model that incorporates the voices, concepts and concerns of the diverse social actors who are involved in the process of health care (Hunt *et al.* 1998). That is, it is felt from this perspective that perhaps things would be better if all parties participated in the construction of alternatives. In the case of diabetes in Mexico, in particular, the authors believed that including the perspectives of poor individuals who attribute their illnesses to their material, economic and emotional circumstances might have a dramatic effect on the provision of health care in Mexico and, indeed, the rest of the world.

Concept formulations, then, can be seen as powerful agents of change. They may reflect the voices, world-views and economic interests of sections of society, some of whom may have hitherto been systematically marginalized in health care research and practice. Thus, the study of lay theories of health and illness, which often begins as a psychological enquiry, may lead to sociological issues and from there to political and ethical concerns.

The question of where the various lay theories or concepts of a health issue will lead is even more acute when we look at the situation within the UK. As the diversity of cultures, experiences and world-views intermingle, this presents enormous challenges in providing a health care system that is geared to the diversity of the population. In addition, when we consider how this culturally diverse population is also shot through with inequality, racism and misogyny, the problems appear even more intractable. If we take the issue of mental health, it is worth noting that this is one area where there has been acute controversy. Let us illustrate the issue by looking at the disproportionate number of young black men who are diagnosed as suffering from schizophrenia (Harrison et al. 1984; Jones and Gray 1986; Lewis et al. 1990). There are concerns that this over-representation of young black men in this category may result from the attitudes and values of psychiatrists (Lewis et al. 1990), or that the kinds of experiences and practices of this group, particularly of a religious nature, place them at risk of being diagnosed with schizophrenia when judged against a white, middle-class, Euro-American nosological system (Kiev 1964; Pote and Orrell 2002). Indeed, in Kiev's classic study in the early 1960s, of 100 Afro-Caribbean youths questioned, almost all had some experience of religious or magical experiences that could be called 'delusional' when judged against psychiatric criteria. In the light of these concerns, Pote and Orrell (2002) examined the ideas of different ethnic groups in the UK about mental health and illness in a study of lay representations in an ethnically and culturally diverse sample. Compared with the white population, participants of Bangladeshi origin were less likely to identify suspiciousness or hallucinations as signs of mental illness and people of Afro-Caribbean origin were the least likely to view unusual thought content as indicative of mental illness. This difference between people of Afro-Caribbean origin and the majority white population, the authors argued, is important in making sense of the former's higher rate of diagnosis. Moreover, if a client's and psychiatrist's fundamental concepts of mental disorder differ, it will be that much more difficult for productive therapeutic alliances to be formed. Indeed, by looking at case notes, Johnson and Orrell (1996) detected that psychiatrists were much more likely to say that their white patients had 'insight' whereas their black ones did not. This was independent of the severity of symptoms and reflects, the authors surmised, the differing world-views of mental illness held by psychiatry on the one hand and the Afro-Caribbean population on the other. Thus, looking at the concepts held by different groups in the arena of health care could have some important implications for how we address clients themselves and how we address the larger-scale structure of health inequalities within which they are embedded.

The reader might wish to contrast this example with the case of cranial osteopathy we mentioned earlier. There, the fact that the practitioner and the clients seemed to be at loggerheads in terms of how they conceptualized what was going on didn't seem to matter. Indeed, it might have even made the social business of therapy easier. In the case of psychiatry and ethnicity though, it appears that the lack of commonality between the service providers and some client groups may contribute to the latter's disadvantage in the mental health care system. Certainly, there is a good deal of literature to suggest that consensus and coherence is an important issue. For example, Kitson (1993) argued that the best concepts are those which result when 'all the different concepts of a thing coincide'. Certainly, this might make communication easier but is consensus always a good thing? What if the young black men diagnosed with schizophrenia and those who cared for them shared the same concept formulations as the largely white psychiatric establishment? What if they believed that they were indeed mad and required treatment? A lack of consensus perhaps offers the possibility that concepts might be formulated differently and less oppressively.

What does it mean for us? Philosophy and research in practice

After having considered all these different ideas that have impacted on the conceptualization of nature, the formulation of research questions, research design and making sense of the results, it is appropriate to examine what it means for our lives as researchers, practitioners and theorists.

One of the important features of present-day life is that it is often possible to detect intriguing contradictions between different belief systems, moralities, styles of life and compartments of experience. To make sense of this and explain what it means in more detail, let us take some examples from our own lifeworlds as scholars and citizens to help identify some of these disjunctures and contradictions. Thus, let us consider what we three authors think we are doing as we conduct research, attempt to get it published, and sustain positions in UK universities.

One of us, Brian Brown, is in his spare time an amateur engineer and metallurgist as well as a would-be performance artist, yet in his academic life he describes himself as a 'nosebleed antifoundationalist' and subscribes to analytic positions that challenge the very physical substrate on which he works. His experiments with physical materials and objects are motivated by a kind of curiosity as to the kinds of forces they will sustain, yet the emotional and perceptual effects on the audience are important too. In his exhibition work as an artist, he tries to create visual effects with architectural materials that mix up the audience and juxtapose things that are usually seen in different parts of buildings and include images of rejuvenation with images of decay. Doing research and getting things published is about playing a kind of game whose rules are largely opaque but which are implemented by people like journal editors and referees as well as people on RAE panels, all of whom have to be satisfied, but at the same time it is important to install something of oneself in published work too. Especially if it is an idea which is subversive or which has not appeared in print before. There is a great deal of satisfaction to be had in smuggling things past the gatekeepers.

Carolyn Hicks, who has perhaps been the most successful academically, being the only one of the three of us to have achieved a professorship, has this to say about the relationship between her work as a researcher and her awareness of philosophy:

> I could not honestly say that the philosophical principles underpinning the scientific method consciously impinge on my research activities. Despite my theoretical commitment to Popper's theory of falsification, my aim usually is to find support for the hypothesis; I certainly rarely think of submitting an article for publication unless I have significant results. In view of this mismatch, there is a clear dissonance between my values, what I do and what I say. I have been

pressured by the RAE to publish, publish, publish and seduced by the implicit journal rules that state that publication is more likely if the results are significant. Therefore, because I am bound by the political, organizational and occupational contexts that place these demands on academics, I do exactly the opposite of what Popper would claim is the real route to truth. I am therefore subverting the proper scientific process and my own principles to boot. There is also, of course, the human need for affirmation. To proceed down the route towards falsification is a negative human experience, even if it is ultimately positive for scientific truth. Despite my constant reassurances to my postgraduate students that getting non-significant results is just as valuable as getting significant ones, their anxiety about obtaining support for the hypothesis is a constant reminder that despite all Popper's logic, it doesn't hold much sway for the researcher, and especially the novice researcher. Indeed, my experience suggests that obtaining non-significant results can act as a serious deterrent to conducting any more research. In an era of evidence-based health care, where the corpus of sound research needed to inform all levels and types of practice is woefully inadequate, this would seem to be counterproductive. It is philosophical dilemma, with philosophy and health/academic research seemingly serving two different masters.

Another of us, Paul Crawford, has a variety of different backgrounds. A one-time trainee Roman Catholic priest, he has also been a nurse and is a novelist who is currently working in fields as diverse as nursing, English literature and journalism. One of his pieces of fiction may soon become a film or television drama. Again, this diversity of interests brings with it new insights as well as frustrations. He is constrained by the needs of the nursing degree curriculum in a university context but at the same time is attracted to teaching literature, developing new courses exploiting new media. Overall, the need to attract external funding if one is to succeed these days in a UK university is a powerful one and seems to be the key to career advancement and promotion.

These brief biographical fragments of what we do and how we sustain our lives in the UK university context are also tempered by the increase in student numbers, the sight of so many of our colleagues becoming ill with stress-related cardiovascular disorders and the difficulty in coping with increasing numbers of directives from within both the university system and the health care system. The difficulty in putting down roots and making links with other bodies such as health care providers and service users is complicated even further by the high turnover of personnel and the frequent reorganizations. One of Brown's PhD students has seen the health care organizations she is studying transform out of all recognition in the space of three years. This, then, places additional constraints on the kinds of research we can do. Yet at the same time it opens up opportunities for research designs and forms of understanding that have yet to be invented.

Despite all this disruption and fragmentation, it appears to us that the ideology of the health care services remains relentlessly modernist and continues to be dominated by medically trained practitioners and researchers whose perspective on life is usually modernist too. It is easy to gain the impression that as far as they are concerned, theirs is the only truth; that they are the ones with the privileged expert knowledge base; and that their preferred methodology is the scientific one. In other words, health care and health care research still have a prevailing ethos that there is only one view and only one true, objective perspective. On the other hand, nursing, along with the other non-medical professions, embraces the notion of multiple perspectives more readily and, in this way, is certainly more postmodernist than the medical professions. This predilection for multiple perspectives and methodologies also challenges more readily the grand narrative of the medical profession. Two of us (B.B. and C.H.) were originally taught in the modernist scientific spirit and have more or less wandered off the path. From an early attachment to the scientific method, C.H. has moved to a multiple methodology and multiple-perspective viewpoint, going for method triangulation where possible, because she believes it provides the richest picture and the most accurate information. B.B. disputes that anything can be 'accurate' in any simple sense because the notion of accuracy itself is subject to judgement and relies on very many assumptions and taken-for-granteds concerning how the world should be conceptualized, seen and measured. Thus, he would see the knowledge creation process itself as a topic of enquiry. In this view, the interesting things about nature are created by humans doing things together, rather than simply heating things and hammering them.

All three of us would probably agree that experience cannot easily be quantified or broken down into fragments about which one can generate meaningful hypotheses or collect numerical data, because it is too varied, complicated and subjective. Yet it is this very experience that seems to provide the insights and explanations needed to interpret the quantitative data that we generate. The process of making the numbers mean something is much more difficult to explain. So, in some ways our own research approaches fit neatly with the postmodernist agenda, though we have not necessarily moved in that direction because postmodernism was persuasive, but rather because of the circumstances within which we work and an affinity with the belief that in complex systems there can be multiple solutions and answers and, therefore, our understanding may be enriched if we use multiple approaches.

It is also apposite to consider whether there are any implications here for teaching the value of a philosophical approach to research in the academy, the clinic, the community or on a training course. In a sense, people are adroit at adjudicating between competing truth claims. An exercise one of us (B.B.) sometimes uses with students is to say to them, 'A funny thing happened to me yesterday. I saw a flying saucer and the aliens came out and abducted me and took me back into the spaceship and did experiments on me and stuck probes in my you-know-what. Now if someone said that to you, would you believe it?' Most people say no. Then we attempt to generate some discussion as to why this is a difficult thing to believe, what would make it convincing (part of the spaceship perhaps?) and what other explanations there are for this kind of experience. The aim is to mobilize and examine the kinds of folk epistemologies that students bring to the educational encounter. In this way, we are perhaps coming close to the educational process that Northrop Frye envisaged:

> The teacher, as has been recognized at least since Plato's Meno, is not primarily someone who knows instructing someone who does not know. He [sic] is rather someone who attempts to re-create the subject in the student's mind, and

his strategy in doing this is first of all to get the student to recognize what he already potentially knows, which includes breaking up the powers of repression in his mind that keep him from knowing what he knows.

(Frye 1982, p. xv)

Part of generating this kind of philosophical awareness on the part of students and beginning researchers, then, is to get them to recognize what they are already doing in evaluating knowledge, making inferences and creating credible stories of their own.

One of the fundamental techniques that underlies traditional variants of positivism and falsificationism and has also played a key role in realist and postmodernist philosophies, is reformulating what we know as a set of questions or problems that we can then go on to solve. Whether we treat these as research questions from which we can deduce testable hypotheses or use them as more speculative thought experiments – as 'what if' and 'as if' statements – will play a key role in our enquiry. Getting people to think of the world around them in terms of questions is perhaps the breakthrough that turns them into thinkers. This centrality of questions to the educational and research processes has been recognized by other thinkers on educational topics too. Here is Neil Postman, writing in his book *Teaching as a Conserving Activity*:

all our knowledge results from questions, which is another way of saying that question-asking is our most important intellectual tool. I would go so far as to say that the answers we carry about in our heads are largely meaningless unless we know the questions which produced them . . . What, for example, are the sorts of questions that obstruct the mind, or free it, in the study of history? How are these questions different from those one might ask of a mathematical proof, or a literary work, or a biological theory? What students need to know are the rules of discourse which comprise the subject, and among the most central of such rules are those which govern what is and what is not a legitimate question.

(Postman 1979, p. 23)

In other words, it is not so much the solutions we come up with but the kinds of questions we ask that creates us as thinkers. Thus, the ability to turn experience into questions is the hallmark of the kind of mindset we are trying to convey. Perhaps among these final words it would be apposite to quote the late C. Wright Mills, who had a firm grasp on the possibilities inherent in human enquiry. What he had to say about sociological research has a good deal in common with what we are encouraging:

Neither the life of an individual nor the history of a society can be understood without understanding both. Yet men [*sic*] do not usually define the troubles they endure in terms of historical change and institutional contradiction . . . The sociological imagination enables its possessor to understand the larger historical scene in terms of its meaning for the inner life and the external career of a variety of individuals . . . The first fruit of this imagination – and the first lesson of the social science that embodies it – is the idea that the individual can understand his own experience and gauge his own fate only by locating himself within this period, that he can know his own chances in life only by becoming aware of those of all individuals in his circumstances . . . We have come to know that every individual lives, from one generation to the next, in some society; that he lives out a biography, and that he lives it out within some historical sequence.

(Mills 1959, pp. 3–10)

The details of individual experience and individual biographies, from heart transplants to ingrowing toenails, and from mild disaffection to florid psychosis, are intelligible in this view if we examine the context and look at the experience as part of an individual's biography. They also become understandable if we step back and look at them in the general context of the society and the culture where the troubles are taking place. In this way, perhaps the experience of ill health can be made meaningful by the researcher and hence to the sufferer too. The concluding words concerning what we are trying to advocate within health care research should perhaps go to Arthur Kleinman (1988; Schweizer 1995), taken from his book *The Illness Narratives*:

clinical and behavioural science research . . . possess no category to describe suffering, no routine way of recording this most thickly human dimension of patients' and families' stories of experiencing illness. Symptom scales and survey questionnaires and behavioural checklists quantify functional impairment and disability, rendering the quality of life fungible.

(Kleinman 1988, p. 17)

Medical – or even nursing – categories however are woefully insufficient to account for the experience of illness:

[A]bout suffering they are silent. The thinned out image of patients and families which perforce must emerge from such research is scientifically replicable but ontologically invalid; it has statistical, not epistemological significance; it is a dangerous distortion.

(Kleinman 1988, p. 17)

Kleinman himself, as a practitioner, sees his job as to *delay* the naming of the illness so as to 'legitimiz[e] the patient's illness experience – authorizing that experience, auditing it empathetically' (p. 17). Indeed, 'we should be willing to stop at that point where validity becomes uncertain' (p. 74).

Or, as one of the major twentieth-century thinkers who tried to understand inhumanity and suffering, Theodor Adorno puts it, capturing a final paradox:

Reason can subsume suffering under concepts, it can furnish means to alleviate suffering; but it can never express suffering in the medium of experience, for to do so would be irrational by reason's own standards. Therefore, even when it is understood, suffering remains mute and inconsequential.

(Adorno 1984, p. 27)

There is a great deal yet to be understood.

References

Abbott, S., Johnson, L. and Lewis, H. (2001) Participation in arranging continuing health care packages: experiences and aspirations of service users, *Journal of Nursing Management*, 9: 79–85.

Adorno, T.W. (1984) *Aesthetic Theory* (translated by C. Lenhardt). London: Routledge.

Aspis, S. (1997) Self-advocacy for people with learning difficulties: does it have a future?, *Disability and Society*, 12(4): 501–11.

Benner, P. (1982) Issues in competency-based testing, *Nursing Outlook*, May, pp. 303–9.

Benner, P. (1984) *From Novice to Expert: Excellence and Power in Clinical Nursing*. Menlo Park, CA: Addison-Wesley.

Benner, P. (1992) *From Beginner to Expert: Clinical Knowledge in Critical Care Nursing*. Athens, OH: Fuld Institute for Technology in Nursing Education (video).

Benner, P. and Tanner, C. (1987) Clinical judgement: how expert nurses use intuition, *American Journal of Nursing*, 87(1): 23–31.

Benner, P. and Wrubel, J. (1989) *The Primacy of Caring Stress and Coping in Health and Illness*. Menlo Park, CA: Addison-Wesley.

Bonner, G., Lowe, T., Rawcliffe, D. and Wellman, N. (2002) Trauma for all: a pilot study of the subjective experience of physical restraint for mental health inpatients and staff in the UK, *Journal of Psychiatric and Mental Health Nursing*, 8: 465–73.

Carper, B. (1978) Fundamental patterns of knowing in nursing, *Advances in Nursing Science*, 1(1): 13–23.

Darling, H. (1995) Satisfying a hunger: a personal journey of self discovery through further nursing education, *Nursing Praxis*, 10(1): 12–21.

Davies, D. (2000) Sex and the relationship facilitation project for people with disabilities, *Sexuality and Disability*, 18(3): 187–94.

Dreyfus, H.L. (1979) *What Computers Can't Do*. New York: Harper & Row.

Dreyfus, H.L. and Dreyfus, S.E. (1985) *Mind Over Machine: The Power of Human Intuition and Expertise in the Era of the Computer*. New York: Free Press/Macmillan.

Frye, N. (1982) *The Great Code: The Bible and Literature*. New York: Harcourt Brace & Co.

Furnham, A. (1988) *Lay Theories: Everyday Understanding of Problems in the Social Sciences*. Oxford: Pergamon Press.

Furnham, A. and Cheng, H. (2000) Lay theories of happiness, *Journal of Happiness Studies*, 1(2): 227–46.

Furnham, A. and Murao, M. (2000) A cross cultural comparison of British and Japanese lay theories of schizophrenia, *International Journal of Social Psychiatry*, 46(1): 4–20.

Furnham, A., Pereira, E. and Rawles, R. (2001) Lay theories of psychotherapy: perceptions of the efficacy of different cures for specific disorders, *Psychology, Health and Medicine*, 6(1): 77–84.

Gardner, H. (1983) *Frames of Mind: The Theory of Multiple Intelligences*. London: Heinemann.

Garro, L. (1995) Individual or societal responsibility? Explanations of diabetes in an Anishinaabe (Ojibway) community, *Social Science and Medicine*, 40(1): 37–46.

Gerth, H. and Mills, C.W. (1964) *Character and Social Structure*. New York: Harbinger.

Goffman, E. (1961) *Asylums*. New York: Anchor.

Harrison, G., Ineichen, B., Smith, J. and Morgan, H.G. (1984) Psychiatric hospital admissions in Bristol. II. Social and clinical aspects of compulsory admission, *British Journal of Psychiatry*, 145: 605–11.

Herzlich, C. (1973) *Health and Illness: A Social Psychological Analysis*. London: Academic Press.

Holden, D. and Smart, D. (1999) Adding value to the patient experience in emergency medicine: what features of the emergency department visit are most important to patients?, *Emergency Medicine*, 1: 3–8.

Hunt, L., Valenzuela, M. and Pugh, J. (1998) *Porque me toco a mi*? Mexican American diabetes patients' causal stories and their relationship to treatment behaviours, *Social Science and Medicine*, 46: 959–69.

Jodelet, D. (1991) *Madness and Social Representations*. Hemel Hempstead: Harvester Wheatsheaf.

Johns, C. (1995a) The value of reflective practice for nursing, *Journal of Clinical Nursing*, 4(1): 23–30.

Johns, C. (1995b) Framing learning through reflection with Carper's fundamental ways of knowing in nursing, *Journal of Advanced Nursing*, 22(2): 226–34.

Johnson, S. and Orrell, M. (1996) Insight, psychosis and ethnicity: a case note study, *Psychological Medicine*, 26: 1081–4.

Jones, B.E. and Gray, B.A. (1986) Problems in diagnosing schizophrenia and affective disorders amongst blacks, *Hospital and Community Psychiatry*, 37: 61–5.

Kay, M. (1979) Health and illness in a Mexican American barrio, in E. Spicer (ed.) *Ethnic Medicine in the Southwest*. Tuscon, AZ: University of Arizona Press.

Kiev, A. (1964) *Magic, Faith and Healing*. New York: Free Press.

Kitson, A. (ed.) (1993) *Nursing Art and Science*. London: Chapman & Hall.

Kleinman, A. (1988) *The Illness Narratives: Suffering, Healing and the Human Condition*. New York: Basic Books.

Lathlean, J. and Vaughan, B. (1994) *Unifying Nursing Practice and Theory*. Oxford: Butterworth Heinemann.

Lewis, G., Croft Jeffreys, C. and David, A. (1990) Are British psychiatrists racist?, *British Journal of Psychiatry*, 157: 410–15.

Lumby, J. (1991) Threads of an emerging discipline: praxis, reflection, rhetoric and research, in G. Gray and R. Pratt (eds) *Towards a Discipline of Nursing*. Melbourne, VIC: Churchill-Livingstone.

Mercado-Martinez, F.J. and Ramos-Herrera, I.M. (2002) Diabetes: the layperson's theories of causality, *Qualitative Health Research*, 12(6): 792–806.

Mills, C.W. (1959) *The Sociological Imagination*. New York: Oxford University Press.

Moscovici, S. (1973) Foreword, in C. Herzlich, *Health and Illness: A Social Psychological Analysis*. London: Academic Press.

Moscovici, S. (1976) *La Psychoanalyse: Son Image et Son Public* (revised edition). Paris: Presses Universitaires de France.

Moscovici, S. (1984) The phenomenon of social representations, in R.M. Farr and S. Moscovici (eds) *Social Representations*. Cambridge/Paris: Cambridge University Press/ Maison des Sciences de l'Homme.

Moscovici, S. (1988) Notes towards a description of social representations, *European Journal of Social Psychology*, 18: 211–80.

Moscovici, S. and Hewstone, M. (1983) Social representations and social explanation: from the naive to the amateur scientist, in M. Hewstone (ed.) *Attribution Theory: Social and Functional Extensions*. Oxford: Blackwell.

Paterson, B. (1991) *Excellence and Expertise in Nursing*. Melbourne, VIC: Deakin University Press.

Peplau, H. (1952) *Interpersonal Relations in Nursing*. New York: GP Putnam's Sons.

Popper, K.R. ([1935] 1959) *The Logic of Scientific Discovery*. London: Hutchinson.

Postman, N. (1979) *Teaching as a Conserving Activity*. New York: Bantam Dell Doubleday.

Pote, H.L. and Orrell, M.W. (2002) Perceptions of schizophrenia in multi-cultural Britain, *Ethnicity and Health*, 7(1): 7–20.

Potter, J. and Edwards, D. (1999) Social representations and discursive psychology: from cognition to action, *Culture and Psychology*, 5(4): 447–58.

Rew, L. (1988) Intuition in decision making, *Image: The Journal of Nursing Scholarship*, 20(3): 150–4.

Rosen, R.D. (1977) *Psychobabble: Fast Talk and Quick Cure in the Era of Feeling*. New York: Athaneum Press.

Rubel, A., O'Nell, C. and Collado, R. (1992) *Introduccion al susto*, in R. Campos (ed.) *La anthropologia medicia en Mexico*. Mexico: Instituto Mora/Universidad Autonoma Metropolitana.

Schraeder, B. and Fischer, D. (1986) Using intuitive knowledge to make clinical decisions, *Maternal Child Nursing*, 2: 161–2.

Schweizer, H. (1995) To give suffering a language, *Literature and Medicine*, 14(2): 210–21.

Wagner, W., Duveen, G., Themel, M. and Verma, J. (1999) The modernisation of tradition: thinking about madness in Patna, India, *Culture and Psychology*, 5(4): 413–45.

Warelow, P. (1997) A nursing journey through discursive praxis, *Journal of Advanced Nursing*, 26(6): 1020–7.

White, J. (1995) Patterns of knowing: review, critique, and update, *Advances in Nursing Science*, 17(4): 73–86.

Wilkes, L. (1991) Phenomenology: a window to the nursing world, in G. Gray and R. Pratt (eds) *Towards a Discipline of Nursing*. Melbourne, VIC: Churchill Livingstone.

Index

acquaintance knowledge, 20
actor network theory, 64–6
Advanced Nurse Practitioner, 162
advice giving, 227–8
Aggressive Research Intelligence Facility
    (ARIF), 85
AIDS, thalidomide, 96
Alexander, Franz, hypertension, 67
alternation as allocation means, 127
ambiguous genitalia, 203
anatomy of human body, 10–16,
    161–2
  Descartes, René, 13, 15
  Fallopius, Gabriele, 13
  Galen, 14, 16
  Gray's Anatomy, 13–14
  Hippocrates, 14, 16
  Hume, David, 16
  Leonardo Da Vinci, 12–15
  Locke, John, 16
  Michelangelo, 12
  Vesalius, Andreas, 14–15
anchoring, 270
anorexia, 131
anti-foundationalism, 237
antipsychiatry, 242
Aristotle
  heavenly bodies, 10–11
  induction, 21
Asch's Central Trait Theory, 121
asthma, 238
astronomy, 10–12
asylum, Tuke, 51

attention deficit hyperactivity disorder
    (ADHD), 247, 252
  Ritalin, 247
auras, 235
autobiography and self-conceptualization,
    203–5
Ayer, A.J., 42
  basic statements, 26

Bacon, Francis, knowledge is power, 22, 239
Bacon, Roger, lenses, 11
bad news delivery, 225–7, 237
Bakhtin, M.M., grotesque body, 250–1
Baudrillard, J.
  melancholy, 246
  reality, 239–40
  symptoms, 252
Becker, Howard, 199–200, 206
  Boys in White, 212–13
  ethnography, 210
Beddoe, John, phrenology, 218–19
behaviour, explanation, 194–5
Bell Laboratories, 102
Bennett, Deborah, randomization, 146–7
Benviste, Jacques, water with memory, 235
Berkeley, Bishop
  perception, 201
  perception theories, 21–2
Bernard, Claude, 29
  laboratory work, 2
  organ systems, 2
Bertillion, Alphonse, 28
Bhaskar, Roy, realism, 5

bias sources in research, 120–2
  Asch's Central Trait Theory, 121
  Research Assessment Exercise, 121–2
biomedical reductionism, 4
Biotechnology and Biological Sciences
    Research Council, GM foods, 100
Black, Douglas, poverty and ill health, 99–100
Blair, Tony, GM foods, 100
bleeding, 16–17, 52, 149
blood pressure monitoring, 119–20
Bloor, David, 62–4
body
  as communication system, 59
  and illness, 250–1
Bolivia, trepanning, 7
Booth, Charles and Mary, poverty in, 19th
    century, 29
borderline personality disorder, 154
Boring, Edward, psychology, 79
bracketing, 214
brain function, localization, 219–20
brain and skull shape, 217–18
Breast Cancer Coalition, random allocation,
  128
breast screening, 125
Bridgman, Percy, 78–82
  Feigl, Herbert, 81
  Logic of Modern Physics, 78
Bristol Cancer Help Centre, 124
British Anthropological Institute, 218
Broca, Paul, trepanning and Broca's area, 9
Brown, Dr John, 51–3
  Bruonian system, 51–3
Brown, Brian, 277
Burt, Cyril, 11-plus exam, 101
Butler, Josephine, 33

Caen, Antonie, black swan, 22
Calvin, John, 194
cancer, 145–6
  breast, 251
  thalidomide, 96
Cannon, Walter, 67
cardiovascular system, 67
caring work, 41
Carnap, Rudolf, 36, 38, 41
  operationalism, 81
  Vienna Circle, 26
Catholic Church, heliocentric theories, 10–12
cerebral dualism, 271

Chadwick, Edwin, poverty in, 19th century,
  28
Chamberlain, Geoffrey, ectopic paper, 64–6
Changing Childbirth, 132
characteristics of good theory, *see* theory
Charcot, Jean Martin, hysteria, 251
Chemie Grunenthal, thalidomide, 100
childbirth, Caesarean section, 249
China
  trepanning, 8–9
  Western medicine, 56
  yin and yang, 55–6
Chomsky, Noel, linguistics, 188
chronic fatigue syndrome, 252
Chuengsatiansup, Komatra, 184
  Suzuki Disease, 184
  Yamaha Disease, 184
circulatory system, 58
Civil War, 16
clinical governance, 152–4
  definition, 152
clinical hermeneutics, 186–96
  behaviour, 194–5
  deconstruction, 189–90
  hermeneutic phenomenology, 195–6
  historicism, 191–3
  interpretation of history, 189
  interpretivism, 194
  language difference, 187–9
  positivism, 194
  postmodernism, 188–91
  power issues, 189
  textual readings, 186
Cochrane, Archie, 84–5
  Cochrane Collaboration, 85, 97, 155
Coleridge, Samuel Taylor, Bruonian system,
  52
Combe, George, phrenology, 218
complementary therapists, 251
complexity science, 133
Comte, Auguste, 7, 35, 41, 112
  atheism, 39
  history of science theory, 24
  positivism, 5, 23–6, 112
  sociology, 19, 25–6
concept formulations, 50–5
  asylum, 51
  Bruonian theory, 51–2
  disease, 51
  health, 51

Hippocrates, 50–1
Hufeland, 52
humoral theory, 51
life force, 54
medical model, 53
vitalism, 55
concepts in health sciences, 46–77
    concept formulations, 50–5
    contexts of discovery and verification,
        61–4
    cultures, concepts and communication,
        55–6
    immune system, 57–61
    personalities, diseases and stress, 67–72
    science, actors and networks, 64–6
concepts origination, 46–50
    concept definition, 47
    concept formulation, 50
    concepts and theories, 48
    conceptual mix, 49
    cultural diversity, 48
    health care, 47
    script formulation, 49–50
    sick person, 46
    theory building, 48
concepts, theories and philosophy of science,
    72–4
constructivism, 5
consumers, 151–3
contexts of discovery and verification, 61–4
    Bloor, David, 62–4
    Latour, Bruno, 63–4
    scientific knowledge, 63–4
    strong programme of sociology of science,
        61–4
control groups, 122–4
    Bristol Cancer Help Centre, 124
    hysterical conversion symptoms, 123
    mind-body relationship, 122–3
    placebo, 122–3
    psychoneuroimmunology (PNI), 122
    random factors, 123–4
    stress, 123
conversation analysis, 221–8, 237
    advice giving, 227–8
    bad news delivery, 225–7
    examination commentary, 224–5
    getting started, 223–4
Cooper, David E., liberation vs. enslavement,
    159

Copernicus
    astronomical investigations, 11
    heliocentrism, 3
coronary heart disease (CHD), 68
cranial osteopathy, 276
    Sutherland, William Garner, 248
craniology, 218–19
Crawford, Paul, 278
Crick, Francis, DNA, 166
criminality, 219–20
criminology, 220–1
critical realism, 5
crock, 199–200
cultural diversity, 48
cultures, concepts and communication, 55–6
    yin and yang, 55–6
Cunningham, Jack, GM foods, 100

Dante, 25
Darwin, Charles, 2
    Galapagos Islands, 114
    positivism, 24
deconstructionism, 6, 189–90
deduction, 36–7
Dee, John, 220
degradation ceremony, 228–31
    Garfinkel, Harold, 229
    Goffman, E., 229
DeMoivre, A., normal distribution, 24
Department of Health, typology of evidence,
    143
depravity, 30–5
    feeblemindedness, 30
    gynaecology, 32–3
    homosexuality, 31
    nymphomania, 31–5
    sexuality, 31
depression, 252
Derrida, Jacques
    deconstructionism, 6, 188
    language, 189–90, 238, 241
    logocentrism, 238
    postmodernism, 234
    university of the future, 254–5
Descartes, René, 21–2
    I think therefore I am, 21
    rationalism, 22
    reflexes, 15
    seat of soul, 14, 15
description, see philosophies of description

diabetes, 124
    lay theories and everyday explanations, 275
Dickens, Charles, poverty in, 19th century, 29
Dilthey, Wilhelm, 180–1
diphtheria, 145–6, 252
disability and sexuality, 265–6
dissection, 9–10
dissociative identity disorder, 176, 252
DNA, 166
    criminal, 220
Doctrine of Signatures, 220
Doll, Richard, 144, 150
    randomization, 144
    smoking and cancer, 93
dominant paradigm, 4–5
domination, 208–9
Doyle, Arthur Conan, cocaine, 17
drugs, opiate, 17
Durkheim, Emile, 112
    crime is a disease, 27
    positivism, 112
    suicide rates, 24

eating disorders, 131, 133
economy, fertility and problem solving, 95–6
    Occam's Razor, 95–6
Eddington, Arthur, operationalism, 78
Edwards, Derek, script formulation, 49–50
Einstein, Albert, 94
Eliot, George, positivism, 24
Ellis, Havelock, sexology, 34–5
empiricism, 4, 22, 39–40
Enlightenment, theology, 11
enrolment, 66
epiphanies, 183
episiotomy, 159–60
epistemic enslavement, 159
epistemology definition, 20
    acquaintance knowledge, 20
    procedural knowledge, 20
    propositional knowledge, 20
ethics, 125–6
    breast screening, 125
    human volunteers, 125
    Tuskegee Syphilis Study, 125
ethnography, 209–12
    definition, 209–10

ethnographers as co-actors, 210
    origin, 211
    value, 211–12
Euro-American enlightenment, 2
Evidence-based Health Care, 132
evidence-based health care (EBHC), 83–6, 96–104, 131–5
    advantages, 84
    objective observation, 119–20
    research, 121–2
    see also experiments in medicine and health sciences
examination commentary, 224–5
experimentation, *see* philosophy of experimentation
experiments in medicine and health sciences, 141–73
    cancer, 145–6
    clinical governance, 152–4
    consumers, 151–3
    diphtheria, 145–6
    DNA, 166
    Doll, Richard, 144
    episiotomy, 159–60
    epistemic enslavement, 159
    experimentation growth, 161–2
    Fibiger, Johannes, 145–6
    Hacking, Ian, 165
    individual empowerment, 155
    informed consent, 150–3
    language and culture changes, 154
    liberation, 159
    lifestyle management, 160–1
    lobar pneumonia, 147
    mental health care, 154
    mumps, measles and rubella (MMR), 163–8
    nursing profession, 162
    Pearson, Karl, 145
    Pierce, Charles Sanders, 146
    prostate cancer, 155–7
    public health improvements, 142
    randomization, 146–51
    role of medicine, 141–2
    severe acute respiratory syndrome (SARS), 163
    trials, 152
    tuberculosis, 141, 148–9
explanation levels, 134–5
external funding, 103–4

Fallopius, Gabriele, 13
falsificationism, 42–3, 91
feeblemindedness, 30
Feigl, Herbert, Bridgman, Percy, 81
feminist perspectives, 48, 236
Feyerabend, Paul, 116–17
Fibiger, Johannes, 145–6
    antidiptheria serum, 123
fight or flight response, 67
figuration, 270
figure/ground phenomenon, 118–19
Fleming, Alexander, penicillin, 88
Fodor, Jerry, psychology, 79
Food and Drug Administration, 104
Foucault, Michel
    genealogy of ideas, 16
    history, 189, 236
    power, 189, 239
Framingham Study, 68
Frank, Philipp, Vienna Circle, 26
Frederick the Great, 25
Frege, Gottlob, mathematical logic, 38
Frenkel-Brunswick, Else, 119
Freud, Sigmund, 178, 238
    sexuality, 34

Gadamer, Hans-Georg, 181–2
    fusion of horizons, 182
Galen, 14, 17
    humours, 16–17
Galileo, 21
    astronomical investigations, 10–12
Gall, Franz Joseph, brain and skull size,
    217–20
Galton, Francis, psychology, 24
Garfinkel, Harold, degradation ceremony,
    229
Gauss, C.F., 10
    normal distribution, 24
Geertz, C., thin and thick description,
    210–11
general relativity, 3
genetic code, Nirenberg, Marshall, 166
geometry of good and evil, 6
Gershon, Richard, 57
getting started, 223–4
Giddens, Anthony, double hermeneutic,
    176
    duality of structure, 5
global migration, 1

Goethe, Bruonian system, 52
Goffman, E.
    Asylums, 209
    degradation ceremony, 229
    symbolic interactionism, 206–9
Gould, Stephen J., phrenology, 219
governmentality, 154
Gray, John, Mars and Venus, 35
Gray's Anatomy, 13–14, 58
Greece
    battlefield wound care, 2
    madness, 51
    trepanning, 8–9
Griffiths Report, 99
grounded theory, 200, 215–16
Gulf War Syndrome, 1
gynaecology, 32–3

Habermas, 117
Hacking, Ian, 165
Haeckel, Ernst, 180
Hahn, Hans, Vienna Circle, 26
Hansen, G.A., leprosy, 162
Haraway, Donna, 57–61
    sexuality, 35
hardy personalities, 71–2
Harrison, John Heslop, hoaxes, 100
health care
    concepts, 47
    conceptual mix, 49
    history, 27
    knowledge, 260–1
    language, 243
    organizations, 1
    philosophy of science, 1–18
    postmodern approach, 252–5
    research, 92–3, 237–9, 244
    tragedy/truth relationship, 183
    see also experiments in medicine and health
        sciences
health care provision, 242
    postmodern approach, 252–5
health care users, 203–16
    ambiguous genitalia, 203
    autobiography and self-conceptualization,
        203–5
    ethnography, 209–12
    grounded theory, 215–16
    Howard Becker's Boys in White, 212–13
    illness pleasures, 214–15

phenomenology, 214
symbolic interactionism, 206–9
health sciences, 40
hypothetico-deductive model, 111
postmodernism, 234
see also experiments in medicine and health sciences
heart-sink patient, 200
Heisenberg, uncertainty principle, 43
hermeneutic inquiry, 200
hermeneutic phenomenology, 195–6
hermeneutic/interpretivist stance, 40
see also interpretation and hermeneutics
Hicks, Carolyn, 277–8
Hill, Austin Bradford
patient information, 152
randomization, 148–9
Hippocrates, 14, 17
humours, 16–17
physical explanations and concepts, 50–1
trepanning, 9
well-being, 51
historicism, 191–3
histories of reason, 21–8
Aristotle and induction, 21
Bacon, Francis, 22
Berkeley, Bishop, 21–2
Bertillion, Alphonse, 28
Comte, Auguste, 23–6
Descartes, René, 21–2
Durkheim, Emile, 24
empiricism, 22
Galileo, 21
health care, 27
Hume, David, 22–3
Jastrow, Joseph, 27
Kant, 21
Locke, John, 22–3
Newton, Isaac, 21
Plato, 21
Popper, Karl, 26
Quetelet, Adolphe, 23–4
rationalism, 21
sociology, 25–6
Vienna Circle, 26
history, 16–18
genealogy of ideas, 16
of the head, 221
HIV, 1, 253
holistic clinical care, 92–3

homosexuality, 31
human volunteers, 125
Hume, David, 16
empiricism, 22–3
humours, 16–17, 51–2
hunger, 1
Husserl, Edmund, phenomenology, 175, 214, 266
Huxley, Thomas, 116
hypertension, Alexander, Franz, 67
hypothetico-deductive process, 109–18
hysterical conversion symptoms, 123

iatrogenic problems, 1
idealism, 21
Illich, Ivan, medicine's role, 141
illness
narrations, 250–2
patterns, 46–7
pleasures, 214–15
spiritual dimensions, 211
imagery, 57–9
immune system, 57–61, 164, 252
bodies as communication systems, 59
definition, 57
Gershon, Richard, 57
Haraway, Donna, 57–61
imagery, 57–9
Matzinger, Polly, 60
as orchestra, 58
Pasteur, Louis, 57, 60–1
Incas, trepanning, 8
individual empowerment, 155
individualism, 4
induction, 36–7, 109
inductive method, 87–90
industrial revolution, 16
information theory, Shannon, Claude, 59
informed consent, 150–3
innatism, 21
institutions, 207–9
intentionality, 214
interpretation and hermeneutics, 174–98
clinical hermeneutics, 186–96
Dilthey, Wilhelm, 180–1
epiphanies, 183
Gadamer, Hans-Georg, 181–2
hermeneutics definition, 175–6
interpretivism, 175–96
pain interpretation, 184–6

positivism, 182–3
  soundscapes of everyday life, 184
  validation, 179
interpretation of history, 189
interpretivism, 175–96
  see also interpretation and hermeneutics
intersubjectivity, 214
intuition, 266–8

James, William, 73
  psychological approaches, 67
Jastrow, Joseph, psychology, 27–8
journal articles, 110
Jung, Carl, intuition, 267

Kant, Immanuel, 21
  knowledge acquisition, 21
  life force, 54
Kennedy, Donald, 102
Kepler, J., astronomical investigations, 11
Kings Fund, 98
kleptomania, 82
knowledge, 239–40
  foundations, 38, 236–7
  status, 39
knowledge acquisition, Kant, Immanuel, 21
knowledge, experience and new social
    objects, 263–6
  disability and sexuality, 265–6
  mental health care, 263–5
knowledge representation and becoming
    expert, 266–8
  intuition, 266–8
Koch, Robert, 61, 149
  cholera and tuberculosis, 2
Kuhn, Thomas, 73–4, 111–12
  history, 189
  language use, 187
  paradigm shifts, 3–4, 166

Lacan, Jaques, language, 238–9
language
  and culture changes, 154
  in action, 245
  Speech Act Theory, 245
  difference, 187–9
Latour, Bruno, 63–4
  on Louis Pasteur, 60–1
Lavater, Johann, *Physiognomic Fragments*,
  217

lay theories and everyday explanations,
  275–7
  concept formulations, 275
  diabetes, 275
  schizophrenia, 275
Lee, De, 160
Leibniz, G.W., 10
Lemaitre, Georges, theory of universe, 11
Leonardo Da Vinci, anatomy, 12–15
leprosy, 1, 96, 162
leukaemia, 133
Lévi-Strauss, Claude, structuralism, 188
Lewis, Thomas, randomization, 147–8
liberation, 159
life force, 54
  Medicus, 54
  psychotherapy, 54
lifestyle management, 160–1
liminality, 250–1
Lipperhay, lenses, 11
liturgy of the clinic, 236
lobar pneumonia, 147
Local Protocol Developments, 97
Locke, John, 16
  empiricism, 22–3
  inner world, 200
  tabula rasa, 22
logical positivism, 90
  Vienna Circle, 26
Lombroso, Cesare, phrenology, 219–20
Luther, Martin, Copernican cosmology, 11
Lyotard, Jean-Francois, 190
  grand narratives, 188, 239
  postmodernism, 234
Lyte, Henry Francis, health, 53

Machiavelli, 22
mad pride, 242
Marx, Karl, 5, 178
  positivism, 24
Marxist perspectives, 48, 110, 236
masturbation, 32, 239
mathematics, 10–12
Matzinger, Polly, 60
Maudsley, Henry, madness, 220
Mayhew, Henry, ethnography, 211
measles, mumps and rubella (MMR) vaccine,
  94–5
Medawar, Peter, hypothetico-deductive
  stance, 109

Medical Research Council
  consumer liaison groups, 151
  MMR, 164
  streptomycin, 148–50
medicine, 27
  language, 240
  role, 141–2
  see also experiments in medicine and health
    sciences
Medicines Control Agency, MMR, 164
Medicus, life force, 54
Mendel, Gregor, objective observation, 118
mental health care, 154
  and madness, 271–3
  violence and restraint, 263–5
Merton, Robert, scientific good practice, 39
Michelangelo, anatomy, 12
microcosm and macrocosm, 12
Middle Ages, theology, 10–12
Mill, John Stuart, 33, 109, 113
  positivism, 24
Mills, C. Wright, interpretive social science,
    182–3
mind-body relationship, 122–3, 167
Minnesota Multiphasic Personality
    Inventory, 70
modernism and postmodernism, 245–55
  language, 246
  nursing thinking, 246–7
  positive attitude, 248–9
moral philosophy, 27
Morton, Samuel
  Crania Americana, 7
  skull collection, 218
Moscovici, S.
  anchoring, 270
  objectification, 270
  social representations, 268–70
multicultural perspectives, 48
mumps, measles and rubella (MMR), 163–8
Muybridge, Eadward, photographic studies,
    201–3
myocardial infarction (MI), 68

National Institute for Clinical Excellence
    (NICE), 97, 155
National Service Frameworks (NSF), 97
natural philosophy, 23, 144
Nature, 102
nature/nurture controversy, 101

near death experience, 7
Neolithic battleaxe people, trepanning, 8–9
Neurath, Otto, 38, 42
  theory of knowledge, 20
  Vienna Circle, 20, 26
Newton, Isaac, 10, 21
Newtonian mechanics, 3, 43
NHS Centre for Reviews and Dissemination,
    85
NHS Direct, 46–7
NHS Research and Development money,
    103
Nicholas of Cusa, moving earth, 11
Nietzsche, F.W., 41, 178
  truth, 239
Nightingale, Florence, 121
Nirenberg, Marshall, genetic code, 166
noise pollution, 184
normal distribution, 24
Northampton mortality tables, 23
nurse
  conceptual map, 49
  qualitative methodology, 174
  research, 120–2
nursing
  aesthetic way of knowing, 262
  empirical knowledge, 261
  ethical or moral knowledge, 261
  interpersonal process, 242–3
  language, 240
  personal knowledge, 261–2
  philosophy, 243
  process, 132, 174
  profession, 162
  socio-political knowledge, 262
  typology, 260
  ways of knowing, 261–3
nymphomania, 31–5, 220, 239

objectification, 270
  figuration, 270
  ontologization, 270
  personification, 270
objective observation, 118–20
  evidence-based health care, 119–20
  figure/ground phenomenon, 118–19
  Mendel, Gregor, 118
  Popper, Karl, 118
observer role, 199–200
occupational therapy, language, 240

ontologization, 270
operationalism, 78–108
   Bridgman, Percy, 78–82
   characteristics of good theory, 90–6
   Cochrane, Archie, 84–5
   definition, 78
   Eddington, Arthur, 78
   evidence-based health care (EBHC), 83–6
   history, 78–86
   Peirce, Charles, 78
   and positivism, 79–81
   principles and philosophy of scientific
      method, 87–90
   randomized controlled trial and
      experimental design, 86–7
   scientific research and philosophies of
      power, 96–104
opium, 52
Orseme, Nicholas, moving earth, 11
Osler, William, 69
   angina, 67
Owen, John, heliocentric astronomy, 11

pain interpretation, 184–6
paradigm shifts, 3–5, 7, 111–12, 239
paranormal phenomena, Randi, James,
   234–5
Pare, 123
Pasteur, Louis, 57, 60–1, 149
patient, 1–2
   as consumer, 1–2
patient treatment preference, 127–9
Pearce, Malcolm, 64–6
   ectopic paper, 64–6
Pearson, Karl, 146
   Chi-square test, 145
Peirce, C.S., 41–2, 73, 109, 78
   abduction, 36
   operationalism, 78
Peking Man, 115
peptic ulcer, falsification process, 91–2
perineal trauma, 129–30
personalities, diseases and stress, 67–72
   cardiovascular system, 67
   fight or flight response, 67
   Framingham Study, 68
   hardy personalities, 71–2
   Minnesota Multiphasic Personality
      Inventory, 70
   stress, 67–72

   trusting heart, 71
   type A behaviour pattern, 68–72
   type B behaviour pattern, 68–72
   vital force, 70
   Western Collaborative Group Study, 69
personality disorder, 154
personification, 270
Peru, trepanning, 7
pharmaceutical companies, 104
phenomenology, 214, 235
   bracketing, 214
   Derrida, Jacques, 238
   intentionality, 214
   intersubjectivity, 214
philosophies of description, 199–201
   conversation analysis, 221–8
   degradation ceremony, 228–31
   grounded theory, 200
   health care users, 203–16
   hermeneutic inquiry, 200
   observer role, 199–200
   phrenology and physical maps of mind,
      216–21
   reflection theory and realism, 201–3
   reflexivity, 200–1
philosophy of experimentation, 109–40
   Comte, Auguste, 112
   control groups, 122–4
   Durkheim, Emile, 112
   ethics, 125–6
   hypothetico-deductive process, 109–18
   Kuhn, Thomas, 111–12
   objective observation, 118–20
   Popper, Karl, 109–11, 114, 117
   positivism, 109, 112–13
   random allocation, 126–9
   randomized controlled trial and health care
      research, 114, 131–5
   sources of bias in research, 120–2
   statistics, 129–30
   Thomas Maxim, 116
philosophy and research design, 260–84
   knowledge, experience and new social
      objects, 263–6
   knowledge representation and becoming
      expert, 266–8
   lay theories and everyday explanations,
      275–7
   philosophy and research in practice,
      277–81

social representations, 268–75
ways of knowing: nursing, 261–3
philosophy and research in practice,
    277–81
philosophy of science, 2–3, 7
    positivism, 19–45
phrenology and physical maps of mind, 32,
    216–21
    brain and skull shape, 217–18
    craniology, 218–19
    criminality, 219–20
    history of the head, 221
    history of phrenology, 217–19
    localization of brain function, 219–20
physics, 10–12, 42–3
physiognomy, 32
physiotherapy, language, 240
Piaget, Jean, childhood stages, 235
Pierce, Charles Sanders, 146
Piltdown Man, 100, 115
placebo, 122–3
Plato
    rationalism, 21
    reality, 201
Pope Clement VII, 11
Pope Paul III, 11
Popper, Karl, 26, 74, 153, 183
    falsificationism, 26, 42–3, 73, 91
    hypothesis testing, 149
    and inductive approach, 88–90
    objective observation, 118
    philosophy of experimentation, 109–11,
        114, 117
    scientific theory, 38–9
positivism, 4–5, 19–45, 109, 112–13, 182–3,
    194
    depravity, 30–5
    empiricism, 39–40
    epistemology definition, 20
    histories of reason, 21–8
    and operationalism, 79–81
    and postmodernism, 42–3, 234
    poverty in, 19th century, 28–30
    social issues as physical problems,
        40–2
    theorizing visibility, 36–40
postmodernism, 5–6, 48, 188–91,
    234–59
    approach, 252–5
    definition, 191, 241

foundations of knowledge, 38, 236–7
geometry of good and evil, 6
health care provision, 242, 252–5
health care research, 237–9
knowledge, 239–40
language, 234, 238–43
language in action, 245
liturgy of the clinic, 236
modernism and postmodernism, 245–55
paradigm shift, 239
and positivism, 42–3
qualitative research, 234, 237–9
social world, 235–6
poststructuralism, 188
Potter, Jonathan, concepts, 49
poverty in, 19th century, 28–30
    Booth, Charles and Mary, 29
    Chadwick, Edwin, 28
    Dickens, Charles, 30
    Mayhew, Henry, 28–9
    Thackeray, William Makepeace, 29
power issues, 189, 208–9, 236
predictive power of theory, 93–5
primacy effect, 90–1
procedural knowledge, 20
propositional knowledge, 20
Propp, Vladimir, 188
prostate cancer, 155–7
Protestant work ethic, 181
psychoanalysis, Popper, 110
psychology, Galton, Francis, 24
psychoneuroimmunology (PNI), 122
psychotherapy, life force, 54
Ptolemy
    cosmology, 3
    planets, 10–11
public health improvements, 142
purging, 16–17, 51, 149
Pusztai, Arpad, GM foods, 100, 104

qualitative research, 234, 237–9
quality of life, 39–40, 206
quantum physics, 3, 43
Quetelet, Adolphe, 27, 220
    mass body index, 23–4
    mortality rates, 23–4
    normal distribution, 24
    social mechanics, 24
Quine, W. Van O., 41–2, 73
    translation, 187–8

Randi, James, paranormal phenomena, 234–5
random allocation, 123–4, 126–9
    alternation, 127
    Breast Cancer Coalition, 128
    patient treatment preference, 127–9
    white coat compliance, 128
randomization, 146–51
randomized controlled trial, 85–7, 92–3,
        96–104, 114, 260
    deficiencies, 101–2
    health care research, 131–5
    see also control groups; ethics; experiments
        in medicine and health sciences
rationalism, 16, 21–2
    Plato, 21
realism, 5
    and postmodernism, 234
    see also reflection theory and realism
reality, 206–9
reflection theory and realism, 201–3
    Muybridge's photographic studies, 202–3
reflexivity, 200–1
relapse profile, 158
relativity, 43
Renaissance, 161–2
    anatomies, 10–12
    theology, 11
research
    in health care, 1–2
    selectivity, 90–1
    sources of bias, 120–2
    see also scientific research and philosophies
        of power
Research Assessment Exercise, 102–3, 121–2
Ridley, Harold, cataract operation, 88
Roger of Salerno, trepanning, 9
Rorty, Richard, 42, 73
    epistemology, 20
    history, 189
Rush, Benjamin, Bruonian system, 52
Russell, Bertrand, 27
    atomic propositions, 26
    mathematical logic, 38
Ryle, Gilbert, thin and thick description,
        210–11

Salisbury, David, immunization, 167
Saussure, Ferdinand de, Saussurean
        linguistics, 59
scarlet fever, 252

schizophrenia, 131, 206–7, 236
    grounded theory, 216
    lay theories and everyday explanations, 275
Schlick, Moritz, 36, 38
    Vienna Circle, 26
Scholein, Johann Lucas, medical model, 53
Schon, Jan Hendrik, data falsification, 100–2
Schopenhauer, 89, 92
Schrödinger, cat attest, 43
Science, 102
science
    definition, 82–3
    theories, see theories of science and society
science, actors and networks, 64–6
    actor network theory, 64–6
    enrolment, 66
    Pearce, Malcolm, 64–6
    translation strategy, 66
scientific good practice, Merton, Robert, 39
scientific knowledge, 38–9, 63–4
scientific method, principles and philosophy,
        87–90
scientific research and philosophies of power,
        96–104
    Cochrane Centre, 97
    evidence-based health care (EBHC),
        96–104
    external funding, 103–4
    Food and Drug Administration, 104
    Griffiths Report, 99
    Kings Fund, 98
    Local Protocol Developments, 97
    National Institute for Clinical Excellence
        (NICE), 97
    National Service Frameworks (NSF), 97
    NHS Research and Development money,
        103
    pharmaceutical companies, 104
    randomized controlled trial, 96–104
    Research Assessment Exercise, 102–3
    Thatcher, Margaret, 98–9
    therapeutic relationship, 96
script formulation, 49–50
    Edwards, Derek, 49–50
self-conceptualization, see autobiography and
        self-conceptualization
Selye, Hans, 70
    stress and cardiovascular system, 67
severe acute respiratory syndrome (SARS),
        163, 253

sexuality, 31, 220, 236
Shakespeare, 25
Shannon, Claude, information theory, 59
Sharp, Jane, genitourinary medicine, 2
Shipman, Harold, 193
sick person, 46
Skinner, Quentin, history, 189
Smith, Adam, 25
Snow, John, cholera, 92
social behaviour, *see* interpretation and
    hermeneutics
social issues as physical problems, 40–2
    caring work, 41
social mechanics, Quetelet, Adolphe, 24
social representations, 268–75
    action, 274
    cerebral dualism, 271
    cognition, 274
    communication, 274
    language, 274
    mental health and madness, 271–3
    Moscovici, S., 268–70
    perception, 274
    representation, 274
social science, 234
social world, 235–6
society, theories, *see* theories of science and
    society
sociology, 19, 25–7
sociology of science, *see* strong programme
soundscapes of everyday life, 184
Spearman, Charles, statistical techniques,
    146
Speech Act Theory, 245
Spencer, Herbert, phrenology, 218
spirituality in health care, 4
statistics, 129–30
    see also control groups
stress, 123
    see also personalities, diseases and stress
strong programme of sociology of science,
    61–4, 236
structuralism, Lévi-Strauss, Claude, 188
suicide rates, Durkheim, Emile, 24
Sutherland, William Garner, cranial
    osteopathy, 248
symbolic interactionism, 206–9
    description in social settings, 206–9
    Goffman, E., 206–9
syphilis, 53

tabula rasa, 22
Taylor, F.W., scientific management,
    153
Terman, Lewis, feeblemindedness, 30
textual readings, 186, 188–9
Thackeray, William Makepeace, poverty in
    19th century, 28–9
Thai Tshang Kung, trepanning, 9
Thales, flat earth astronomy, 11
thalidomide, 96, 100
Thatcher, Margaret, 98–9
theories of science and society, 1–18
    anatomy of human body, 12–16
    Bernard, Claude, 2, 7
    Bhaskar, Roy, 5
    biomedical reductionism, 4
    Comte, August, 5, 7
    constructivism, 5
    critical realism, 5
    Darwin, Charles, 2
    deconstructionism, 6
    Derrida, Jacques, 6
    dominant paradigm, 4–5
    empiricism, 4
    Euro-American enlightenment, 2
    Giddens, Anthony, 5
    history, 16–18
    individualism, 4
    Koch, Robert, 2
    Kuhn, Thomas, 3–4
    Marx, Karl, 5
    paradigm shifts, 3–5, 7
    patient, 1–2
    philosophy, 2–3, 7
    positivism, 4–5
    postmodernism, 5–6
    realism, 5
    Renaissance anatomies, 10–12
    research in health care, 1–2
    Sharp, Jane, 2
    spirituality in health care, 4
    trepanning and reconstruction of health
        care histories, 7–10
theorizing visibility, 36–40
    deduction, 36–7
    empiricism, 39–40
    health sciences, 40
    hermeneutic/interpretivist stance, 40
    induction, 36–7
    positivism, 36–40

quality of life, 39–40
  scientific knowledge, 38–9
  Vienna Circle, 36, 38
  well-being, 39–40
theory building, 48
theory characteristics, 90–6
  economy, fertility and problem solving,
    95–6
  predictive power, 93–5
  verification *vs.* falsification, 90–3
therapeutic relationship, 96, 195–6
Thomas Maxim, 116
transplant, 251
trepanning and reconstruction of health care
    histories, 7–10
  Bolivia, 7
  Broca, Paul, 9
  China, 8–9
  Greece, 8–9
  Incas, 8
  Morton, Samuel, 7
  Neolithic battleaxe people, 8–9
  Peru, 7
  Roger of Salerno, 9
  Thai Tshang Kung, 9
trials, 152
trusting heart, 71
Truth, Sojourner, 33
tuberculosis, 53, 141, 148–9, 252
Tuskegee Syphilis Study, 125, 150
type A behaviour pattern, 68–72
type B behaviour pattern, 68–72

United Kingdom Co-ordinating Committee
    on Cancer Research, consumer liaison
    groups, 151
United Nations, 40
user-led perspectives, 48

validation, 179
Vane, John, 89

verification *vs.* falsification, 90–3
Vesalius, Andreas, 14–15
  De Humanis Corporis Fabrica, 14
Vienna Circle, 20, 26–7, 36, 38
  logical positivism, 26, 42, 109
  operationalism, 81
  protocol statements, 26
Virchow, Rudolf, disease, 53
Visible Human Project, 202
vital force, 70
vitalism, 55
Vlamingh, Willem de, black swan, 22–3
vomiting, 16–17, 51

Wakefield, Andrew, MMR immunization,
    163–8
warfare, 1
watchful waiting, 47, 155–6
Watson, James, DNA, 166
ways of knowing: nursing, 261–3
Weber, Max
  Protestant work ethic, 194–5
  social sciences, 174
  Verstehen, 181, 194
well-being, 39–40
Wesley, John, heliocentric astronomy, 12
Western Collaborative Group Study, 69
white coat compliance, 128
Whitehead, Alfred North, 11
Williams' Obstetrics, 159–60
Wittgenstein, Ludwig, 27, 56, 79
  elementary propositions, 26
  language, 189
  meaning, 187
Wollstonecraft, Mary, 33
World Health Organization, 40
  quality of life, 206
world view, 187, 200, 237

Ziemelis, Karl, 102
zone of complexity, 133

THINKING NURSING

Tom Mason and Elizabeth Whitehead

- Important new nursing theory textbook

This major new text seeks to provide nursing students with an accessible overview of the theory which informs the application of nursing activity. The key disciplines that contribute to the nursing curriculum – such as sociology, psychology, public health, economic science and politics – are comprehensively discussed, with each chapter offering both a theoretical discussion and a section showing how the topic in question applies to nursing practice. Particular attention has been paid to pedagogy with brief boxed case studies, chapter summaries, glossaries of key words and further reading lists enabling easy use by students.

Contents:
Introduction – Thinking Sociology – Thinking Psychology – Thinking Anthropology – Thinking Public Health – Thinking Philosophy – Thinking Economics – Thinking Politics – Thinking Science – Thinking Writing – Conclusions – References – Index.

432pp   0 335 21040 6 (Paperback)   0 335 21041 4 (Hardback)

RESEARCH METHODS IN HEALTH
INVESTIGATING HEALTH AND HEALTH SERVICES

Ann Bowling

Praise for the first edition of *Research Methods in Health*:

> . . . a brilliantly clear documentation of different philosophies, approaches and methods of research about health and services. Laid out in an accessible and manageable way, it covers an enormous amount of material without sacrificing thoroughness . . . I would recommend it to a broad readership.
>
> *MIDIRS Midwifery Digest*

> . . . This major research textbook is as good as an introduction to the field as you are likely to find.
>
> *The International Journal of Social Psychiatry*

> . . . an easy to read book with excellent background information on the theory and practice of research. A summary of main points, key terms and recommended reading follows each chapter and there is a useful glossary of terms at the end of the book for quick reference . . . I particularly liked the checklists when undertaking literature reviews and writing research proposals.
>
> *British Journal of Health Care Management*

This new edition of Ann Bowling's well-known and highly respected text has been thoroughly revised and updated to reflect key methodological developments in health research. It is a comprehensive, easy to read guide to the range of methods used to study and evaluate health and health services. It describes the concepts and methods used by the main disciplines involved in health research, including: demography, epidemiology, health economics, psychology and sociology.

The research methods described cover the assessment of health needs, morbidity and mortality trends and rates, costing health services, sampling for survey research, cross-sectional and longitudinal survey design, experimental methods and techniques of group assignment, questionnaire design, interviewing techniques, coding and analysis of quantitative data, methods and analysis of qualitative observational studies, and types of unstructured interviewing.

With new material on topics such as cluster randomization, utility analyses, patients' preferences, and perception of risk, the text is aimed at students and researchers of health and health services. It has also been designed for health professionals and policy makers who have responsibility for applying research findings in practice, and who need to know how to judge the value of that research.

Contents
Part one: Investigating health services and health: the scope of research – Part two: The philosophy, theory and practice of research – Part three: Quantitative research: sampling and research methods – Part four: The tools of quantitative research – Part five: Qualitative and combined research methods, and their analysis – Index.

512pp   0 335 20643 3 (Paperback)   0 335 20644 1 (Hardback)

KEY CONCEPTS AND DEBATES IN HEALTH AND SOCIAL POLICY

Nigel Malin, Stephen Wilmot and Jill Manthorpe

This book identifies key social policy concepts and explores their relevance for health and welfare policy, and for the practice of professionals such as nurses and social workers who are involved in the delivery of services and provision. The text adopts ideologies of welfare approach using examples of recent policy shifts to illustrate theoretical and political tensions. This shift in emphasis away from the traditional approach of documenting policy areas is an important feature of the book. The concepts are organized in terms of doctrinal contests. This allows the authors to explore the tension between different approaches and ways of defining social policy. The aim is to help professionals identify these tensions, to be aware of the strategic choices which have been made in national and agency policy, and to locate their own practice in relationship to these choices. It draws upon the continuing debate around the Third Way and New Labour policies as they apply to health and social welfare; and identifies tensions within a non-ideological, pragmatic set of practices.

Key Concepts and Debates in Health and Social Policy has been written with students and practitioners in mind. It is a valuable resource for a wide range of health and welfare professionals, especially in nursing, social work and occupational therapy. It is also suitable for use on professional training courses, and with students of social policy and health studies.

Contents
Introduction – The Third Way: a distinct approach? – Identifying the Health Problem: need or risk? – Responsibility and Solidarity – Consumerism or Empowerment? – Central Planning and Market Competition – Controlling Service Delivery: professionalism versus managerialism – Community Care and Family Policy – Evaluating Services: quality assurance and the quality debate – Prioritizing and Rationing – Conclusion – Index.

176pp   0 335 19905 4 (Paperback)   0 335 19906 2 (Hardback)

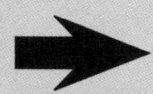
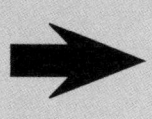